Communication in Me

This new and pa... us-sion of communication ... care consultations. The first of its kind for ... years, ... brings together a team of leading contributors from the fields of linguistics, sociology, and medicine to describe each phase of the primary care consultation, identifying the distinctive tasks, goals, and activities that make up each phase of primary care as social interaction. Using conversation analysis techniques, the authors analyze the sequential unfolding of a visit, and describe the dilemmas and conflicts faced by physicians and patients as they work through each of these activities. The result is a view of the medical encounter that takes the perspective of both physicians and patients in a way that is rigorous and humane. Clear and comprehensive, this book will be essential reading for students and researchers in sociolinguistics, communication studies, sociology, and medicine.

JOHN HERITAGE is Professor of Sociology at the University of California, Los Angeles, working in the field of communication and interaction with particular reference to health care and political communication. His previous books include *Talk at Work: Interaction in Institutional Settings* (co-edited with Paul Drew, Cambridge University Press, 1992) and *The News Interview: Journalists and Public Figures on the Air* (with Steven Clayman, Cambridge, Cambridge University Press, 2002).

DOUGLAS W. MAYNARD is Professor of Sociology at the University of Wisconsin-Madison. He has carried out interaction-based research in a variety of settings, including legal medical, educational testing, and survey interviews. He is author of *Bad News, Good News: Conversational Order in Everyday Talk and Clinical Settings* (2003) and co-editor of *Standardization and Tacit Knowledge: Interaction and Practice in the Survey Interview* (2002).

Studies in Interactional Sociolinguistics

1. *Discourse Strategies* John J. Gumperz
2. *Language and Social Identity* John J. Gumperz
3. *The Social Construction of Literacy* edited by Jenny Cook-Gumperz
4. *Politeness: Some universals in language usage* Penelope Brown and Stephen C. Levinson
5. *Discourse Markers* Deborah Schiffrin
6. *Talking Voices: Repetition, dialogue, and imagery in conversational Discourse* Deborah Tannen
7. *Conducting Interaction: Patterns of behaviour in focused encounters* Adam Kendon
8. *Talk at Work: Interaction in institutional settings* Paul Drew and John Heritage
9. *Grammar in Interaction: Adverbial Clauses in American English Conversations* Cecilia E. Ford
10. *Crosstalk and Culture in Sino-American Communication* Linda W. L. Young and John J. Gumperz
11. *AIDS Counselling: Institutional Interaction and Clinical Practice* Anssi Peräkylä
12. *Prosody in Conversation: Interactional Studies* Elizabeth Couper-Kuhlen and Margret Selting
13. *Interaction and Grammar* Elinor Ochs, Emanuel A. Schegloff, and Sandra A. Thompson
14. *Credibility in Court: Communicative Practices in the Camorra Trials* Marco Jacquemet
15. *Interaction and the Development of Mind* A. J. Wootton
16. *The News Interview: Journalists and Public Figures on the Air* Steven Clayman and John Heritage
17. *Gender and Politeness* Sara Mills
18. *Laughter in Interaction* Philip Glenn
19. *Matters of Opinion: Talking about Public Issues* Greg Myer

Communication in Medical Care

Interaction between Primary Care Physicians and Patients

Edited by
JOHN HERITAGE
University of California, Los Angeles

and

DOUGLAS W. MAYNARD
University of Wisconsin-Madison

CAMBRIDGE
UNIVERSITY PRESS

CAMBRIDGE UNIVERSITY PRESS
Cambridge, New York, Melbourne, Madrid, Cape Town, Singapore, São Paulo

Cambridge University Press
The Edinburgh Building, Cambridge CB2 2RU, UK

Published in the United States of America by Cambridge University Press, New York

www.cambridge.org
Information on this title: www.cambridge.org/9780521628990

First published 2006

Printed in the United Kingdom at the University Press, Cambridge

A catalogue record for this book is available from the British Library

Library of Congress Cataloguing in Publication data
Communication in medical care : interaction between primary care physicians and patients / edited by John Heritage and Douglas W. Maynard. – 1st ed.
p. cm. – (Studies in interactional sociolinguistics)
Includes bibliographical references and index.
ISBN-13 978-0-521-62123-6 hardback
ISBN-10 0-521-62123-2 hardback
ISBN-13 978-0-521-62899-0 paperback
ISBN-10 0-521-62899-7 paperback
1. Physician and patient. 2. Communication in medicine. 3. Physicians (General practice). 4. Interpersonal communication. 5. Social interaction. 6. Discourse analysis. I. Heritage, John. II. Maynard, Douglas W. III. Series.
[DNLM: 1. Physician–Patient Relations. 2. Communication. W 62 C7343 2006]
R727.3.C66 2006 610.69′6 – dc22 2005012928

Contents

Figures

Tables

Contributors

Professor Elizabeth Boyd, Department of Clinical Pharmacy, University of California, San Francisco, USA

Professor Paul Drew, Department of Sociology, York University, UK

Professor Richard Frankel, Department of General Internal Medicine, Indiana University School of Medicine, USA

Professor Virginia Teas Gill, Department of Sociology, Illinois State University, USA

Professor David Greatbatch, Department of Education, University of Nottingham, UK

Dr. Markku Haakana, Department of Finnish, University of Helsinki, Finland

Professor Timothy Halkowski, Department of Communication, State University of New York at Albany, USA

Professor Christian Heath, Centre for Work, Interaction and Technology, King's College, University of London, UK

Professor John Heritage, Department of Sociology, University of California, Los Angeles, USA

Professor Douglas W. Maynard, Department of Sociology, University of Wisconsin-Madison, USA

Professor Anssi Peräkylä, Department of Sociology, University of Helsinki, Finland

Dr. Liisa Raevaara, Research Institute for the Languages of Finland, Helsinki, Finland

Professor Jeffrey D. Robinson, Department of Communication, Rutgers University, USA

Professor Debra Roter, School of Public Health, Johns Hopkins University, USA

Dr. Marja-Leena Sorjonen, Research Institute for the Languages of Finland, Helsinki, Finland

Dr. Tanya Stivers, Max Planck Institute for Psycholinguistics, Netherlands

Dr. Tuukka Tammi, Department of Sociology, University of Helsinki, Finland

Professor Candace West, Department of Sociology, University of California, Santa Cruz, USA

Foreword

Debra Roter

This very thoughtful volume, assembled by two of the field's leading conversation analysts, is a notable contribution to the literature on medical communication by taking the reader through the examination room door to the heart of the medical dialogue. The book is expressly conversation-analytic in orientation and presents authentic dialogue from patients and physicians as it unfolds, thus capturing the social and medical dynamic within which medicine is practiced. The book also presents chapters in which quantitative analyses are built upon conversational analytic material. By doing this, the significance of the book goes beyond the contribution of its individual chapters. It provides support for the development of a new kind of interaction study – one with the potential for rich and meaningful synthesis of the medical dialogue derived from an integration of qualitative and quantitative methods.

The integration of quantitative and qualitative approaches in a study of medical dialogue is not without controversy. Indeed, a debate of longstanding intensity has centered on the perception that these approaches reflect incompatible scientific paradigms. Advocates of each have not only argued their own relative merits, but have maintained unusually critical and polarized positions. These positions are reflected in a well-worn list of attributes that are widely used to characterize quantitative and qualitative approaches, as well as their practitioners. The quantitative perspective is characterized as hypothetico-deductive, particularistic, objective, and outcome-oriented; its researchers are logical positivists. In contrast, the qualitative approach is characterized as social-anthropological, inductive, holistic, subjective, and process-oriented; its researchers are phenomenologists (Reichardt and Cook 1969).

The paradigmatic schism so apparent in the well-established areas of scientific inquiry described above is also evident in studies of the medical dialogue. Association with a particular paradigm not only implies a worldview, but also a paradigm-specific method of inquiry and even different styles of presentation. Quantitative studies of medical interaction are characterized as narrowly reflecting the biomedical model's emphasis on deductive methods and a tendency to translate observations of patient and provider behavior into statistical summaries. Qualitatively inclined researchers, on the other hand, record data in the language of their subjects, almost always presenting actual speech through verbatim transcripts of audio- and videotape recordings and rarely assigning numerical values to their observations. Despite obvious overlap in the questions asked and problems tackled, the two approaches are seldom combined.

In lamenting the advances and insights lost to intellectual isolation, my good colleague and friend Richard Frankel and I began a series of conversations pertaining to the research traditions and the professional circles that placed each of us, and our work, within opposing paradigm camps (Roter and Frankel 1992). In doing so, we found a parallel may be drawn between the systems of open-sea navigation described by the cultural anthropologist Thomas Gladwin, and the debate among researchers of the medical encounter over qualitative and quantitative methods (Gladwin 1964). The system of navigation represented by the European tradition is characterized by the plotting of a course prior to a journey's beginning that subsequently guides all decisions regarding location. The extent to which the journey "stays the course" is a testament to the European navigator's skill. The islanders of Truk face the problem of managing long distances over uncertain conditions in a very different manner than the Europeans. The Trukese navigator has no pre-established plan of any kind; rather, experience from previous voyages and information at hand during the current sailing trip account completely for Trukese navigational expertise.

The paradigmatic perspective which promotes mutual exclusivity is in error; there is no inherent logic in the limitations established by the traditions, other than tradition itself. Much of the debate in medical interaction research has focused on comparing methods independent of particular contexts, questions, or outcomes. Although it is quite clear that the methods used by Gladwin's navigators differ in both kind and degree, it is also the case that they both solve the same practical problem successfully. The value of Gladwin's analysis is that it includes both context and outcome as determinants of methodological utility. The presence or absence of map-making skills is essentially irrelevant to the Trukese navigator, as is the ability or inability of European navigators to read local wave patterns. Methods of research, like those of navigation, are open to description in their own terms, and should be judged on the extent to which they succeed in answering the questions which they raise in the context in which they were raised. However, respect for alternative methods does not preclude combining methods to maximize discovery and insight.

In this book, Douglas Maynard and John Heritage have assembled a thoughtful collection of papers in which the richness of the communication experience is reflected in a variety of ways. In doing so, this book makes a meaningful contribution to the literature and begins to address the formidable challenge of breaking paradigmatic boundaries.

Transcript symbols

The transcript notation used in this book, and in conversation analytic research more generally, was developed by Gail Jefferson. It is designed to capture the details of talk in interaction as it actually occurs, and is a system that continues to evolve in response to current research interests and needs.

Temporal and sequential relationships

A. Overlapping or simultaneous talk is indicated in a variety of ways.

[[	Separate left square brackets, one above the other on two successive lines with utterances by different speakers, indicates a point of overlap onset, whether at the start of an utterance or later.
]]	Separate right square brackets, one above the other on two successive lines with utterances by different speakers, indicates a point at which two overlapping utterances both end, where one ends while the other continues, or simultaneous moments in overlaps which continue.
// *	In some older transcripts or where graphic arrangement of the transcript requires it, a double slash indicates the point at which a current speaker's utterance is overlapped by the talk of another, which appears on the next line attributed to another speaker. If there is more than one double slash in an utterance, then the second indicates where a second overlap begins, the overlapping talk appearing on the next line attributed to another speaker, etc. In transcripts using the // notation for overlap onset, the end of the overlap may be marked by a right bracket (as above) or by an asterisk.

So, the following are alternative ways of representing the same event: Bee's "Uh really?" overlaps Ava's talk starting at "a" and ending at the "t" of "tough."

```
Ava:   I 'av [a lotta  t]ough cou:rses.
Bee:         [Uh really?]

Ava:   I 'av // a lotta t*ough cou:rses.
Bee:   Uh really?
```

= B. Equal signs ordinarily come in pairs – one at the end of a line and another at the start of the next line or one shortly thereafter. They are used to indicate two things:

1) If the two lines connected by the equal signs are by the same speaker, then there was a single, continuous utterance with no break or pause, which was broken up in order to accommodate the placement of overlapping talk. For example,

```
Bee:   In the gy:m? [(hh)
Ava:                [Yea:h. Like grou(h)p
       therapy.Yuh know [half the grou]p thet=
Bee:                    [ O h : : : . ] ·hh
Ava:   =we had la:s' term wz there en we [jus'=
Bee:                                     [ ·hh
Ava:   =playing arou:nd.
```

Ava's talk is continuous, but room has been made for Bee's overlapping talk (the "Oh").

2) If the lines connected by two equal signs are by different speakers, then the second followed the first with no discernable silence between them, or was "latched" to it.

(0.5) C. Numbers in parentheses indicate silence, represented in tenths of a second; what is given here in the left margin indicates 5/10 second (half a second) of silence. Silences may be marked either within an utterance or between utterances, as in the two excerpts below:

```
Bee:   ·hhh Uh::, (0.3) I don'know I guess
       she's aw- she's awright she went to
       thee uh:: hhospital again tihda:y,

Bee:   Tch! .hh So uh I don't kno:w,
       (0.3)
Bee:   En:=
```

(.) D. A dot in parentheses indicates a "micropause," hearable but not readily measurable; ordinarily less than 2/10 of a second.

((pause)) E. In some older or less carefully prepared transcripts, untimed silences may be indicated by the word "pause" in double parentheses.

Aspects of speech delivery, including aspects of intonation

.
?
,
?,
¿

A. The punctuation marks are *not* used grammatically, but to indicate intonation. The period indicates a falling, or final, intonation contour, not necessarily the end of a sentence. Similarly, a question mark indicates rising intonation, not necessarily a question, and a comma indicates "continuing" intonation, not necessarily a clause boundary. In some transcript fragments in your readings you may see a combined question mark and comma, which indicates a rise stronger than a comma but weaker than a question mark. Because this symbol cannot be produced by the computer, the inverted question mark (¿) is used for this purpose. Sometimes completely "level" intonation is indicated by an "empty" underline at the end of a word, e.g., *"word_".

: : B. Colons are used to indicate the prolongation or stretching of the sound just preceding them. The more colons, the longer the stretching. On the other hand, graphically stretching a word on the page by inserting blank spaces between the letters does *not* necessarily indicate how it was pronounced; it is used to allow alignment with overlapping talk. Thus,

```
Bee:  Tch! (M'n)/(En ) they can't delay much
      lo:nguh they [jus' wannid] uh-·hhh=
Ava:               [ O h   :  . ]
Bee:  =yihknow have anothuh consulta:tion,
Ava:  Ri::ght.
Bee:  En then deci::de.
```

The word "Ri::ght" in Ava's second turn, or "deci::de" in Bee's third are more stretched than "Oh:" in Ava's first turn, even though "Oh:" appears to occupy more space. But "Oh" has only one colon, and the others have two; "Oh:" has been spaced out so that its brackets will align with the talk in Bee's ("jus' wannid") turn with which it is in overlap.

C. A hyphen after a word or part of a word indicates a cut-off or self-interruption, often done with a glottal or dental stop.

word — D. Underlining is used to indicate some form of stress or emphasis, either by increased loudness or higher pitch.

word — The more underlining, the greater the emphasis. Therefore, underlining sometimes is placed under the first letter or two of a word, rather than under the letters which are

WOrd — actually raised in pitch or volume. Especially loud talk may be indicated by upper case; again, the louder, the more letters in upper case. And in extreme cases, upper case may be underlined.

° — E. The degree sign indicates that the talk following it was markedly quiet or soft. When there are two degree signs, the

°° — talk between them is markedly softer than the talk around it.

F. Combinations of underlining and colons are used to indicate intonation contours, as follows:

_: — If the letter(s) preceding a colon is underlined, then there is an "inflected" *falling* intonation contour (you can hear the pitch turn downward).

: — If a colon is itself underlined, then there is an inflected *rising* intonation contour (i.e., you can hear the pitch turn upward).

So, in

```
Bee:  In the gy:m? [(hh)
Ava:               [Yea:h. Like grou(h)p
      therapy.Yuh know [half the grou]p thet=
Bee:                   [ O h : : : . ]˙hh
Ava:  =we had la:s' term wz there en we [jus'=
Bee:                                    [˙hh
Ava:  =playing arou:nd.
Bee:  Uh-fo[oling around.
Ava:       [˙hhh
Ava:  Eh-yeah so, some a' the guys who were
      bedder y'know wen' off by themselves so
      it wz two girls against this one guy en
      he's ta:ll.Y'know? [˙hh
Bee:                     [ Mm hm?
```

the "Oh:::." in Bee's second turn has an upward inflection while it is being stretched (even though it ends with falling intonation, as indicated by the period). On the other hand, "ta:ll" at the end of Ava's last turn is inflected downward ("bends downward," so to speak, over and above its "period intonation").

↑ ∧ ↓ ∨	G. The up and down arrows mark sharper rises or falls in pitch than would be indicated by combinations of colons and underlining, or may mark a whole shift, or resetting, of the pitch register at which the talk is being produced.
>< <> <	H. The combination of "more than" and "less than" symbols indicates that the talk between them is compressed or rushed. Used in the reverse order, they can indicate that a stretch of talk is markedly slowed or drawn out. The "less than" symbol by itself indicates that the immediately following talk is "jump-started," i.e., sounds like it starts with a rush.
hhh (hh) ·hh	I. Hearable aspiration is shown where it occurs in the talk by the letter "h" – the more "h"s, the more aspiration. The aspiration may represent breathing, laughter, etc. If it occurs inside the boundaries of a word, it may be enclosed in parentheses in order to set it apart from the sounds of the word (below). If the aspiration is an inhalation, it is shown with a dot before it (sometimes a raised dot).
# £/$	J. Some elements of voice quality are marked in these transcripts. A rasping or "creaky" voice quality is indicated with the "#" sign. Similarly, a "smile voice" – a voice quality which betrays the fact that the speaker is smiling while speaking – is normally indicated with the "£" (or "$") sign.

Other markings

(( ))	A. Double parentheses are used to mark transcriber's descriptions of events, rather than representations of them. Thus ((cough)), ((sniff)), ((telephone rings)), ((footsteps)), ((whispered)), ((pause)), and the like.
(word) ( )	B. When all or part of an utterance is in parentheses, or the speaker identification is, this indicates uncertainty on the transcriber's part, but represents a likely possibility. Empty parentheses indicate that something is being said, but no hearing (or, in some cases, speaker identification) can be achieved.
(try 1) (try 2)	C. In some transcript excerpts, two parentheses may be printed, one above the other: these represent alternative hearings of the same strip of talk. In some instances this format cannot be printed, and is replaced by putting the alternative hearings in parentheses, separated by a single oblique or slash, as in

```
Bee:   °(Bu::t.)=/°(Goo:d.)=
```

Here, the degree marks show that the utterance is very soft. The transcript remains indeterminate between "Bu::t." and "Goo:d." Each is in parentheses and they are separated by a slash.

1

Introduction: Analyzing interaction between doctors and patients in primary care encounters

John Heritage and Douglas W. Maynard

In 1976, Patrick Byrne and Barrie Long published a path-breaking study of the doctor–patient relationship. Based on some 2,500 tape-recorded primary care encounters, *Doctors Talking to Patients* anatomized the medical visit into a series of stages, and developed an elaborate characterization of doctor behaviors in each of them. Drawing on Michael Balint's (1957) proposal that the primary care visit has therapeutic value in its own right, Byrne and Long focused on the ways in which its therapeutic possibilities were attenuated by the prevalence of doctor-centered behaviors in the encounters they studied. The study was also conceived as an intervention: physicians were invited to use its coding framework to evaluate their own conduct, and to modify it in a more patient-centered direction. Not surprisingly, given these goals, *Doctors Talking to Patients* was itself somewhat doctor-centered. The authors had little to say about patients' contributions to the encounter or the sociocultural context of social interaction in primary care.

In the present volume we revisit Byrne and Long's project of anatomizing the primary care visit, doing so from a primarily sociological and interactional perspective. We begin from the standpoint that physician and patient – with various levels of mutual understanding, conflict, cooperation, authority, and subordination – jointly construct the medical visit as a real-time interactional product. Within this orientation, we consider some of the social, moral, and technical dilemmas that physicians and patients face in primary care, and the resources that they deploy in solving them. Our objective is to open the study of doctor–patient relations to a wide range of social and interactional considerations.

We begin this Introduction with a sketch of recent approaches to the analysis of the physician–patient relationship, before going on to describe the methodological underpinnings of our research. The objective is to set out the conceptual context of the studies making up this volume, and to consider what they might contribute both to the social scientific investigation of primary care and, in keeping with Byrne and Long's original objective, to its practice.

Studies of doctor–patient interaction: a brief overview

Sociological concern with the doctor–patient relationship received its classic formulation in a chapter of Parsons' (1951) theoretical work, *The Social System*. Working within the functionalist perspective that he did much to develop, Parsons conceptualized the institution of medicine as a social system's mechanism for assisting those who fall ill and returning them to their regular contributory capacities. Rather abstract and generalized, the role-based model that Parsons formulated did not generate much empirical investigation. Instead, starting in the 1960s, research on doctor–patient interaction has increased greatly according to two main approaches: process analysis, and the microanalysis of discourse (Charon et al. 1994).

Process analysis

Process analysis was introduced into medicine in a series of path-breaking studies by Barbara Korsch and associates on interaction in a pediatric emergency room (Francis et al. 1969; Korsch et al. 1968; Freemon et al. 1971; Korsch and Negrete 1972). Using the "interaction process analysis" coding scheme which had been developed by Robert Bales (1950), these studies demonstrated that mothers, desiring more information than they actually obtained from the physicians, were reticent about asking questions, disappointed at the amount of information they received, and frequently (one-fourth of the subjects) did not mention their most important concern to the physician. These observations were linked to adherence: patients whose needs for information were least satisfied were also least cooperative with treatment recommendations and also less satisfied with the outcome of the visit. Such findings made a powerful case for the study of physician–patient interaction, because they showed that systematic study in the field is achievable, and that the results can be significant for patient health outcomes.

As noted, the original Korsch studies quantified interaction using Bales' interaction process analysis, which had been developed for classifying role behavior in task-oriented small groups in terms of a contrast between task-oriented behaviors and socio-emotional categories. The Bales scheme had real strengths, including the attempt to be exhaustive and to facilitate administration so that a trained Bales researcher can code interaction in real time, without the need even of a tape recorder. As an approach to doctor–patient interaction, however, the scheme also had significant drawbacks. Its categories are exceedingly general, yielding a picture of the physician–patient encounter that is fuzzy at best. Nor were they adapted to the specificities of doctor–patient communication and the phases of the medical encounter.

Subsequently, coding schemes have undergone progressive refinements over the years to address these problems, becoming adjusted to dyadic interaction and to the specific content of physician–patient interactions (for overviews, see Inui et al. 1982; Wassermann and Inui 1983; Inui and Carter 1985; Roter et al. 1988; Roter and McNeilis 2003). By far the most influential is that developed by Roter and colleagues. The current Roter interaction analysis system (RIAS) contains 39 categories, broadly subdivided into socio-emotional (15 categories) and task-focused (24 categories) (Roter 2004). Like the Bales system, RIAS (Roter and Larson 2001, 2002) is designed to implement an exhaustive classification of the events of the medical visit, while using categories that are compatible with the three-function model of the medical visit described by Cohen-Cole and Bird (Cohen-Cole 1991; Cohen-Cole and Bird 1991).

The RIAS framework has opened up the physician–patient relationship to a significant degree, accommodating a wide range of contents and circumstances beyond primary care, including oncology, obstetrics and gynecology, end-of-life discussions, well-baby care, and specific diagnostic categories such as asthma, hypertension, and diabetes (Roter and Larson 2002). Related studies showed that eliciting the patient's view of the illness increased recall, understanding, and commitment to following a physician's advice (see Stewart [1995] and Brown et al. [2003] for overviews of outcomes related to physician–patient interaction). Shown by comparative studies to be superior to other coding systems (Inui et al. [1982]; see also Thompson [2001] for a broad overview of systems), it has revealed important differences in how men and women (both physicians and patients) interact in the medical visit and how these interaction patterns are related to physician and patient satisfaction (Hall et al. 1994a, 1994b; Roter and Hall 1992). It has formed the basis for a valuable empirical specification of the main styles of primary care visits (Roter et al. 1997), and it has been used in nearly a hundred empirical investigations of a wide variety of medical contexts (Roter and Larson 2002).

Although the Roter system has served as the backbone for the study of the physician–patient relationship over the past twenty years, it is not without controversy. Criticisms of the RIAS system have focused on the very features that have contributed to its success – its capacity to deliver an exhaustive and quantified overview of the medical encounter. Critics of the RIAS system argue that its categories fail to address issues of content, context, and meaning in medical interaction, sacrificing these for an overview across medical encounters in which the interactivity – the capacity for one party to influence the behavior of another, or to adjust behavior in response to another – becomes invisible (Charon et al. 1994; Mishler 1984; Stiles 1989). Many of these criticisms have been developed from the microanalysis perspective, to which we now turn.

Microanalysis

At the opposite pole of the analytic continuum lie studies that focus on the microanalysis of medical discourse. Originating within anthropology and sociology, these studies deploy an essentially ethnographic and interpretive methodology to disclose the background orientations, individual experiences, sensibilities, understandings, and objectives that inhabit the medical visit. In sociology, microanalytic studies have a heritage that includes the "Chicago School" of ethnography and Hughes' (1963) work on occupations and professions. Hughes was among those in sociology to note the professionalization of work and occupations, but because of this focus, shared by Freidson (Hughes' student) and others, an astute observation by Fox (1989:38) still holds true: "Sociologists have written more about health professionals – especially about physicians – than they have about patients."

We would add that, besides patients themselves, the physician–patient *relationship* is also much neglected. In recent years, ethnographers have included discourse analysis as part of their investigation of doctoring, investigating patients' experiences, sensibilities, understandings, and objectives to suggest that patients' subjectivity resides, like an iceberg, mainly below the surface of talk. It is maintained in this submerged condition by a combination of patient diffidence and self-censorship (Strong 1979), and practitioner disattention and obfuscation. Practitioner suppression of patient experience, investigators argue, is due to status and authority as built from educational, socioeconomic, ethnic, gender, and other differences between patients and physicians (Atkinson 1995; Clair and Allman 1993; Davis 1963; Fisher 1984; Todd 1989; Zola 1964, 1973). Ethnographic research in this vein is consistent with the perspective of social constructionism (Brown 1995; Miller and Holstein 1993; Spector and Kitsuse 1977). Where process techniques like those of Roter concentrate on what is present in medical conversations, the microanalytic approach, in highlighting absences in the dialogue, imparts a strongly critical edge to appraisals of medical practice.

Elliot Mishler's (1984) *The Discourse of Medicine* is a most compelling implementation of microanalysis. Mainly focusing on the medical history, Mishler observes that physician and patient often pursue distinct, and sometimes conflicting, agendas in the medical visit: the doctor's medical agenda focuses on biomedical evaluation and treatment, and the patient's "lifeworld" agenda concentrates on personal fears, anxieties, and other everyday lifeworld circumstances. Implementing the medical agenda, physicians recurrently suppress the patient's concerns, even though they can be important resources for understanding medical problems.

In the context of history-taking, the basic mechanism of this suppression is the simple three-part sequence of actions through which history-taking is recurrently transacted:

Doctor:	Symptom question
Patient:	Response
Doctor:	Evaluation or acknowledgment (e.g., "OK") and/or Next question

Mishler observes that this interaction sequence, while ordinary and unremarkable, is in fact a mechanism by which the physician controls three important matters: initiation of particular topics, extent of their development, and the degree to which patients can respond. Although a patient may "leak" lifeworld concerns into the interview by offering "surplus information" in response to medically focused questions, regularly physicians' subsequent questions avoid taking up the moral, social, and existential issues the patient raises in favor of a narrowly focused medical agenda (Mishler 1984:85).

Mishler's observations were expanded in Howard Waitzkin's *The Politics of Medical Encounters*, where he (1991:231–2) argues that the underlying, and largely unrecognized, structure of medical discourse militates against the expression of personal troubles including "difficulties with work, economic insecurity, family life and gender roles, the process of aging, the patterning of substance use and other 'vices,' and resources to deal with emotional stress." Instead, the medical management of patients' contextually generated problems focuses on technical solutions, reinforces ideologically dominant outlooks and prohibitions, and contributes to social control by reinforcing the patient's accommodation to the social contexts from which illness arises. Waitzkin observes that these dysfunctional features of the medical visit emerged in 70 per cent of the 336 cases he examines. Similar findings are reported in microanalytic studies involving women's reproductive choices (Fisher 1986; Todd 1989; see also Fisher and Todd 1993), which also address a variety of other aspects of the medical visit.

Taking stock

It is now time to take stock of these two traditions of interaction research: the Bales-based RIAS coding model and the microanalytic approach. In principle, the strengths and weaknesses of the two approaches are complementary, and combining them should result in a greatly enhanced view of the medical encounter (Roter and Frankel 1992; Waitzkin 1990). In practice, this has not come about (Roter and McNeilis 2003). Process approaches have resulted in findings about the medical encounter that are systematic and replicable. The most robust findings have centered on relationships between interaction variables and patient and provider characteristics, and to a lesser extent with patient satisfaction and adherence outcomes. Process approaches have not developed associations between interaction variables and medical decision-making (surely one of the core areas of medical practice), nor in relation to patients' treatment preferences or physicians' perceptions of those preferences.

Such deficiencies are probably associated with the kinds of coding categories used in process analysis. In the effort to generalize across practice contexts, coding categories are pitched at a very general level. This is a well-rehearsed criticism of process analysis (see Mishler 1984; Inui and Carter 1985; Tuckett et al. 1985; Tuckett and Williams 1984; Pendleton 1983), and it is associated with two related problems. The first is that, in the course of coding, the *content* of the medical encounter is largely washed out. What the physician and patient were talking about is lost, often irretrievably, when the original tapes are destroyed and the coded material effectively becomes "the data" (Mishler 1984; Charon et al. 1994). A second problem is that coding expunges the *context* of utterances and actions – their location in a phased activity within the encounter such as history-taking or counseling, and their placement in a specific and autochthonously intelligible sequence and course of action. It is precisely these aspects of context that give utterances and actions the meaning they have.

On the other side of the ledger, microanalytic approaches have retained crucial elements of medical sense-making and interpretation, but issues remain. One of these is how to integrate ethnographic inquiry (interviews and observations) with the study of interaction and language use (Maynard 2003: Chapter 3). Even when that integration is successful, many small-scale quasi-ethnographic studies of discourse have not been able to establish a non-interpretive evidential base for associations between meaningful communicative practices on the one hand, and medical outcomes on the other.

Of course, many studies in this tradition, including those in this book, analyze generic practices of talk-in-interaction, and thereby are able to make recommendations about specific practices for enhancing the medical interview. In delivering diagnostic news, for instance, it is demonstrable from interactional evidence that, and how, physicians can enhance the understanding and acceptance of patients or other recipients. Or in making treatment recommendations, it is also clear that proposing particular therapies in one fashion rather than another can decrease the likelihood of patient resistance. Each of our chapters, on the basis of the conversation-analytic methodology employed, has implications for medical practice, whether it is how to open the interview, take an effective and sensitive history, conduct the physical exam, explain illness and convey diagnostic news, make treatment recommendations and prescribe medicine, deal with lifestyle matters, or close the encounter.

Nonetheless to extract robust outcome-based conclusions about how physicians (or patients) should conduct themselves in specific moments in the flow of the medical encounter, it is important to find a meeting point between the two methodologies of coding and microanalysis (Roter 2000; Roter and Frankel 1992; Roter and McNeilis 2003). In other words, beyond the intrinsic worth of analytical framework responsive to very granular, individual moments in the physician–patient encounter, we need one that simultaneously supports coding at a broader level of granularity sufficient to reach beyond individual cases to generate findings at a statistical evidential standard. For example, qualitative studies of pediatric interactions involving patients who present with upper respiratory tract infections (Stivers 2002b, 2005a, 2005b, this volume; Heritage and Stivers 1999) have resulted in quantitative studies that show how these various conversational actions are associated with the perception of demand for antibiotics and inappropriate prescribing (Stivers et al. 2003) and parent resistance to treatment recommendations. These studies identify communicative resources that physicians can deploy to resist these negative outcomes (Mangione-Smith et al. 2003, 2004). In addition to their generic implications for medical practice, accordingly, the chapters of this book offer a framework for granular *and* quantitative, outcome-oriented analyses. In the remainder of this Introduction, we provide an overview of the theory of interaction and its methodology as they provide for clinical implications of our individual chapters, and as they allow for connections between microanalysis and coding operations for overall assessment of medical communication.

Conversation analysis as an approach to medical communication

In this section, we will first give a brief preview of the orientation of conversation analysis (henceforth CA) to social interaction in general. Second, we will sketch several levels of application of CA to the medical interview, and address the relationship of qualitative and quantitative analysis. Finally we will give a thematic overview of the contents of this book.

(1) Conversation analysis: a brief introduction

Conversation analysis emerged as a field in the 1970s from pioneering research by Harvey Sacks, Emanuel Schegloff, Gail Jefferson, and others. Initially focused on ordinary conversations between relatives, friends and acquaintances, and (later) on interactions in more formal or institutional settings such as medical clinics, the field coalesced around a set of fundamental theoretical assumptions: (1) social interaction is an autonomously organized domain – an "interaction order" (Goffman 1983) – that exists independently of particular motivational, psychological, or demographic (race, class, gender, ethnic) characteristics of participants; (2) gestures, utterances, turns of talk, and their subcomponents perform recognizable actions that are both context-shaped and context-renewing; (3) these first two properties inhere in the very minutiae of interaction, which means that no order of detail in conversation is to be dismissed a priori as disorderly, accidental, or irrelevant to participants' concerted endeavors; (4) appreciating the sequential organization of conversation could mean an important methodological advance in the analysis of everyday talk that would make that analysis both "reliable" and "valid" in the terms of normal social science.

(1) The bedrock upon which conversation analysis stands is sequencing, which was explored in early papers on turn-taking (Sacks et al. 1974) and the organization of adjacency pairs – turns of talk like questions and answers that are two utterances long and have other regular characteristics (Schegloff and Sacks 1973). To start analysis with a focus on turn-taking and adjacency pairs translates in the medical context into a concern with everything from

"how are you" questions and their replies, to history-taking questions and answers, to diagnostic announcements and their receipts, to treatment proposals and their acceptance or rejection, to many other kinds of sequences (as the chapters in this volume show). The analysis of turn-taking and adjacency pairs permits the appreciation of how parties to conversation make it possible to coordinate understanding and joint actions at all, whatever the sociodemographic backgrounds or psychological dispositions of these parties may be. This approach is taken, for example, in studies of interruptions by men and women in conversation and medical interviews (Kollock et al. 1985; West and Zimmerman 1983; Zimmerman and West 1975; West 1984).

(2) Spoken utterances (as well as nonvocal gestures and other embodied behavior) accomplish activities. In one of his early lectures, Sacks proposed that the most banal and familiar conversational utterances are social objects that *do* actions and activities without necessarily formulating them as such. He noted that with "This is Mr. Smith," a call recipient at a suicide prevention center can unofficially ask a caller to identify himself and to do so with the same mode of address (Sacks 1992a:3). With "I was trying you all day and the line was busy for, like, hours," a caller can "fish" for information as to her caller's whereabouts by giving her own version of things, which invites the recipient to tell hers (Pomerantz 1980). Conversation analysis represents the attempt to describe and analyze a host of ordinary activities – informing, describing, criticizing, insulting, complaining, giving advice, requesting, apologizing, joking, greeting, and many more. These activities are rarely announced in so many words. Nor does the syntactic structure of an utterance often convey its force as an action. For example, we use question forms to align with a speaker's talk ("Oh, isn't he dreadful?"), we use declarative forms to make requests ("It's cold in here."), and we use imperatives to invite ("Come in."). The production and understanding of an utterance as an action derives from *features of the social context*, most especially an utterance's place in an organized sequence of talk. Sequencing is what conversation analysts regard as an utterance's fundamental context.

Any participant's communicative action is doubly contextual. First, the action is *context-shaped*. Its contribution to an ongoing activity derives in part from the immediately preceding utterance or set of utterances in which it occurs. Second, conversational actions are *context-renewing*. Every current utterance will itself form the primary framework for some next action in a sequence. In this sense, the context of a next action is inevitably renewed with each current action. To put it differently, the local sequencing of utterances is significant both because *speakers* routinely draw upon it as a resource in designing their current utterances and because, correspondingly, *hearers* draw upon it in order to make adequate sense of what is said. Moreover, sequencing functions to recondition (i.e., maintain, adjust, or alter) any broader or more generally prevailing sense of context which is the object of the participants' orientations and actions. That is, the doubly contextual quality of utterances contributes to the "larger" interactional environment or overall activity (such as the medical interview) within which these utterances make their step-by-step appearance.

(3) Research in conversation analysis has shown that there are no aspects of interaction that are disorderly or insignificant "noise." Another reason why conversation analysts avoid initial considerations of how attributes like race, class, and gender affect conversational interaction is that any initial dealing with these kinds of abstractions eviscerates the detail that is involved in the orderly achievement of mutual understanding. As a sociologist, Sacks turned to conversation as a domain of inquiry because mechanical devices were available for recording interactions and thus preserving the minutiae and particulars of everyday talk. Drawing on Garfinkel's (1967) ethnomethodological sensibility, conversation analysts realized that it was within this detail that the orderliness of action and meaning-making were to be found. Thus a working principle of CA is that "No scale of detail, however fine, is exempt from interactional organization, and hence must be presumed to be orderly" (Zimmerman 1988:415). This implies an interest not just in what participants say but also in silences, in overlapping talk, in sound stretches, breathing, and so on. Hence, conversation analysts transcribe tape recordings to be used in conjunction with the recordings and to show as many of these features as possible in orthographic form.

(4) An important methodological consequence flows from this theoretical perspective. As a feature of a turn of talk in conversation, a current speaker will display an understanding of the talk in

previous turns (Sacks et al. 1974:728). Hence, speakers can look to the next turn after their own to find an analysis of what they have just said. If the displayed understanding in that next turn does not align with the speaker's own, then the *next* turn of the speaker can be devoted to correcting the matter. By and large, *repair* of all kinds of conversational trouble exhibits sequentially systematic properties (Schegloff et al. 1977), which means that conversation has in-built procedures for its maintenance as a mechanism of social action and interaction. This is *local determination*, whereby participants manage the course of conversational interaction on a turn-by-turn basis. And because of the requirement that participants display their understanding on this local, turn-by-turn basis, analysts have a "proof criterion" and a "search procedure" for the analysis of any given turn, to see how recipients construct their understanding of it.

The CA perspective aims to develop claims about systematic structural organization in interaction. However, such claims can only be supported by substantial accumulations of instances of a practice, each instance of which the investigator examines as an individual "case." For example, if it is to be claimed that responses to Yes/No questions should ordinarily begin with the word "Yes" or "No," large numbers of instances need to be collected and examined with each instance examined individually. When departures from this practice occur – by qualifying an answer or, indeed, by avoiding the words "Yes" and "No" altogether – the investigator needs to see if something special or distinctive is happening. For example, a participant may be rejecting the presuppositions embedded in the form of the question (Raymond 2003). Related to examining departures from an interactional regularity is the analysis of "deviant" cases, which allows researchers to move from the observation of the regularity to capture what a practice achieves in terms of the meaning-making process and the assembly of social actions. Along the way, deviant case analysis also contributes to the validation of empirical findings.

These features of conversation analysis theory and method imply a systematic approach to the organization in interaction that distinguishes it from studies that rely on anecdote, educated intuition, or sophisticated prior theorizing to make propositions about how talk operates for the people who produce it. In addition, once structural organization in talk is explicated, it can function as an "internally validated" basis on which to base quantitative analysis that connects interactional practices to the social, psychological, and motivational characteristics of individuals and to the contexts and outcomes of interactions.

We will not labor these points further. However, there are three important conclusions to be drawn about the application of CA to the medical interview. First, interactional practices through which persons conduct themselves elsewhere are not abandoned at the threshold of the medical clinic. That is, the organization of interaction described in CA studies is largely carried forward from the everyday world into the doctor's office. Second, and connected with our first point, practices for effecting particular kinds of actions – for example, describing a problem or trouble (Jefferson 1980b, 1988) or telling bad or good news (Maynard 2003) – are also carried across the threshold of the doctor's office and affect how doctors and patients go about addressing particular interactional tasks. Third, the organization of interaction is fundamentally geared to the joint management of self–other relations (Goffman 1955; Brown and Levinson 1987; Heritage and Raymond 2005; Maynard and Zimmerman 1984). Departures from this organization, as in the interruption of one speaker by another, represent violations of this joint management process, though there are practices for dealing with these violations (Schegloff 2000c; Jefferson 2004b). These issues of interaction order, communicative practices in the clinic, and the management of social relations, emerged in early conversation-analytic research on doctor–patient interaction (Frankel 1984a, 1984b, 1990), and will appear repeatedly in the studies making up this volume.

The primary care interview: levels of analysis

In this section of our CA overview, we review three levels through which investigators can conduct the analysis of medical conversations. These include: (1) the overall structure of the primary care visit, (2) the sequence structures through which its particular component activities and tasks are realized, and (3) the designs of the individual turns at talk that make up those sequences. As will be apparent, these three levels of analysis are interrelated: turn design

I <u>Opening</u>: Doctor and patient establish an interactional relationship.

II <u>Presenting Complaint:</u> The patient presents the problem/reason for the visit.

III <u>Examination</u>: The doctor conducts a verbal or physical examination or both.

IV <u>Diagnosis</u>: The doctor evaluates the patient's condition.

V <u>Treatment</u>: The doctor (in consultation with the patient) details treatment or further investigation.

VI <u>Closing</u>: The consultation is terminated.

Figure 1.1 Overall structure of acute primary care visits

is a feature of sequence organization, sequences are compiled into particular activities which, finally, compose the visit as a whole.

Overall structural organization

Most kinds of interactions have some overall structural features. In ordinary conversation, these structural features include specific located activities such as openings and closings, and slots for "first topics" (Schegloff 1968, 1986; Schegloff and Sacks 1973; Button 1987; Button and Casey 1984, 1985), whose absence may be noticeable and accountable. However, within the "body" of an ordinary conversation, matters are comparatively fluid and free to vary with the inclinations of the participants. In contrast, the medical visit has a more specific internal shape or overall structural organization, in which physicians are trained in medical school and with which patients are ordinarily familiar as a matter of repeated experience. This structural organization is built from component phases or activities which characteristically emerge in a particular order.

Acute care doctor–patient interactions (interactions involving the presentation of a new medical problem) thus have a highly structured overall organization (Byrne and Long 1976; Robinson 1998, 2001b, 2003).

Although this structure is a great deal more complex than the structure of some other kinds of task-focused interactions – for example, 911 emergency calls (Zimmerman 1992) – and is subject to a great deal more variation, doctors' and patients' conduct can be examined for how they orient and negotiate the boundaries of each of the main activity components (Heritage 1997). For example, the ways in which patients handle history-taking questions may clearly exhibit an analysis of their purpose, and even of the progress of a differential diagnosis. Or again, particular behaviors during problem presentation pointing towards the physical examination, diagnosis, or treatment (Robinson 2003; Robinson and Stivers 2001; Ruusuvuori 2000; Robinson and Heritage 2003) may be used to indicate that, from the patient's point of view, the problem presentation is complete. In these ways, the overall structure of an encounter may be evoked as a resource for moving the encounter forward.

Using this structural framework, it can be relatively easy to identify the relevant sections of the acute primary care encounter (follow-up and routine visits are often less clearly structured). However, the purpose of these classifications is not to identify each section of a medical visit exhaustively. And it is not to claim that each of these sections will always occur in the same order in each and every acute primary care visit. Still less should it be an objective to force the analysis in terms of these sections, not least because, for example, the parties may well break out of and return to particular activities, reopen them and reinstate task orientations that they had previously treated as complete. However, these very possibilities testify to the lively sense that the participants have, and exhibit for one another, of the existence and relevance of specific task-focused activities within the medical visit. Accordingly, investigating the overall structural organization of the medical visit is not aimed at the creation of a Procrustean taxonomy. Rather, it is valuable in providing access to understandings about the nature of the medical visit which are drawn upon by physicians and patients in their joint management of its progress.

Sequence organization

Sequence organization is the "engine room" of interaction. It is through sequence organization that the activities and tasks central to the medical visit are managed. Sequence organization is the primary means through which context-bound utterances achieve their sense, and interactional identities and roles (storyteller, news deliverer, sympathizer) and larger social and institutional identities (woman, grandparent, Latino, physician, patient, etc.) are established, maintained, and manipulated. This role for sequence organization is true for both ordinary conversation and the medical visit. To illustrate this role for sequence organization, we will focus on sequences in which physicians offer diagnoses and make treatment recommendations.

A substantial body of CA research has shown that physicians and patients treat the management of diagnosis and treatment discussions in sequentially distinctive ways. Diagnoses tend to be offered and accepted "on authority" and ordinarily do not attract significant overt acknowledgment or "acceptance" by patients (Heath 1992; Peräkylä 1998, 2002, this volume; Stivers 2000, 2005a, 2005b, this volume), although when diagnostic news is bad, silence also may be a patient's exhibit of stoicism (Maynard 2003). Moreover, patients may view the diagnosis as a precursor to treatment proposals (Freidson 1970a) and tend to withhold a response in light of that consideration (Robinson 2003). In sequential terms, this manifests itself in little or no patient responsiveness to clinicians' diagnostic statements.

Treatment proposals, by contrast with diagnostic announcements, tend to receive some form of acknowledgment, most often in the form of a fully overt acceptance (cf. Heritage and Sefi 1992). Underlying this sequential variation are profound differences in the social, epistemic, and interactional foundations of the two actions. Diagnoses are produced and recognized as actions performed by an expert who is licensed to perform medicine and render authoritative judgments about the nature of medical conditions. However, in orienting to treatment recommendations as *proposals*, physicians and patients treat these sequences as complete only when some exhibit of *acceptance* is produced. The contrasting properties of diagnostic announcements and treatment proposals offer different affordances to patients who wish to resist diagnoses, by comparison with those who wish to resist treatment recommendations (Stivers this volume). Diagnoses that the patient views as undesirable must be resisted *actively* (e.g., "You don't think it's strep?"). Treatment recommendations, by comparison, can be resisted *passively*: patients, by withholding acceptance to a treatment recommendation, can pressure clinicians into elaborate justifications of a recommendation and, not infrequently, to alter or reverse it.

Before leaving the topic of sequence organization, it is also relevant to note that physicians often systematically and strategically manipulate sequence structures to achieve rather specific objectives. For example, in a series of papers Maynard (1991c, 1991d, 1992, 1996) has identified practices involved in the perspective-display sequence (PDS) whereby clinicians prepare recipients for the delivery of adverse medical diagnoses. In pre-sequential fashion, patients are invited to describe their own view of the medical problem before clinicians present their own diagnostic conclusions. At one level, use of these practices can seem like a grotesque manipulation of medical authority: what possible value can the lay person's view be in a context where a professional medical judgement is about to be expertly rendered? But Maynard shows that, among other things, the PDS facilitates "forecasting" the news, not only preparing the patient for the difficult information they must receive, but also establishing an auspicious interactional environment in which the professional can build on the patient's perspective through agreement rather than confrontation. The patient's perspective is *co-implicated* in the diagnostic presentation. The PDS does involve a strategic manipulation of the asymmetric relations between doctor and patient, but in a displayed benign way and with consequences which are often beneficial to the patient's understanding and acceptance (Maynard 1996).

Turn design

Sequences are made up of turns and, therefore, require analysis of turn design. This is a massive topic and only glimpses of its ramifications can be presented in a short review. Among the contributions to this volume, Robinson shows that physicians' phrasing of questions that open the business of the medical visit index whether the physician believes that the patient is presenting for a new, follow-up, or chronic concern. Similarly, Boyd and Heritage observe that medical questioning is shaped by the twin principles of "optimization" and "recipient design" (see also Heritage 2002a; Stivers and Heritage 2001). "Optimized" questions embody presuppositions and preferences that favor "best-case" or "no-problem" responses. These question designs are departed from when mandated by the particulars of the recipient's circumstances. And in his contribution, Peräkylä describes the different ways in which the articulation of diagnoses can manage the balance between authority and accountability that is intrinsic to the practice of contemporary medicine.

Just as clinicians' questions are designed with sensitivities to the medical and interactional exigencies "in play," so too are patients' responses. Heritage and Robinson show that problem presentations are designed with distinctive trajectories that are sensitive to whether the problem is new, recurrent, or routine. Halkowski analyzes the ways in which patients manage descriptions of how they became aware of particular symptoms so as to convey that they are not excessively preoccupied with their bodily functions. Gill and Maynard observe ways in which patients present etiological hypotheses so as not to require an immediate response. Boyd and Heritage describe ways in which answers to questions can be designed with a brevity aimed at collaborating in the production of "checklist" questioning. And Drew describes ways in which patients, who find themselves giving "no problem" responses to questions that pursue a particular diagnostic outcome, engage in what he terms "dramatic detailing" of somewhat related symptoms.

This section began with the suggestion that turn design is a massive and complex subject. But it is clear that its investigation can be enormously fruitful, with strong potential for large-scale analysis of data. For example, in a follow-up to Robinson's contribution, it has been shown that openings which invite the patient to confirm symptoms previously disclosed to other practice staff (e.g., "So fever and headache for three days huh?") strongly curtail patient problem presentations, though this format is associated with presenting concerns, such as upper respiratory infections, which are highly routine (Heritage and Robinson forthcoming). Consider also how patients (as opposed to clinicians) offer explanations for disease. Patients produce them in hesitant and disguised ways, while doctors are more forthright and declarative (Gill 1998a; Gill and Maynard this volume). And Stivers (2002b; Stivers et al. 2003) has shown that a patient's initial problem presentation that offers a candidate diagnosis (e.g., "I think I have an ear infection"), is frequently understood by physicians as indexing a desire for antibiotic treatment, whereas a simple description of symptoms (e.g., "I have a fever and my ear hurts") is not understood in this way. Also in the realm of diagnosis, Maynard (2003) and Maynard and Frankel (this volume) show that physicians alter the design of announcing turns depending on whether their news is bad or good. When the news is good, the announcement *exposes* the diagnosis and its valence, whereas with bad news the diagnosis and valence are *shrouded* in various ways (see also Stivers 1998; Heritage and Stivers 1999; Leppänen 1998).

More generally, turn design is a vehicle for dealing with dilemmas that the physicians and patients often face on a fairly recurrent basis. Accordingly, turn design is an arena in which participants to the medical interview unavoidably exhibit the trade-offs to be made between getting medical tasks done while paying attention to issues of knowledge and authority (Peräkylä, 1998, this volume), solidarity and distance, understanding and misunderstanding, and many other features.

Conclusion

In constructing this volume, we have attempted to replicate Byrne and Long's (1976) pioneering study by bringing together contributions that address most of the major aspects of the primary care visit from beginning to end. While far from exhaustive, our studies address a variety of dilemmas inhabiting the medical visit as an occasion that is simultaneously social *and* medical. These dilemmas are, then, sociomedical, and they take different forms during different phases of the medical visit. Moreover, they involve a variety of procedural solutions that are sensitive to many particular contingencies in the visit's content.

The chapters making up this volume depart from the Byrne and Long (1976) approach and other studies in one very specific and important way. Where previous research has concentrated primarily on the conduct of doctors, or on patients, the "co-constructive" approach in this book emphasizes the conduct of *both* parties. It is by acting together that doctor and patient assemble each particular visit with its interactional textures, perceived features, and outcomes. Our approach is not just a research imperative. The theme of co-construction derives from a complex interplay of theoretical, methodological, and ethical considerations.

Analyzing co-construction is a direct research embodiment of patient-centeredness, because it includes physicians and patients both within the nexus of communication through which medicine is practiced.

If this book has a single message, however, it is that ordinary norms and practices of language use and social interaction exert a powerful and systematic influence on the texture and features of medical visits, and do so in fine detail. For example, patients may hedge their disclosure of troubles in the medical interview according to generic interactional and cultural practices that favor a stoic, "troubles-resistant," or "stiff-upper-lip" stance. Such practices, and the orientations they reflect (Jefferson 1980b, 1988; Jefferson and Lee 1992), profoundly shape social dynamics in the clinic in ways that practitioners of technical medicine have not been trained to handle.

Medical practice is similarly laminated onto the sociocultural base of interaction and cannot be separated from it (Heritage 1984a; Maynard 1991c, 2004), and this creates many difficulties and paradoxes. Though every medical practitioner should remember that a patient may understand the "occult blood test" to involve magic rather than a search for hidden blood, remedying difficult interactional problems is not simply a matter of being careful with abstruse terminology. Nor does it mean knowing how to confront the sometimes "overeducated" but naive understandings patients bring to the interview – when they claim that an "ear infection" is present, they are not necessarily lobbying for antibiotic medication (Stivers et al. 2003). As important as these terminological matters are, we believe there is something more fundamental to problems and paradoxes in the medical interview. This concerns how interaction works: becoming aware of the inexplicit tactics by which patients approach physicians on various topics, and the taken-for-granted ways by which physicians deploy their specialized knowledge through conversational means whose effects they may not fully comprehend. Without such awareness, doctors and patients may jointly produce the appearance of shared understanding rather than the reality.

Detailed analysis of physician–patient interaction can tease apart perplexing difficulties, lay bare the multiple paradoxes and dilemmas that inhabit the medical interview, and suggest valuable remedies. If interaction analysis can show the ways in which physicians and patients, distanced in terms of official expertise yet bound in the communicational sphere, manage the practice of primary care, then much can be done not only to improve the scientific understanding of medical practice but also to improve it.

2

Soliciting patients' presenting concerns

Jeffrey D. Robinson

Although patients may have multiple concerns, their visits with primary care physicians are typically arranged for, and organized around, particular reasons. These reasons are referred to as patients' chief complaints or *presenting concerns*. After visits are opened (Heath 1981; Robinson 1998),[1] physicians typically solicit patients' presenting concerns with questions such as *What can I do for you today?*[2] These questions are an important locus for research because different question designs/formats (i.e., different wordings) can differentially shape and constrain patients' answers (for review, see Boyd and Heritage, this volume). Physicians' solicitations of patients' presenting concerns directly affect the manner in which patients present their problems, and this can have a variety of medical consequences (e.g., for diagnosis and treatment, Fisher, 1991; Larsson et al. 1987; Lipkin, Frankel et al. 1995; McWhinney 1981, 1989; Mishler 1984; Sankar 1986; Todd 1984, 1989). In order to improve health care, both researchers and medical educators have advised physicians to use open-ended questions (Bates et al. 1995; Cohen-Cole 1991; Coupland et al. 1994; Frankel 1995b; Swartz 1998). However, this is a very general dictum, and very little is

[1] During openings, before physicians solicit patients' presenting concerns, they commonly greet patients, sit down, identify patients, and read patients' medical records (Heath 1981; Robinson 1998); many other types of actions can also occur (Byrne and Long 1976; Coupland et al. 1994; Robinson 1999).

[2] Patients' presenting concerns can be established in other, less common ways. For instance, physicians can treat patients' concerns as having already been established (in prior interactions with medical staff) by simply beginning to take the history of patients' concerns, with questions such as *How long has this cough been going on?* (Stivers 2000). Alternatively, patients can initiate the presentation of their concerns (Heath 1986; Robinson 1999; Stivers 2000).

known about physicians' solicitations of patients' presenting concerns, per se.

This chapter advances research in two ways. First, it demonstrates that even subtle differences in how physicians design questions can change the action that questions perform (Coupland et al. 1994; Frankel 1995b; see Boyd and Heritage this volume). The distinction between open- and closed-ended questions is not sufficient to capture these differences. For instance, although the question formats *What can I do for you?*, *How are you?*, and *What's new?* can all be characterized as being open-ended, this chapter demonstrates that they each perform a different social action. Insofar as differently formatted questions perform different actions, they can communicate different things and thus be understood, and responded to, differently by patients.

Second, this chapter demonstrates that physicians and patients orient to the existence of at least three different types of reasons for visiting physicians: to deal with (1) relatively *new* concerns (i.e., ones that are being presented for the first time to a particular physician or clinic, or for the first time since previously being "cured"); (2) *follow-up* concerns (i.e., ones that were raised and dealt with during previous visits and are now being followed up on in terms of patients' recoveries); and (3) *chronic-routine* concerns (i.e., ones that are generally ongoing but under control, such as blood pressure and diabetes, and that are dealt with on a regular basis). This observation is neither new nor unexpected – the National Ambulatory Medical Care Survey (http://www.cdc.gov/nchs/about/major/ahcd/ahcd1.htm) has long coded patients' reasons for visiting physicians into similar categories.[3] Each of these different reasons make relevant different types of medical goals and activities, and thus different interactional trajectories, for visits (Byrne and Long 1976; Robinson 2003).[4] This chapter demonstrates that the question

[3] The 1999 version of the National Ambulatory Medical Care Survey includes codes for five major reasons that patients visit physicians: (1) acute problem (30.3 percent of all visits to primary-care physicians); (2) chronic problem (routine) (34.9 percent of all visits); (3) chronic problem (flare-up) (9.6 percent of all visits); (4) pre- or post-surgery, injury follow-up (11.8 percent of all visits); and (4) non-illness care (11.2 percent of all visits). The remaining 2.2 percent of all visits are coded as blank or unknown.

[4] For example, medical textbooks suggest that there are at least four different types of medical histories that physicians can take: complete, inventory, problem

formats that physicians use to solicit patients' presenting concerns communicate physicians' understandings of patients' reasons for visiting physicians. As such, physicians design, are understood to design, and are held accountable for designing, their solicitations so as to address, or be fitted to, the specific reasons why patients are visiting physicians.[5] As will be argued, this accountability has implications for both the content and shape of ensuing communication, as well as for patients' perceptions of physicians' competence and credibility.

This chapter (1) describes question formats that are designed to index *new, follow-up*, and *chronic-routine* reasons for visiting; (2) describes question formats that do *not* index patients' institutionally relevant concerns; (3) describes cases in which physicians' question formats are inappropriately fitted to patients' reasons for visiting; and (4) discusses the implications of physicians' question formats for medical care.

Data

The data include 182 audio- and videotapes of actual, primary care, physician–patient visits. Seventy-three visits were collected from community-based clinics in Southern California, 23 from hospital-based clinics in Southern California and Texas, and 86 from a community-based clinic in Britain.[6] The data consist of 77 new visits, 15 follow-up visits, and 90 chronic-routine visits. Data were transcribed by the author according to the conventions developed

(or focused), and interim (Seidel et al. 1995). Each of these histories is tailored to different types of presenting concerns and their interactional contingencies. For instance, the problem (or focused) history "is taken when the problem is acute, possibly life threatening, requiring immediate attention so that only the need of the moment is given full attention" (Seidel et al. 1995:32).

5 This is in accordance with the general principle of *recipient design*, which refers to the "multitude of respects in which the talk by a party in a conversation is constructed or designed in ways which display an orientation and sensitivity to the particular other(s) who are the coparticipants" (Sacks et al. 1974:727). Part of this accountability may stem from the fact that patients' reasons for visiting physicians are almost always institutionalized. That is, although patients may have a variety of distinct concerns when they visit physicians, they generally make an appointment for a particular concern, which is typically documented in their medical records, and thus available to physicians, prior to consultations (Heath, 1982b).

6 I would like to thank Peter Campion, Virginia Elderkin-Thompson, Sarah Fox, John Heritage, Tanya Stivers, and Howard Waitzkin for making their data available.

by Gail Jefferson (Atkinson and Heritage 1984). Names and identifying characteristics of the participants have been changed. Data collection was approved by university human-subjects' protection committees.

Analysis

Question formats designed to solicit new concerns

New-concern question formats, which can be either open- or closed-ended, are designed to communicate physicians' understandings that patients are visiting to deal with *new* (vs. follow-up or chronic-routine) concerns. Some examples of open-ended formats are, *What can I do for you today?*, *What brings you in to see me?*, *How can I help you today?*, *What's going on today?*, and *What's the problem?* These formats are designed to communicate that the concerns being solicited are unknown to physicians. It is in this way that they communicate physicians' *lack* of knowledge of patients' concerns and thus that, for physicians, the concerns are new (see Heath 1981).

For example, see Extract (1). In response to the physician's "So what can I do for you today." (line 18), the patient produces her presenting concern: "W'll- (.) I have (.) som:e shoulder pa:in a:nd (0.2) a:nd (.) (from) the top of my a:rm." (lines 19–21).

Extract 1: SHOULDER PAIN

18	DOC:	So what can I do for you today.
19	PAT:	W'll- (.) I have (.) som:e shoulder pa:in
20		a:nd (0.2) a:nd (.) (from) the top of my
21		a:rm. a:nd (0.2) thuh reason I'm here is
22		because >a couple years ago< I had frozen
23		shoulder in thee other a:rm, an' I had to
24		have surgery. and=( ) this is starting to
25		get stuck, and I want to stop it before it
26		gets stuck.
27		(0.4)
28	DOC:	A[d h e : s i]ve capsuli[tis.]
29	PAT:	[I'm losing] [Ri:gh]t.
30	PAT:	I'm losi:ng (0.4) range of motion in my
31		a:rm.
32		(2.2)
33	DOC:	We:ll. (.) .hh (ng)- ( ) can't you tell

me: thuh=w:asn't there some trau:ma,
er s[omethin'‗ you=(w-) s:]:wung at
PAT: [I've ha:d]
DOC: [some]b[ody [er [.hhhh
PAT: [No.] [I've [had [a history of
DOC: [s:: fe[:ll]
PAT: [bursitis [fer-]=
DOC: =er:=uh n-=there's n:o r:ecent >thing
thet ya< s:ma:shed it, an[ything] you
PAT: [(No)]
can tell me thet .hhh mi:ght've,
DOC: .hh So: it's been bothering you now
since whe:n.
PAT: 'Bout two weeks.
DOC: Just two wee:[ks:.]
PAT: [It's get]ti:ng a little bit
stiffer: an' stiffer.
DOC: .tch Whe[:re.]
PAT: [I wa]ke up in the morning.
Right here:=in thuh shoulder joint.

There is evidence that the patient understands that the physician's question at line 18 solicits a new concern. For instance, Terasaki (1976) argued that speakers do not normally tell recipients news that speakers figure that recipients already know. When the patient informs the physician "I have (.) som:e shoulder pa:in a:nd (0.2) a:nd (.) (from) the top of my a:rm." (lines 19–21), she presents her concern as if the physician does not already know about it (i.e., as if it were new for him). Furthermore, the patient describes her concern as if it were new by saying that it is "starting" (line 24) to get stuck and indicating that it has only existed for "'Bout two weeks." (line 47). There is also evidence that this problem is new for the physician. For example, after the patient finishes presenting her concern, the physician proceeds to ask a series of questions about the concern's cause (see lines 33–39 and 41–44), duration (lines 45–46), and location (line 51). All of these questions display the physician's lack of prior knowledge of the concern and thus that, for him, it is new.

Two examples of closed-ended, new-concern question formats are *You have a problem with your index finger?* and *Your ears are popping, huh?* Physicians frequently produce these questions while reading patients' medical records and thus communicate that they are addressing a concern that was documented by a nurse prior to the visit. Although closed-ended formats communicate that physicians have some idea about the nature of patients' concerns, they nonetheless communicate that such concerns are new to physicians.

For example, in Extract (2), while the physician reads the records, he solicits the patient's presenting concern: "Your ear's ('re) poppin'. huh," (line 14).

Extract 2: EAR PROBLEM

14 DOC: Your ear's ('re) [pop]pin'. huh,
15 PAT: [(I)]
16 (0.7)
17 PAT: Yeah it's like- (.) (either)/(maybe) there's
18 f:luid er wax build up.
19 (0.2)
20 PAT: °But° (.) tuhday's not as ba:d.
21 (1.5)
22 PAT: Actually it started like- (.) week- two weeks
23 ago:=uh week,=h
((19 lines deleted))
43 DOC: Any drainage at a:ll,
44 (0.3)
45 PAT: Only with cue tips.
46 (0.2)
47 DOC: What color is that stuff.
48 (1.7)
49 PAT: .hhh Dark o:range,

There is evidence that the patient's concern is new for the physician. First, the physician's question (line 14), which is produced while reading the patient's medical records, is designed as what Labov and Fanshel (1977) termed a *b-event* statement. *B-event* statements are statements by one speaker (e.g., the physician) that include events (e.g., medical concerns) that another speaker (e.g., the patient) has primary authority over, including access, knowledge, and so on. Stated negatively, *b-event* statements communicate that their speakers (e.g., the physician) do not have primary authority (including knowledge) concerning the event. Physicians' *b-event* solicitations typically seek confirmation or disconfirmation by patients and thus communicate that, for physicians, the concern

Table 2.1 *The relationship between new-concern visits and different question formats*

	New-concern question format	Follow-up-concern question format	"Other"-concern question format	Total
New-concern Visits	68 (88.3%)	0 (0%)	9 (11.7%)	77 (100%)

is new.[7] Second, by proceeding to ask a series of questions about the problem (lines 43 and 47), the physician displays his lack of knowledge about the concern and thus that, for him, the concern is new. There is also evidence that the patient understands that the physician's question solicits a new concern. Similar to the patient in Extract (1), by informing the physician of when the concern started, "Actually it started like- (.) week- tw<u>o</u> weeks ago:=uh week,=h" (lines 22–23), the patient displays an orientation to both the recency of the problem and to the physician not already knowing about the problem (Terasaki 1976).

Quantitative results for new-concern question formats

The data contain 77 cases where patients are visiting physicians with new concerns. Table 1 displays the relationship between visits in which patients had new concerns (i.e., new-concern visits) and the types of question formats that physicians used to solicit those concerns (i.e., new, follow-up, or other).

In 68 out of 77 visits (88.3 percent) in which patients had new concerns, physicians used new-concern question formats. In no cases did physicians use follow-up formats (which are discussed below). In nine cases (11.7 percent), physicians used some other question format. Table 2.1 shows that, in visits where patients had new presenting concerns, physicians were much more likely to use new-concern question formats than they were to use follow-up formats or other formats. This supports the previous, qualitatively supported claim that new-concern formats communicate physicians' understandings that patients have new concerns.

[7] This is supported by the fact that the physician uses the *tag question* "huh," (line 14) to pursue confirmation/disconfirmation (for tag questions, see Sacks et al. 1974) and that the patient produces a confirmation: "Yeah" (line 17).

Question formats designed to solicit follow-up concerns

Follow-up-concern question formats tend to share three features. First, they display physicians' knowledge of a particular concern. Second, they frequently perform the action of soliciting an evaluation or assessment of, or an update on, a particular concern. Third, in doing so, they embody physicians' claims to have had prior experience with the concern in question. (Thus, the concern is specifically *not* new to physicians.) As their name implies, follow-up formats are designed to communicate physicians' understandings that patients have follow-up (vs. new or routine) concerns. For example, Extract (3) is drawn from a follow-up visit for a sore arm.

Extract 3: SORE ARM

DOC: How is it?
(0.5)
PAT: Its fi:ne=its: (0.8) >still a bit< so:re.
but s: alright now.

The physician's question, "How is it?" (line 6), solicits an update or evaluation of a particular concern, which is referenced by "it". By using the reference form "it" – rather than others, such as "the arm" – the physician displays an assumption that his knowledge of the concern is shared by the patient (Schegloff 1996c).[8] In his response, the patient uses the word "still" (line 8) to describe his arm as continuing to be "a bit so:re" relative to a prior point in time. Additionally, he uses the word "now" (line 9) to contrast the current condition of his arm with that during a prior point in time. The prior point in time is the patient's prior visit with the physician. Here, the patient's relative evaluations display his orientation to the concern as being *old* (i.e., non-new) and his presumption that the physician already knows about the concern.

How are you feeling?

It is not too difficult to see that question formats such as "How is it?" solicit follow-up concerns. However, there are other, less obvious formats. In particular, this subsection focuses on the format *How are*

[8] According to Schegloff (1996c), the patient's "it" is a *locally subsequent reference form* located in a *locally initial reference position.*

you feeling? Researchers have included *How are you feeling?* in the category of *How are you?*-type questions, including *How are you?* and *How are you doing?* (Frankel 1995b; Jefferson 1980b). Despite the fact that these question formats all contain lexical and grammatical similarities (e.g., they all begin with *how are you*), all can occur as solicitations of patients' presenting concerns, and all can relevantly be receipted with a range of identical evaluative responses (e.g., *Great, Fine*, and *Terrible*) (Jefferson 1980b; Sacks 1975), they nonetheless accomplish different actions (Button and Casey 1985; Coupland et al. 1994; Jefferson 1980b; Schegloff 1986). On the surface, *How are you feeling?* may appear to be open-ended and social (vs. medical). In contrast, this chapter argues that *How are you feeling?* is narrow and biomedically focused. The question format *How are you feeling?* holds special interest because, unlike other follow-up-concern formats, such as *How's the dizziness?*, the nature of the object that it solicits an evaluation of is less clear (to analysts, but not to participants). Because of this opacity, the action accomplished by *How are you feeling?* is more likely to be misinterpreted by researchers, whose findings are being used to train physicians. What follows is an analysis of the action accomplished by *How are you feeling?* in mundane and medical contexts, respectively.

"How are you feeling?" in mundane conversation. In their analysis of mundane conversation, Button and Casey (1985) included *How are you feeling?* in a category of turns they called *itemized news inquiries*, which are designed to accomplish topic nomination. According to Button and Casey, itemized news inquiries display: (1) a speaker's orientation to a particular event; (2) a speaker's orientation to the event as *live* or *ongoing*; (3) that a speaker has some access to, and knowledge of, the event; (4) a speaker's orientation to the event as being known about by the recipient; (5) that a speaker's knowledge is only partial relative to that of the recipient and thus that there may be news to tell since last time; and (6) a speaker's "'willingness' to hear recipient's news, thereby shaping some part of the conversation around co-participant" (Button and Casey 1985:48). In sum, itemized news inquiries are "requests to be brought up to date on developments concerning an ongoing recipient-related activity or circumstance, and are oriented to finding out about the latest developments, the latest news about

the activity or circumstance" (1985:8). Button and Casey described *How are you feeling?*-type utterances specifically as "solicitous enquiries into troubles which recipients are known to have" (Button and Casey 1985:8; see also Jefferson 1980b) and noted that *How are you feeling?* contrasts "with enquiries into personal states – such as 'How are you' – which do not presume a trouble" (1985:9).

Extending previous research, this chapter argues that, in both mundane and medical contexts, *How are you feeling?* performs the action of soliciting an evaluation of a particular, recipient-owned, currently experienced condition that is known about by the speaker and typically related to physical health. For example, Extract (4) is drawn from a dinner conversation between friends. At line 1, John, the husband of one couple, asks Ann, the pregnant wife of another couple, "How are you feeling. (.) these da:ys."

Extract 4: FAT

1 JOHN: How are you feeling. (.) these da:ys.
2 ANN: Fa:t.
3 JOHN: ((nods for 1.3 seconds while chewing food))
4 ANN: ( ) I can't- I don't have a waist anymore

Ann initially responds with "Fa:t." (line 2). At line 3, John nods while chewing a piece of food, and Ann continues her response with "( ) I can't- I don't have a waist anymore" (line 4). Ann's response of "Fa:t." and her subsequent complaint about losing her figure constitute both negative self-descriptions and negative evaluations concerning one particular aspect of being pregnant – that of gaining weight. In sum, Ann displays her orientation to John's "How are you feeling. (.) these da:ys." as a solicitation of an evaluation of a particular and ongoing, physical-health related condition (in this case, pregnancy).[9] Although the argument being made is for the question format *How are you feeling?*, Ann is admittedly responding to "How are you feeling. (.) these da:ys." (line 1). Turn-terminal,

[9] Researchers have described *How are you feeling?* as inquiring into "troubles" (Button and Casey 1985; Jefferson 1980b). Although pregnancy is not generally considered to be a trouble per se, it is notable that Ann responds with troubling features of her pregnancy and, in that sense, orients to it as a trouble. Nonetheless, this chapter errs on the side of caution when it describes *How are you feeling?* as inquiring into "conditions."

temporal modifications, such as "these da:ys," do not change the action accomplished by *How are you feeling?*, but rather further specify and/or clarify the conditions being inquired into.

For another example, see Extract (5), drawn from a mundane telephone conversation between two friends, Helen and Joyce.

Extract 5: EVERYTHING'S ALRIGHT

1	HELEN:	How are you feeling Joyce.=
2	JOYCE:	=Oh fi:ne.
3	HELEN:	'Cause- I think Doreen mentioned that
4		you weren't so well? A few [weeks ago:?]
5	JOYCE:	[Ye:ah,]
6	JOYCE:	Couple of weeks ago.
7	HELEN:	Ye:ah. And you're alright no: [w?
8	JOYCE:	[Yeah.

Prior to this conversation, Helen has been informed by a third party, Doreen, that Joyce is ill. However, by the time of this conversation, Joyce has recovered (see line 8, where Joyce agrees with Helen's proposal that Joyce is "alright no:w?"). When Helen asks, "How are you feeling Joyce." (line 1), she solicits an evaluation of an ongoing physical-health condition that no longer exists. Thus, Helen's question embodies an incorrect presumption that Joyce is currently ill, and presents Joyce with an interactional conundrum. That is, it makes relevant an evaluative response, but any such response will tend to be heard as an evaluation of a particular and ongoing health condition, which is no longer relevant for Joyce. Heritage (1998) argued that prefacing responses to questions with the particle *Oh* can be a practice for indicating that such questions are inapposite. Joyce's "Oh fi:ne." (line 2) claims that she is not currently experiencing an ongoing, physical-health condition (i.e., she is "fi:ne") and that Helen's "How are you feeling Joyce." (line 1) is inapposite for making such a presumption. Helen displays her understanding that her question was inapposite by going on to explain that her "How are you feeling Joyce." (line 1) was asked based on the presumption that Joyce was ill – with "'Cause- I think Doreen mentioned that you weren't so well? A few weeks ago:?" (lines 3–4), Helen accounts for, and defends, the asking of her question. Furthermore, Joyce agrees with this presumption with "Ye:ah," (line 5). Thus, both Helen and Joyce display that Helen's "How are you feeling Joyce." was indeed designed to solicit an evaluation of a particular and ongoing physical-health condition.

"How are you feeling?" in physician–patient visits. In the previous section, it was argued that, in mundane conversation, *How are you feeling?* performs the action of soliciting an evaluation of a particular, recipient-owned, currently experienced condition that is known about by the speaker and typically related to physical health. As such, as a solicitation of patients' concerns, *How are you feeling?* is suited to the solicitation of follow-up concerns.[10] Initially, this is supported by anecdotal evidence from medical textbooks. For instance, regarding how to begin a medical interview in a hospital context, where patients have known-about and continuing illnesses, medical textbooks advise physicians to first "inquire how the patient is *feeling*" (Bates et al. 1995:12; emphasis added). One suggested solicitation is: "Before I ask you about your illness itself [note the presumption of a preexisting illness], I want to check how you're *feeling* right now?" (Cohen-Cole 1991:56; emphasis added).

Evidence also comes from actual physician–patient communication. For example, in Extract (6), the patient is visiting the physician to follow up on a severe sinus infection.

Extract 6: SINUSES

```
DOC:  Hi mister A[nderso:n. [How are y]ou:::.=
PAT:             [Hi::      [(        )]
PAT:  =Oka::y,
DOC:  How are you feelin' to[da:y. ]
PAT:                        [.hhhh]h Better,
DOC:  And your sinu[se[s?]
PAT:               [.h[.h] ((two 'sniffs'))
      (.)
PAT:  (W)ell they're still: they're about
      the same.
```

[10] Talk in institutional contexts often involves a reduction in the range of interactional practices that participants deploy in mundane contexts and a specialization and respecification of the mundane practices that remain (Drew and Heritage 1992). In physician–patient visits, this does not appear to be the case for *How are you feeling?*, which is a mundane practice that just happens to accomplish an action perfectly suited to physicians' goals of following up on old concerns.

At line 4, the physician asks, "How are you feelin' toda:y." The addition of "toda:y" invites the patient to evaluate the current state of his condition relative to its previous state (presumably during the prior visit). The patient responds with "Better," (line 5), which is a report of improvement on, and thus a positive evaluation of, the state of a particular and ongoing health condition (i.e., his general, sinus-related condition). This is partially supported by the physician's subsequent question, "And your sinuses?" (line 6). By prefacing her question with the word "And," the physician communicates that it is a next question in a series of agenda-related questions begun with "How are you feelin' toda:y." (Heritage and Sorjonen 1994). Insofar as this question requests an evaluation of a specific aspect (i.e., sinuses vs. headaches or sneezing) of the patient's general, sinus-related condition, the physician displays that her "How are you feelin' toda:y" was designed to solicit an evaluation of a particular, ongoing, physical-health condition.

For another example, see Extract (7). In the previous visit, the patient had been ill due to high blood pressure. During that visit, the physician attempted to control the blood pressure by increasing the patient's prescription of a drug named Chlonadine. The current visit has been arranged to follow up on the patient's blood pressure.

Extract 7: NO ENERGY

DOC: Hi Missis Mo:ff[et,
PAT: [Good morning.
DOC: Good mo:rning.
DOC: How are you do:[ing.]
PAT: [Fi:n]e,
(.)
DOC: How are y[ou fe[eling.]
PAT: [Much [(better.)]
PAT: I feel good.
(.)
DOC: Okay.=so you're feeling
a little [bit better] with thuh
PAT: [Mm hm,]
DOC: three: of thuh [Chlon]adine?
PAT: [Yes.]
(.)
DOC: O:ka:y.

Table 2.2 *The relationship between follow-up-concern visits and different question formats*

	New-concern question format	Follow-up-concern question format	"Other" concern question format	Total
Follow-up-concern visits	4 (26.7%)	10 (66.7%)	1 (6.6%)	15 (100%)

In response to the physician's "How are you feeling." (line 7), the patient says "I feel good." (line 9). After the physician accepts the patient's response with "Okay." (line 11), she goes on to formulate an upshot of the patient's response: "so you're feeling a little bit better with thuh three: of thuh Chlonadine?" (lines 11–14; for formulations, see Garfinkel and Sacks 1970; Heritage and Watson 1979). The physician's formulation seeks to confirm that the patient's response was an evaluation of her high blood pressure condition. At line 15, the patient confirms that formulation. In sum, both physician and patient display an understanding that the physician's "How are you feeling." was designed to solicit an evaluation of a particular, ongoing, physical-health condition.

Quantitative results for follow-up-concern question formats

The data contain 15 cases where patients are visiting physicians for follow-up presenting concerns. Table 2.2 displays the relationship between visits in which patients had follow-up concerns (i.e., follow-up-concern visits) and the types of question formats that physicians used to solicit those concerns.

In 10 out of 15 cases (66.7 percent) where patients had follow-up concerns, physicians used follow-up-concern question formats. In 4 cases (26.7 percent) physicians used new-concern formats. (These *deviant* cases are discussed below.) In 1 case (6.6 percent), physicians used some other question format. Table 2.2 shows that, in visits where patients had follow-up presenting concerns, physicians were considerably more likely to use follow-up-concern question formats than they were to use new-concern or other-concern formats. This supports the previous, qualitatively supported claim that follow-up-concern question formats communicate physicians' understandings that patients have follow-up concerns.

Question formats designed to index chronic-routine visits

There also appear to be questions designed to communicate physicians' understandings that patients are visiting to deal with chronic-routine concerns (e.g., monitoring blood pressure or diabetes). During these visits, physicians are commonly faced with two simultaneous issues. On the one hand, these patients generally visit physicians on regular bases (e.g., monthly). Although patients' routine concerns are often in a state of control, they can become problematic and thus need to be monitored. On the other hand, physicians are simultaneously faced with the possibility that these patients also have new concerns. This section focuses on one question format that simultaneously addresses both issues: *What's new?*[11]

"What's new?" in physician–patient visits. What's new?-type question formats allow patients the opportunity to topicalize new medical concerns as first items of business and display physicians' orientations to new medical concerns as being immediately current, newsworthy events relative to routine concerns. As a result, *What's new?*-type question formats simultaneously communicate physicians' understandings that: (1) patients have routine concerns; (2) patients may have new concerns; (3) there is a distinction between new and routine concerns; and (4) both new and routine concerns are potentially relevant. Additionally, *What's new?*-type question formats project a structure for the ensuing visit by projecting at least two potential interactional trajectories. First, if patients have new concerns (and opt to present those concerns), then they will be dealt with first, and upon completion of dealing with those concerns the visit will proceed to dealing with routine concerns. Second, if patients do not have new concerns (or opt not to present new concerns), then the visit will proceed directly to dealing with routine concerns.

[11] Contrary to *How are you?* and *How are you feeling?*, the question format *What's new?* operates differently in medical versus mundane contexts. For a review of *What's new?* in mundane contexts, see Button and Casey (1984, 1985).

The first of these trajectories can be seen in Extract (8). This routine visit is organized around monitoring a variety of medical issues concerning the patient's lungs, heart, blood pressure, vision, and hearing. After the visit is opened, the physician asks, "anything new?" (line 33).

Extract 8: EAR PAIN

33	DOC:	hh Uh:m (0.8) .mtch=anything new?
34		(0.8)
35	PAT:	Nothing: really too new:, but °uh-°
36		I don' know (I/I've) been havin' a funny
37		pai:n, (0.5) an' it swells up right in
38		he::re, ((referring to her head))
		((12 lines deleted))
51	PAT:	.hh An' I never had that before=uh course
52		I've had trouble with this ear for quite a
53		whi:le . . . ((Patient continues))
		((144 lines deleted – history taking and physical exam))
198	DOC:	Uh:m=hh (3.9) We'll j'st keep an eye on
199		things. >It'll<
200		(1.1)
201	DOC:	Check again la:ter.
202		(0.7)
203	DOC:	Uh:m (.) remind me next time.
204		(1.6) ((DOC prepares stethoscope for use))
205	DOC:	Huh uh:hh That's fine. just like
206		that's good.
207	PAT:	.hhhhh hh[hhh
208	DOC:	[(Dee-) deep breath,

The format of the physician's question, "anything new?" (line 33), shapes the patient's response in at least two ways. First, the use of the negative-polarity item *anything* (Horn 1989) establishes a practice-based preference (Schegloff 1988) for a *No*-type response, or a report of no new concerns (regarding preference, see Pomerantz 1984a; Sacks 1987; Schegloff 1988). Second, the action of soliciting new medical concerns relative to routine concerns may embody a structure-based preference (Schegloff 1988) for a *No*-type response; that is, patients who already have a series of ongoing concerns may not want to be seen as having new concerns (see Heritage and Robinson this volume). Nonetheless, the patient has a new concern to present. The patient's initial, long pause (0.8 seconds at line 34) communicates that she is about to produce a dispreferred response, that being a new concern. When the patient begins with "Nothing: really too new:," (line 35), she simultaneously denies the presence of a completely new concern – thereby partially managing face issues involved with having a new concern (see Brown and Levinson 1987) – yet communicates that she has a relatively new concern.

As projected, the patient ultimately presents a new concern, a pain in the left side of her head (lines 35–38). The patient explicitly orients to the concern as being new when she says, ".hh An' I never had that before" (line 51). The physician and patient spend a long time dealing with the new concern. In fact, after 144 lines of talk, the physician is not able to diagnose the concern (lines 198–203). Note that, upon completion of dealing with the new concern, and in accordance with the interactional trajectory projected by the physician's "anything new?", the physician immediately begins to deal with the patient's routine concerns – at line 204 he prepares his stethoscope for use, and at lines 205–208 he begins checking her lungs.

For an example of the second trajectory, see Extract (9).

Extract 9: BLOOD PRESSURE

3 DOC: (Eh) So what's new.
4 (0.2)
5 PAT: Nuh I just came in fer thuh blood pressure
6 reche:ck,
7 (.)
8 DOC: Mm [hm:,]
9 PAT: [Which I] guess was hi:gh,

Contrary to the physician's "anything new?" in Extract 8, here the physician's "So what's new." (line 3) is grammatically designed so as to prefer a *Yes*-type response, or a report of new concerns (see Sacks 1987; Schegloff 1988). Despite this, the patient does not have a new concern to present. The patient's initial, brief pause (0.2 seconds at line 4) may communicate that she is about to produce a dispreferred response, that being a report of no new concerns. This is partially supported by the patient's subsequent "Nuh" (line 5), which is hearably on its way to *Nothing* and thus to rejecting the existence of new concerns. If so, then, according to the second interactional trajectory, we should expect the patient to continue to deal with her routine concerns. Indeed, the patient continues to present a routine concern as her reason for visiting the physician: "I just came in fer thuh blood pressure reche:ck,". The patient's "just" (line 5) minimizes her routine concern, and this may be motivated by the physician's assumption, built into the design of his "So what's new." that the patient has new concerns.

Question formats that do not index patients' institutionally relevant concerns

New-concern, follow-up-concern, and routine-concern question formats are similar in that they index patients' institutionally relevant concerns. Consequently, these formats communicate that physicians are shifting into the activity of dealing with patients' concerns. However, there is at least one question format that does not, in and of itself, index patients' institutionally relevant concerns: *How are you?* In mundane contexts, *How are you?* regularly functions as a request for an evaluation of a recipient's current and general (i.e., unspecified) state of being, such as *I'm fine* (Jefferson 1980b, 1988; Sacks 1975; Schegloff 1986). *How are you?* functions similarly in the opening phase of visits when physicians produce it *prior* to displaying their readiness to deal with patients' concerns (Frankel 1995b; Heath 1981; Robinson 1999). This does not mean that *How are you?* cannot be produced by physicians, and understood by patients, as a solicitation of patients' concerns, nor does it mean that patient's do not exploit *How are you?* as an opportunity to produce, or refer to, their concerns (Robinson 1999). However, this does mean that how *How are you?* gets produced and understood as a solicitation of patients' presenting concerns and is accomplished by interactional practices other than turn design, such as intonation (Schegloff 1986) and the turn's positioning in sequences and activities (Robinson 1999).[12]

Relevant to the present chapter, *How are you?* performs a different action compared to other apparently similar question formats,

[12] Jefferson's (1980b) data show that, in mundane contexts, the question format *How are you doing?* can solicit a conventional response and thus be treated very similarly to *How are you?* However, Jefferson's data also show that *How are you doing?* can solicit an update on, and thus index, a specific event, in which case it would operate similarly to *How are you feeling?* More research needs to be done on the operation of *How are you doing?*

such as *How are you feeling?* For example, return to Extract (6) above. In response to the physician's "How are you:::." (line 1), the patient responds with "Oka::y," (line 3), which treats the physician's solicitation as a request for an evaluation of his current and general (i.e., unspecified) state of being. However, in response to the physician's subsequent turn, "How are you feelin' toda:y." (line 4), the patient responds with "Better," (line 5), which, as argued earlier, is a report of improvement on, and thus a positive evaluation of, the state of a particular and ongoing health condition. Insofar as the physician produces "How are you feelin' toda:y." as a next action after "How are you:::.", and insofar as the patient produces a different form and type of response to each solicitation, both participants display that the two question formats are produced and understood as accomplishing different actions.[13]

[13] It was argued earlier that the question format *How are you feeling?* performs the action of soliciting an evaluation of a particular, physical-health-related condition. The re-examination of Extract (6) raises the possibility that participants' understandings of *How are you feeling?* are at least partially, if not wholly, shaped by the fact that it is sequentially positioned immediately after a sequence initiated by a *How are you?*-type question, as is the case in Extract (7) (see lines 4–5, 7–9). In other words, it might be argued that patients understand physicians' *How are you feeling?*-type questions as indexing medical concerns in part, or entirely, because they follow questions that do not index medical concerns. Although the sequential positioning of *How are you feeling?* certainly contributes to participants' understandings of the action that it accomplishes, it is important to note that *How are you feeling?*-type questions do not always follow *How are you?*-type questions and are not reliant on such a positioning for their sense. For example, see Extract (A), in which a mother has brought her son (i.e., the patient) in to follow up on a cold.

Extract A: COLD

13	-->	DOC:	Ri:ght. how do you feel no:w?
14	-->	SON:	hhehh ((throat clear)) B't be:tter.
15		DOC:	Bit be:tter. looks a bit [better [doesn't he?]
16		MOM:	[Looks [bri:ghter.]
17			doesn't he:. ye:s.=

At line 13, the physician asks, "how do you feel no:w?" The addition of "no:w" invites the patient to evaluate the current state of a condition relative to that during the prior visit. The patient shows that he understands the action performed by the physician's question by responding with "B't be:tter." (line 14), which is a qualified report of improvement on, and thus a positive evaluation of, the state of a particular and ongoing health condition (i.e., his cold). This analysis is supported by the mom's subsequent assessment of her son, "Looks bri:ghter." (line 16), which is a colloquial assessment of improved physical health and which displays the mom's understanding of the son's "B't be:tter." as an evaluation of a physical-health condition.

Question formats that are inappropriately fitted to patients' concerns

So far, it has been demonstrated that physicians use particular question formats to solicit particular types of presenting concerns. If particular question formats are designed to index particular types of concerns and reasons for visiting physicians, then physicians and patients should orient to the appropriateness or inappropriateness of different question formats for the solicitation of different types of concerns. This is what the data support. Return to Table 2.2. In 4 of the 15 cases where patients had follow-up concerns, physicians used new-concern question formats. *In each of these four cases, physicians are held accountable for inappropriately designing their solicitation.* Three of these cases are presented below. For instance, see Extract (10).

Extract 10: DIZZINESS

5	DOC:	So what can I do for you today.
6		(0.2)
7	PAT:	Uh:m- (0.2)
8	DOC:	Oh yes. yes.
9		(0.2)
10	DOC:	.hhh How's the dizziness.=hhh
11	PAT:	Well I went to a therapi:st . . .

In response to the physician's new-concern question format, "So what can I do for you today." (line 5), the patient: (1) briefly pauses (0.2 seconds at line 6) and thus delays her answer; (2) projects, but again delays, her answer with "Uh:m-" (line 7; see Schegloff 1996d); (3) cuts herself off (denoted by the hyphen after "Uh:m-"), which can be a practice for initiating self-repair (Schegloff et al. 1977); and (4) briefly pauses (0.2 seconds at line 7), which yet again delays her answer. All of these things display that the patient is having trouble producing her answer and, reflexively, that she is having trouble dealing with the physician's question (see Lerner 1996; Schegloff 1979). This analysis is partially supported by the fact that, before the patient produces her answer, the physician, who is reading the records, interjects with "Oh yes. yes." (line 8), which embodies a claim to remember the patient's medical history (Heritage 1998). The physician subsequently resolicits the patient's presenting concern, this time with a *different* question format: "How's the dizziness." (line 10). This question format requests an update on a specific medical concern and displays the physician's revised understanding that the patient is visiting for a follow-up (vs. new) concern. In sum, the patient displays trouble with producing a response to the physician's new-concern question format, the physician holds himself accountable for initially soliciting the patient's concern with an inappropriate question format (i.e., a new-concern format), and the physician reformats his question to solicit a follow-up concern.

For a second example, see Extract (11):

Extract 11: INFECTED FOOT

9	DOC:	An::d what brings you here to see see us
10		in the clinic?
11		(1.0)
12	PAT:	Well my (.) foot (1.0) uhm (1.0)
13	PAT:	I was in here on Sunday night=
14	DOC:	=Mmkay
15	PAT:	It's actually a follow up
16	DOC:	Yeah I read over your report uh: that
17		they dictated from the emergency room
18		on Sunday . . .

In response to the physician's new-concern question format, "An::d what brings you here to see see us in the clinic?" (lines 9–10), the patient: (1) produces an extended pause (1.0 second at line 11); (2) begins her answer with "Well," which projects some lack of fit between her answer and the physicians's question (for review, see Schegloff 1995); and (3) begins her answer with "my (.) foot" (line 12), but then delays its progression with two long (1.0-second) pauses and "uhm". Similar to Extract 10, all of these things display that the patient is having trouble producing his answer and, reflexively, that he is having trouble dealing with the physician's question (see Lerner 1996; Schegloff 1979). This trouble stems from his struggle to respond relevantly to a question format that is *inappropriately* fitted to his follow-up concern. This is supported by the fact that the patient subsequently abandons his description and restarts his answer by informing the physician: "I was in here on Sunday night" (line 13). Here, the patient begins to extricate himself from the relevance of the physician's question by indicating that this is not the first time that he has been seen for this particular concern and thus that he has a follow-up concern. The physician's "Mmkay" (line 14) is unresponsive to the patient's informing in terms of the problems that it communicates about the physician's question. At line 15, the patient informs the physician "It's actually a follow up"; the "It's" refers to the patient's reason for the visit. Here, the patient upgrades his informing at line 13 and corrects the physician's mistaken assumption, embodied in the design of the physician's question format, that he has a new concern.[14] In sum, rather than answering the physician's question, which makes relevant the presentation of a new concern, the patient corrects its presupposition concerning the nature of his concern and thus holds the physician accountable for its production.

For a third example, see Extract (12):

Extract 12: MILDLY ABNORMAL SMEAR

49	DOC:	.h Tell me what thuh problem is. th[en.]
50	PAT:	[Well]
51	PAT:	there isn't a problem it- I jus' got a
52		letter from: I had a sme:ar?
53		(0.2)
54	PAT:	Before Christmas?
55	PAT:	[An' I got a letter]=
56	DOC:	[Oh::]=
57	PAT:	=[saying that you wanted to] discuss the
58	DOC:	=[ri:::ght]
59	PAT:	results,

In response to the physician's new-concern question format, "Tell me what the problem is." (line 49), the patient begins by denying the existence of a problem: "Well there isn't a problem" (lines 50–51). Thus, rather than answering the question, the patient begins by rejecting its presupposition that a problem exists. At line 51, the patient twice starts, and then abandons, an answer. The patient first cuts herself off after "it-" and then says, "I jus' got a letter from:". It is possible that, with the latter, the patient was on her way to

[14] The correction is partially accomplished though the use of "actually" (line 15).

producing something similar to what she produces at lines 55–59, "An' I got a letter saying that you wanted to discuss the results," (for word repetition and its functions, see Schegloff 1996a). If so, then the patient abandons a response that would have overtly corrected the physician's presupposition that she has a new concern; that is, she abandons a response that would have informed the physician that her current concern is a follow-up. The patient abandons this response in favor of one that informs the physician that she had a pap smear, "I had a sme:ar?" (line 52), and thus in favor of one that less explicitly corrects the physician's presupposition by allowing the physician to arrive at it independently (for the preference for self-correction, see Schegloff et al. 1977). Note that the patient produces "I had a sme:ar?" with rising intonation, pauses (line 53), and then produces a rising-intoned increment, "Before Christmas?" (line 54), all of which pursue a response from the physician. It is only when no response is forthcoming that the patient reproduces a version of her previously abandoned response (lines 55–59). Simultaneously, the physician produces "Oh::=ri:::ght" (lines 56–58). The "Oh::" displays both her receipt of the information and her change from an uninformed to an informed state concerning the information. The "ri:::ght", which is produced after the patient has produced "An' I got a letter" but before the patient has completed her informing, prematurely treats the patient's informing as both complete and sufficient (Schegloff 1995). By producing "Oh::=ri:::ght", the physician displays both newfound and early recognition of the patient's concern. In sum, both the patient and the physician hold the physician accountable for soliciting the patient's follow-up concern with an inappropriate (i.e., new-concern) question format.

To review, in each of the four cases where physicians used new-concern question formats to solicit follow-up concerns (see Table 2.2), there was an orientation by both physicians and patients to the *inappropriateness* of those formats. Thus, in 14 out of 15 cases (93.4 percent), physicians and patients displayed their understandings that follow-up concerns are appropriately solicited with follow-up-concern question formats.

Physicians can also be held accountable for using new-concern question formats to begin chronic-routine visits. For example, see Extract (13).

Extract 13: BLOOD PRESSURE

13 DOC: How can I help.
14 PAT: Oh its just for a (.) checkup. thank you,
15 DOC: For the pressure? ((i.e., blood pressure))
16 PAT: Yes.

In response to the physician's new-concern question format "How can I help." (line 13), the patient begins by producing the particle "Oh" (line 14), which claims that the physician's question is inapposite (Heritage 1998). The patient continues to produce "its just for a (.) checkup. thank you," (line 14); the "its" refers to the reason for the visit. The patient's "just" mitigates the nature of this reason relative to that presupposed by the physician's new-concern question format. Here, the patient addresses and corrects the presupposition, indexed by the physician's "How can I help.", that she has a new concern. Rather, she has the routine concern of monitoring her blood pressure.

Discussion

This chapter demonstrated three things. First, when physicians solicit patients' presenting concerns, subtle differences in how physicians design/format their questions subtly change the action that those questions perform. Second, physicians and patients orient to the existence of at least three different types of reasons for visiting physicians: dealing with new, follow-up, and chronic-routine concerns. Third, physicians format, are understood to format, and are held accountable for formatting, their solicitations so as to be appropriately fitted to patients' reasons for visiting, and thus to patients' types of concerns. Along these lines, this chapter described question formats that index new, follow-up, and chronic-routine concerns, such as *What can I do for you?*, *How are you feeling?*, and *What's new?*, respectively. This chapter also described the question format *How are you?*, which does not, in and of itself, index patients' institutionally relevant concerns. Finally, this chapter described cases in which physicians inappropriately format their solicitations relative to patients' types of concerns and the resultant interactional consequences.

These findings have implications for research and training. For example, social scientists and medical professionals alike have considered the question format *How are you feeling?* to be open-ended and sensitive to non-biomedical aspects of patients' concerns (Coupland et al. 1994; Seidel et al. 1995).[15] To the contrary, this chapter demonstrated that, in both mundane and medical contexts, *How are you feeling?* performs the action of soliciting an evaluation of a particular medical condition that is related to physical health. Thus, *How are you feeling?* not only performs a different action from other traditionally open-ended question formats, such as *How are you?*, but it is also more narrow and biomedically focused. This is not to say that *How are you feeling?* cannot be an appropriate or sensitive question format. In contrast to new-concern formats, such as *What can I do for you?*, *How are you feeling?* is especially suited to the goal of soliciting follow-up concerns. Furthermore, *How are you feeling?* is affiliative in at least three ways. With it, physicians claim: (1) to have a relatively intimate level of knowledge of patients' lives; (2) a shared, prior relationship with patients; and (3) a level of concern for patients, and express a willingness to listen to patients' concerns (see Button and Casey 1985).

This level of attention to language in context has consequences for medical care. For example, there is evidence that how physicians solicit patients' concerns can have consequences for patients' perceptions of physicians' competence and credibility, and thus for patient outcomes, such as satisfaction. For example, return to Extract (11) above. In this case, the physician is an intern. The physician's question format, "An::d what brings you here to see see us in the clinic?" (lines 9–10) communicates an incorrect understanding that the patient has a new concern. This is one potential strike against the physician's competence and credibility. After the patient overtly corrects the physician, "It's actually a <u>follow</u> up" (line 15), the physician does not acknowledge the correction, as is often the case (see Jefferson 1987; Schegloff et al. 1977). Rather, he simply agrees with the patient, "Yeah" (line 16). This is a second potential strike. Finally, after agreeing with the patient, the physician goes on to inform

[15] Coupland et al. argued that the question format *How are you feeling?* "allows patients to represent (a version of) their affective responses to a wide variety of personal circumstances, whether traditionally within the bio-medical frame or not" (1994:107).

him that he had, in fact, read his records prior to the visit: "I read over your report uh: that they dictated from the emergency room on Sunday" (lines 16–18). Thus, the physician implicitly admits that his initial question format was produced with the knowledge that the patient had a follow-up concern. This is a third potential strike. It is possible that this intern has been trained to solicit patients' presenting concerns with one, and only one, class of question format (i.e., new-concern) and that he has little conception of the interactional dynamics of this process.

As visit time shrinks, practices of communication, especially those involving first impressions, will have an increasing effect on patients' satisfaction, which correlates with important variables, such as patients' willingness to adhere to medical advice, and – perhaps most importantly for physicians – their willingness to sue for malpractice. One area where training can improve is in how physicians solicit patients' presenting concerns.

3

Accounting for the visit: giving reasons for seeking medical care

John Heritage and Jeffrey D. Robinson

"In order to have the privilege of talking to your doctor, you must fulfil the essential precondition of being sick. Then you may go to him and ask him if he will perform his professional services upon you." Anonymous New Zealand Primary Care Physician.

(Byrne and Long 1976:20)

Introduction

It is a well-established principle of social psychology that, in presenting a description of some state of affairs, a person is simultaneously engaged in a presentation of self. The central aim of this chapter is to apply this observation to the medical visit, focusing on how patients' descriptions of their medical problems are designed to manage the social accountability of their decision to visit physicians and, in particular, to justify the decision to seek medical care.

In this chapter we examine the phase of acute medical visits in which patients give their reasons for seeking medical assistance. This phase is normally initiated by an inquiry of some kind from the physician (Robinson this volume; Heritage and Robinson forthcoming),[1] and it is very often terminated by a course of medical questioning which is physician-centered and driven by the physician's

We would like to thank Steven Clayman, Paul Drew, Tim Halkowski, Douglas Maynard, Tanya Stivers, and many graduate students and conference participants for conversation and comment on the themes of this chapter, and on its several previous incarnations.

[1] Heritage and Robinson (forthcoming) note that, in 15 percent of a sample of 120 acute primary care visits, physicians began the visit with a statement for confirmation (e.g., "So sore throat and fever for three days, huh?") which normally resulted in further physician-directed history-taking, rather than a problem presentation by the patient. This form of opening was concentrated in urban rather than rural practices and in cases where the patient was presenting for an upper respiratory tract infection.

technical expertise and medical-technical agenda (Beckman and Frankel 1984). Though it is often of brief duration (Beckman and Frankel 1984; Marvel et al. 1999; Langewitz et al. 2002), the problem presentation phase is one of the only (and often *the* only) structurally provided-for locations where patients are licensed to present their concerns in their own way and in accordance with their own agendas.

Although patients' problem presentations can sometimes appear to be monologues, this appearance is deceptive. Not only are they normally initiated and terminated by physicians, but their progressive development is shaped by physician behavior (Beckman and Frankel 1984). In this discussion, we will consider patient problem presentation as a co-construction: a phase of interaction in which circumstances recognizable as "problems" are presented with whatever elements of cogency or disorganization, affective expression, and recognizable structure and content. This phase is ordinarily terminated by physicians who, finding the moment to take the initiative with whatever elements of circumspection, fumbling, or precision, begin the history.

In this context, patients have a range of choices concerning both the content and the form of the presenting concern. These choices include questions of how symptoms are to be presented; that is, of portraying how the symptoms came to be discovered as objects of consciousness and investigation (Halkowski this volume), how they were recognized (or not), and how they are to be described. Then there is the matter of what patients theorize about the symptoms, and of whether they have social rights to know and describe the elements they talk about. Patients will find themselves electing ways to describe unfamiliar and perhaps alarming physical sensations in the midst of the anxieties engendered by these sensations, and also deciding whether the anxieties themselves and/or the reasoning behind them should be articulated or not. In addition, in terms of what relevancies should symptoms be described? Should patients describe symptoms in terms of their presumed medico-diagnostic relevance, thereby "second-guessing" the physician's reasoning, or alternatively frame descriptions in more self-oriented ways that focus on pain, inconvenience, or fear? Finally, patients will find themselves selecting particular formats with which to present a problem: for example, a simple enumeration of symptoms, or a chronological narrative of the illness culminating in the patient's here-and-now presence in the physician's office, and deciding between the expression or suppression of diagnostic or etiological hypotheses.

What drives these choices? In what follows we will describe three broad types of acute problem presentation, and suggest ways in which the nature of medical problems creates affordances for, as well as constraints on, presentational decisions. Subsequently, we will describe some presentational practices that occur in a variety of combinations, and consider their sociological background and significance.

Data

The data are primarily drawn from two videotaped corpora of acute primary care interactions conducted in community practices of family and internal medicine in Los Angeles County and a mid-sized town in Pennsylvania. These data comprise some 300 primary care visits. Although many visits were reviewed for the purpose of this chapter, the data analysis offered here is qualitative and conversation-analytic rather than quantitative. All data collection was approved by a university human-subjects' protection committee. Participants provided informed consent to be recorded prior to the study, were aware of being recorded, and gave permission to publish the recordings.

Presenting a concern: initial considerations

In presenting medical concerns, patients often make an initial distinction between what we will call "known" and "unknown" problems. *Known problems* are medical conditions with which patients have had previous experience, and divide into two broad classes: (1) *routine* acute problems, such as upper respiratory infections, with which patients and their associates are generally familiar and which have vernacular names like "colds," "flu," etc. and (2) *recurrences* in which patients believe that the problem they are presenting is similar to a non-routine condition which was previously the object of specifically medical diagnosis and treatment. *Unknown problems*, by contrast, are framed as beyond the patient's previous experience. These different types of problems pose distinctive challenges and offer particular affordances for justifying the medical visit.

Routine acute problems

By routine acute problems we mean illnesses that are relatively frequently experienced by most people – colds, flu, heartburn, and so on – which have vernacular names or medical names that are becoming vernacularized. These illnesses are commonly mild, self-limiting, and of short duration, and patients who present with them often describe them using minimizing qualifications like "just" to display an orientation to the fact that they are ordinarily mild complaints:

(1) [Flu]

DOC: What's been goin' o:n?
PAT: I just got (0.4) chest cold a:nd it's been uh
goin' on for a week- I don't seem to be able to
[shake it-
DOC: [O:kay

Or the patient may simply describe a set of symptoms.

(2) [Sinus Infection]

DOC: Okay, (.) what's been goin' o:n
PAT: Ba:d sinuses_ (0.4) achey. (0.2) cold an' ho:t.
(0.6)
DOC: °Okay.°
PAT: Headaches.
(1.0)
PAT: °You know.° (.) your usual.=
DOC: =When did they start. do you think.
DOC: [Thuh symptoms.
PAT: [Monday.

Here the patient's list of symptoms (lines 2–7) is presented in a monotone which conveys their utter mundanity, and this is underscored with her observation "°You know.° (.) your usual.=", which functions to complete her problem presentation.

In sum, patients' presentations of routine acute problems tend to formulate them both as mild and as basically familiar and recognizable.

Recurrent problems

Patients who believe that their problem is a recurrence of a previously diagnosed condition often state this within the first few moments of the problem presentation. In (3), for example, a statement of recurrence is almost literally the first thing out of the patient's mouth:

(3) [Hair Problems]

```
1  DOC:        [.hh [W'[l what brings you in today.
2   PAT:                 [Yea:h.
3  DOC:        Thuh nurse [wrote down that you're
4   PAT:                    [We:ll
5  DOC:        havin' some trouble with your [ha:ir.
6   PAT:                                      [ Y:ea:h.
7          ->  [Aga:in. I'm [really   [upse:[t.
8  DOC:        [(   )        [(Okay) [.hh  [When was thuh la:st time.
9              It w's- its been a whi: [le.
```

Here, with the single word "Aga:in." (line 7), the patient indicates a description of her condition as recurrent, prompting the physician to begin a search through her chart for the previous episode of her complaint. A similar case is the following, in which the patient also presents the physician with the medication she was previously prescribed (line 10):

(4) [Eczema]

```
 1  DOC:       .hhh So what's goin' o:n today. what brings you i:[n.
 2   PAT:  ->                                                     [Well- I
 3         ->  have this lip thing again:,=
 4  DOC:       =Aga:in. [Huh?
 5   PAT:                [Yes:[:.
 6  DOC:                      [>When was< thuh las' time we
 7             s[aw you (.) for that.
 8   PAT:       [M:arch.
 9  DOC:       (In M:arch.)
10   PAT:      An' you gave me thi:s:. er- prescribed me this:.
```

More consequential self-diagnoses are more elaborated, as in (5), where the patient goes to some lengths to describe her past experience and to develop the parallel with her present condition:

(5) [Frozen Shoulder]

DOC: So what can I do for you today.
PAT: W'll- (.) I have (.) som:e shoulder pa:in a:nd (0.2) a:nd
-> (.) (from) the top of my a:rm. A:nd (0.2) thuh reason I'm
-> here is because >a couple years ago < I had frozen shoulder
-> in the other a:rm, an' I had to have surgery. and=( )
-> this is starting to get stuck, and I want to stop it before
-> it gets stuck.
(0.4)
DOC: Adhe:sive capsulitis.

At line 9, the physician responds with a more "medical" term ("adhesive capsulitis") replacing the "frozen shoulder" mentioned by the patient (line 4).

In a final case the patient, who is dealing with a primary care physician he does not know, begins by detailing a range of symptoms – shortness of breath, a feeling that his blood pressure is rising, dizziness, and tingling feelings – and brings his account to a climax by asserting the similarity of these symptoms to those he experienced in a heart attack the previous year:

(6) [Dizzy and Tingling Sensations]

DOC: How you doing today?
(2.1)
PAT: Well, (·hhh) I'm a hhh short uh: of breath, an' uh like uh (.)
I feel like (1.1) uh (0.4) blood pressure keeps (0.6) going up.
<This's been (a-uh-) (1.2) two weeks.
DOC: [Two weeks.
PAT: [An' I'm
(0.4)
DOC: Okay,
PAT: ((sniff)) O:hh ((sigh-like)) dizzy, < and this side of the head
is hurtin' (0.4) and (0.4) you know like (0.2) tingling on this
-> side. (0.9) (like) (0.2) ( ) (0.2) like it started happening:
-> (.) last year when I first had the- f:irs[t heart attack.
DOC: [Okay so t- u:h (0.7)
so tell me about so you had a heart attack, about a year ago:?

Notable here is the patient's revision of his final remark making reference to the heart attack. At first, with "like it started happening: (.) last year when I first had the-" (lines 11–12), the patient appears to be analogizing between his current symptoms and those preceding an earlier heart attack. However, perhaps because he finds himself using the definite article to refer to a heart attack that is unknown to this physician, he revises the final phrase to become "the- f:irst heart attack." (line 13), thus reinforcing his implied claim that another such attack is imminent.

Unknown medical problems

Unknown medical problems, by contrast, are presented as basically strange and unrecognizable. They involve symptoms, sensations, and effects which cannot easily be "placed" or explained except as departures from normality. This is quite apparent in (7), where the patient struggles to describe a condition which she has never experienced before:

(7) [Costochondritis]

1 DOC: What can I ↑do for you today.
2 (0.5)
3 PAT: We:ll- (0.4) I fee:l like (.) there's something
4 wro:ng do:wn underneath here in my rib area.
5 DOC: Mka:[y,
6 PAT: [I don't uh:m (0.4) I thought I might'a cracked 'em
7 somehow but I have no clue ho:w,
8 (0.4)
9 PAT: An' I don't even know what cracked ribs £f(h)eel like. £ I jus'
10 Know that there's a pa:in there that shouldn't be. ·hh an' as
11 I'm sittin' here its not (.) not as ba:d but when I'm up an'
12 active an' (.) movin' around an' breathin' an' (.) doin' all
13 that (.) you=know (.) extra (.) [heavy breathin' it (w's)
14 DOC: [Mm hm:,
15 really bo:therin' me.
16 DOC: ·tch= ·hh So- (.) when you take a deep
17 brea[th, does that make it wo:r[se.
18 PAT: [Y:eah. [Yeah.

Here the patient's report of her symptoms is initiated with a formulation "something wro:ng do:wn underneath here in my rib area."

(lines 3–4), which projects a description of symptoms as vaguely known and not understood. She then offers a hypothetical diagnosis for her condition the initiation of which (with "I thought") at line 6 suggests that it is already discounted (Jefferson 2004a; Halkowski this volume), and whose subsequent elements only contribute further elements of doubt to the hypothesis. Finally she offers as the primary symptom that she has "a pa:in there that shouldn't be." (line 10), which she subsequently connects to activity. In every way, this problem presentation is a venture into the unknown.

And in the following two cases, patients offer initial characterizations of their problems as "unknown." In (8), sheer uncertainty about a presently undescribed questionable state of affairs is presented as a reasonable and legitimate basis for a medical visit:

(8) [Questionable Mole]

1 DOC: What's ha:ppenin' to ya Clarisse
2 PAT: I don't know sir=if I knew that I wouldn't
3 h[ave [(ta)
4 DOC: [You [wouldn't be here. [hu:h?
5 PAT: [Yeah. This is true. .hh I- I asked . . .

Here the patient is explicit in stating that her reason for the visit has to do with uncertainty. She is there for a medical evaluation of a questionable condition. In this way, her visit will be legitimated even if her condition is not a medical problem and should not be "treated." Unknown problems deserve medical evaluation.[2] And in (9), the patient, having located the problem to her left ear, immediately goes on to state that she doesn't know "What's going on.", and to rule out a "cold" as the cause of her problem.

[2] As a counterpoint to this case, it may be noted that the transposition of this orientation to other agencies, such as 911 emergency, can have adverse consequences. In a telephone to Dallas 911, the caller began in a similar fashion:

911: And whatiz thuh problem there.
CLR: I don't kno:w, if I knew I wouldn't be needin'
[y-
911: [Si:r:, I a- would you answer my questions
please? whatiz thu[h problem?]
CLR: [She is hav]ing difficult in breathing

Here a stance that can be treated as legitimate in the physician–patient context resulted in rejection of the caller's request. The result was that the caller's mother died without assistance ever being dispatched (Whalen et al. 1988).

(9) [Ear Pain]

1 DOC: What's goin' o:n.
2 PAT: .h >Uhm< I'm having som:e <problems with my left ear.>
3 I don't know_ .h uh:m what's going >on. I< don't have
4 a co:ld, I haven't had a cold_ .hhh a:::n' uh:m (0.7)
5 I::: .hh it- it s:tarted . . .

Other presentations of unknown problems may begin with "first thoughts" (Jefferson 2004a; Halkowski this volume) in which patients present understandings of their concerns which are flagged as incorrect. In (10) below, the patient details the emergence of his symptoms some three months prior to the visit by reference to his first notion, now discounted (with "I thought"), that it was an insect bite. Subsequently he details the development of symptoms that are not compatible with this initial conception of the problem, thereby building an extensive depiction of a problem that is presently "unknown."

(10) [Ringworm]

1 DOC: What happened.
2 (.)
3 PAT: Well I got (.) what I thought (.) in Ju:ne (.)
4 uh was an insect bite.=in thuh back of my neck here_
5 DOC: Okay,
6 PAT: An' I (0.2) you know became aware of it 'cause
7 it was itching an'=I (.) scratched at't,

Here the patient can describe his symptoms and their progression well enough, but he is at a loss to understand them (see below).

We conclude by noting that this is a rough classification of problem *presentations*. There is not an automatic one-to-one correspondence between the type of problem that a patient is presenting with and its style of presentation. The patient may be mistaken in proposing a recurrence – as was eventually determined in (4) and (5) above. Moreover, a patient may offer a problem presentation in a misleading fashion:

(11) [Breathless]

1 DOC: =hhhhh So::. What's the problem.
2 hhh[hhhhhhhhhhhhhhhhh
3 PAT: -> [Well, me breathin's shockin'.

4	DOC:		Ri:ght.
5	PAT:	->	As I'm wa::lkin' [ah- (0.3) I 'av ta sto:p.
6	DOC:		[Yeah, (.) Yeah,
7	DOC:		Yeahs.
8			(.)
9	PAT:	->	An' even when- >do you know when ya go< ta
10			shake the pillas up,
11	DOC:		Yeah
12			(0.3)
13	PAT:	->	I ga- I go out a bre:ath.
14	DOC:		Mm
15			. . .
			((12 lines of data omitted))
27	DOC:		·hhhhh (0.4) Th- this isn' something completely
28			new:: you've had it before . . . ((continues))

In (11), the patient presents the problem as if it were new, and with no indication that she had been treated for the problem previously. However, at line 27, her physician determines from chart notes that a colleague in the same practice had treated her for this condition six months previously. It is likely that the patient has presented this problem as "new" because it is new-for-this-physician. Examples like this underscore that we need to maintain a differentiation between the way in which a problem is presented, and the problem itself as it is understood by physician and patient.

Nonetheless, it is useful to distinguish between these three main types of medical problem presentation which, at least in patients' accounts and physicians' responses to them, are treated as relatively distinct. First are routine acute medical conditions in which known minor and self-limiting medical problems with vernacular names are presented, often in association with an enumeration of current symptoms. Second are recurrences in which patients present symptoms in terms of their similarity to the symptoms of previously diagnosed medical conditions in a process that can often amount to self-diagnosis. Finally there are new and unknown conditions in which patients describe symptoms and their development in ways that underscore their doubt and uncertainty about their medical problems.

Accounting for the visit: the problem of legitimate doctorability

By the act of making an appointment and walking into the physician's office, patients commit themselves to the belief that they have a legitimate reason for attending. This can be a fraught moment for a patient. The patient has a condition which is causing concern, and may be anxious to describe it correctly and present it in an appropriate fashion. Moreover, the presentation, as Bloor and Horobin (1975) noted a quarter-century ago, can involve tensions between lay and professional judgment. Prior to visiting the physician, patients must make a judgment that they have a legitimate concern. Yet this judgment will itself be judged over the course of the visit. Under these circumstances, patients may find themselves designing their descriptions of events, experiences, and circumstances so as to communicate "good reasons" that will justify them being in the physician's office (Halkowski this volume; Heath 1992).

Thus, at the beginning of the medical visit, the patients can face the task of presenting their medical concern as "*doctorable*."[3] For patients, a doctorable problem is one that is worthy of medical attention, worthy of evaluation as a potentially significant medical condition, worthy of counseling and, where necessary, medical treatment. Establishing that they have a doctorable problem is a fundamental aspect of patients' justifications for the decision to visit a physician. It is a means for patients to show that they are reasonable people, which in this context means showing that they have a problem or a concern for which seeking medical assistance is a reasonable solution. Alternatively, reasonableness can be claimed by a display of doubt, if indeed patients believe that their symptoms are only matters of marginally legitimate concern. The presentation of a complaint determined to be nondoctorable can deprive the patient of authoritative medical support for their claim to financial and other benefits from entering the "sick role" (Parsons 1951, 1975; Freidson 1970a), and engender a vulnerability to the judgment that they were misguided in seeking medical assistance, are overconcerned about their health, or in illegitimate search of "secondary gains" from the sick role itself. Patients' concerns with doctorability thus center on showing that they are reasonable people, with "good reasons" to present themselves at the physician's office. Providing for

[3] This term is adapted from Jay Meehan's work on calls to 911 emergency. Meehan (1989) noted callers' interests in showing that their calls were about issues that were legitimate subjects of police interest or intervention, i.e., that they were "police relevant" or "policeable." Related studies by Whalen and Zimmerman (1990), Whalen et al. (1988), and Zimmerman (1992) show the complexities that can be involved in conveying the legitimacy of a call to 911.

that reasonableness effectively converges with providing for the doctorability of the concern which they present.

For example, in (12) the patient's preoccupation with justifying her medical visit effectively dominates her entire problem presentation: this patient has previously been treated for a small basal cell carcinoma on the back of her neck, and she has recently discovered a suspicious raised spot (which she refers to as a "mole" [line 7]) at, or close to, the place where she was previously treated:

(12) [Questionable Lesion]

PAT: I'm here on fal[se pre- pretenses.<I think.
DOC: [·hh
DOC: [<Yes.
PAT: [ehh! hih heh heh heh!
((Five lines omitted))
PAT: I asked my husband yesterday 'cause I could feel: (0.8) (cause)
I: could feel this li'l mo:le coming. An:d: uh (0.5) (he) (.) I:
hh thought I better letchya know-<uh well I asked my husband 'f
it was in the same place you took off thuh (0.5) °thee (mm)
thee: °([ )
DOC: [That's why you've come in be[cause of the mo:le.
PAT: [that's why I ca:me, but=
DOC: =H[ow long 'as it been-]
PAT: [t h i s m o r ning-] I: I didn' I hadn't looked yesterday
he said it was in the same place but ·hh but I: can feel it
nah- it's down here an' the other one was up here so I don't
think it's: th'same one at a:ll.
DOC: Since when.
(0.8)
PAT: Y(h)ea(h)h I(h) just felt it yesterday 'n
DOC: Does it hurt?
PAT: No?
(.)
PAT: No it's just a li:ttle ti:ny thing bu:t=I (.) figured I
sh(h)ou(h)ld l(h)et y(h)ou kn(h) ow .hhh i(h)f i(h)t was (on)
the same pla:ce, b't
DOC: So when you push [on it it doesn't hur[t.
PAT: [(Right.) [No it's
PAT: just a little- li:ttle tiny skin: [(tag) really.
DOC: [I: (.) see=
DOC: =Yeah it's different than whatchu had be[fore.
PAT: [Uh huh.
DOC: Your scar is up here,

34 PAT: Yeah that'[s what I figured (an-)
35 DOC: [An'
36 DOC: An' this is down below.
37 PAT: .hh When he s- When he told me it was in the same place I
38 thought Uh: Oh: I better ca:ll a(h)nd te(h)ll yo(h)u .hhh
39 DOC: Ri:ght.
40 (.)
41 DOC: That's- I'm <ve:ry gla:d that you uh> did that.

A number of aspects of this patient's problem presentation exhibit a concern with the doctorability of her complaint:

1. Her initial statement (line 1) explicitly expresses doubts that her complaint is doctorable, and that her visit is justified. At most, the patient presents her problem as a possible problem.
2. At lines 6, 8, 15, and 37, the patient invokes her husband, a third party, to bolster the validity of her decision to come to the physician with her problem, in effect co-implicating him in the decision to make the visit. At the same time, she disaffiliates (lines 15–17) from the judgment that she reports him as having made about the positioning of the "mole" that is worrying her.
3. When the physician starts to question her at line 11–13, she responds to him briefly in overlap, and then continues on with her account, thus effectively bypassing the physician's attempt to redirect her account. It is relatively unusual for a patient to compete in overlap with a physician, and to resist a course of questioning that a physician initiates during the problem presentation (Beckman and Frankel 1984). In this case, the patient competes with the physician specifically to express further doubts about the doctorability of her condition.
4. When the patient, at line 25, reports making her decision to come in for the visit, she inflects her talk at exactly that place with "breathy" laugh particles. Speakers have the capacity to do this very precisely (Jefferson 1985), and the injection of laugh particles into talk is often associated with the reporting of "misdeeds" of some kind (Jefferson et al. 1987), especially in medical consultations (Haakana 1999, 2001).

Up to this point in the patient's account, we have considered the issue of doctorability as a prospective one that can dominate the problem presentation phase of the consultation. While this issue is particularly apparent during problem presentation, it can also resurface at later moments during the consultation. This is also shown in this datum. The patient's preoccupation with doctorability continues after the physician's evaluation at line 31, "Yeah it's different than whatchu had before." In particular:

5. The patient, who has positioned herself as skeptical about the nature of the problem prior to the physician's "no problem" evaluation, exhibits agreement with that evaluation (line 34). This agreement is consistent with her earlier skepticism, but it also underscores that she is attentive to the issue of reasonable and unreasonable grounds for visiting her physician. It is notable that it is couched in the past tense, conveying that her own position is independent of the physician's evaluation.
6. Then, in redescribing the basis of her decision to come in for the consultation, the patient reinvokes her husband's judgment, and again infiltrates her report of the decision to make the appointment with laugh particles (lines 37–38).

Finally,

7. The patient's redescription of the rationale for her decision has the effect of inviting the physician to offer reassurance as to the legitimacy of her decision to make the visit, and he does so at line 41, by saying "That's- I'm <ve:ry gla:d that you uh> did that."

Though dramatic, this case is matched by others which, in a lower-key way, embody the same preoccupations. In (13), for example, the patient is concerned to stress the exceptional nature of her cold symptoms:

(13) [Cold]

1 DOC: What can I do for you,
2 PAT: It's just- I wouldn' normally come with a cold,=but I
3 'ad this: co::ld. (0.4) fer about.hh >m's been< on
4 (Fri:day).=I keep coughin' up green all the time?

Here the patient's claim that she wouldn't "normally" come with a cold is complemented by her description of a symptom ("coughin' up green") that she treats as problematic. In this way, she asserts the legitimacy of the visit.

A similar concern with doctorability is apparent in the following case:

(14) [Pulled Tendon]

1	DOC:		Something wrong with your hand I understand, huh?
2	PAT:	->	I- it's probably something stupid, but I figure I better
3			have it checked out.
4	DOC:	->	It's never stupid. What have you been up to these days? You
5			watch the Penn State game yesterday?
6			. . .
7			. . .
8	PAT:		Uh, the other day I went to get in my truck, and I grabbed hold
9			of the steering wheel, as usual, and jumped up in it. And when
10			I did, I felt something snap, and you could hear it snap inside
11			my hand. And the pain just shot, like right up my arm.

In this case the patient begins his problem presentation with "I-", which was probably going to be the account of how he injured himself getting into his truck (see line 8). However, he abandons this in favor of a turn that disavows the seriousness of the problem he is about to present: "it's probably something stupid, but I figure I better have it checked out."(lines 2–3). The physician immediately moves to reassure the patient at line 4.

In (12) and (14), the physician, alerted to the patient's concern with doctorability, responded by validating the patient's decision to make the visit. But similar acts of validation can occur shortly after problem presentations which have shown no overt preoccupation with doctorability:

(15) [Ear Pain]

1	DOC:	Mkay¿ (.) mtch!.hh So::, you c'n tell me about yer:: head. nhh
2	PAT:	tch! U:m, (0.4) I: woke up last night, an:' ihm- ihm- it hurts
3		tih touch this side uh my fa:ce, and my ear: (.) is really
4		botherin' me,
5	DOC:	M[mh:m.
6	PAT:	[Sometimes it- (.) I can feel thuh pai:n, other times it's just
7		touching it.an' it hurts. .hh An' u:h (0.6) I didn't sleep much
8		last night, so I figured maybe some- yi- maybe had the ear
9		infection.er something.=
10	DOC:	=So this woke you from your sleep.
11	PAT:	Yeah.

12 DOC: -> That's an important enough. Okay.
13 (0.3)
14 DOC: .hhm tch! Do you have a sore throat?

(16) [Inflamed Parotid Gland]

1 DOC: .hhh Sounds like you're uncomfortable hh
2 PAT: Yeah my ear and my- s- one side of my throat hurts.
3 DOC: .hh So when'd all this start?
4 PAT: Started earlier in the week but I just kept thinking it
5 would get better
6 DOC: And it didn't
7 PAT: No I just- I wake up and it's okay and then it starts to
8 DOC: -> So you toughed it out all week?
9 PAT: Yeah
10 DOC: -> You're a tough cookie.

In (15) the physician explicitly validates the patient's medical concern as "important enough.", and in (16) the patient's character and actions are evaluated as "tough" with the implied judgment that the patient showed fortitude in trying to "wait out" the condition and is now making the visit for a "good reason."

In this set of cases patients, or physicians, or both physicians and patients, display an overt preoccupation with whether (or not) the patient has a legitimate reason for making a medical visit. And we will argue that many facets of patient problem presentation address this issue in more covert ways.

Before proceeding, however, we wish to underscore that a substantial subset of problem presentations shows no concern with doctorability. Prominent among these are visits which are motivated by accidental injuries. In (17), for example, the patient's problem presentation is succinct and entirely devoid of circumstantial justification:

(17) [Cat Bite]

1 DOC: .hh (.) What's goin' on toda:y.
2 PAT: I got bit by my neighbor's cat.=
3 ( ): =mhhh hh!
4 DOC: .hh 'At doesn't sound like fun,=How did 'at happ[en.
5 PAT: [.hh O:h,
6 PAT: I was: uh kinda pettin' him outsi:de, 'n: (.) my other

7 neighbor's cat came eover an' I think spooked him,
8 DOC: nOka:y.
9 PAT: So 'e got me pretty good.>An' they were
10 p[retty big punctu[re wo:unds.
11 DOC: [nOkay. [tch! .hh An:d >when did this happen?

Example (18) is similarly devoid of justification, though the patient's formulation ("I wanna get rid") does hint at an extended period of illness, which is, in turn, just what the physician's initial question pursues:

(18) [Bronchitis]

1 DOC: What can we do for you toda:y. What brings ya i:n.
2 PAT: Uh:=I wanna get rid=a this: stuff in my
3 ·lu:ng[s.·
4 DOC: [O:kay, >.hh< how long have you been sick for.
5 (0.5)
6 PAT: Four (weeks.)

In each of these cases, the patient's problem presentation could hardly be less elaborated: there is no orientation to justifying the visit beyond the simple description of the complaint, which is thus presented as requiring no further justification.

If developing their concern as a doctorable problem is a primary task for many patients during the reason-for-the-visit phase of the consultation, that task becomes attenuated, at least to a degree, when the physician asks the first history-taking question. At that point, the patient's concern becomes "medicalized" by being reconstructed within a course of questioning that embodies a medical frame of reference. With the first history-taking question, the patient ceases to build the case for their concern alone and becomes a party to the co-construction of their concern as a medical problem. Thus the first history-taking question embodies a kind of tacit and provisional bargain that validates the patient's belief that the concern is worthy of medical attention. The reason for the visit phase is occupied with a progression towards that bargain. After this point, patients can surrender control of the encounter in exchange for the medical questioning that, by taking the concern seriously, prospectively underwrites the doctorability of their problems.

Practices for justifying medical visits

A patient who is confronting a medical visit, whether in prospect or in actuality, may have a variety of conflicting issues to manage. Prominent among these are the symptoms to be described and addressed. The description of symptoms is ordinarily central to the justification of a medical visit. What are they (Becker et al. 1993)? How long have they lasted? How did the patient come to notice and identify them (Halkowski this volume)? How much does the patient understand about these symptoms and on what authority (Bloor and Horobin 1975; Heath 1992; Peräkylä 1998)? How serious does the patient think they are, and to what extent should concern about that seriousness be communicated (Bergh 1998; Lang et al. 2000)?

In the following sections, we describe three descriptive practices which patients use in contexts where justifying the medical visit seems to be clearly at stake. These involve (1) making diagnostic claims, (2) invoking third parties as part of the decision-making process, and (3) making "troubles-resistant" claims, for example, about the length of time they have waited before seeking medical assistance. All of these elements could emerge "naturally" during the physician-directed medical history. For example, compare (18) above, with (19) below:

(19) [Heel Pain]

DOC:		Now what brought you in this: a:fternoon.
PAT:		tsk I've got a pain on my- on my heel.
DOC:		Yes.
PAT:	->	And it's been goin' on since roughly about February
	->	on and off,
DOC:		Uh huh,
		(1.0)
PAT:		A:nd I finally decided it's gettin' bad enough where I can
		barely walk and it's especially worse in the mornings.

This visit occurred in June, so when the patient describes her problem as going on since February, she is describing a period of pain and discomfort that is certainly long enough to motivate a medical visit. What is significant about this case is that, rather than waiting to have the duration of her problem elicited as a "simple fact" during the history, she volunteers it during the problem presentation.[4] It is the volunteering of this fact that contributes to the sense of its role as a justification, and of a felt need to justify. The bronchitis patient in (18), by contrast, feels no need to volunteer that he has been dealing with his symptoms for four weeks, and this contributes to the sense that he regards his problem as unquestionably doctorable and as not requiring justification.

Making diagnostic claims

One of the most consistent findings from studies of physician–patient interaction is that, although patients often have quite well-developed diagnostic hunches about their illnesses, they are guarded in introducing them into the consultation (Gill 1998a; Gill and Maynard this volume; see also Drew this volume).

Several factors may underlie this disposition. First, the participants may orient to diagnosis as the task of the physician, and as an area in which the physician has legitimate expertise:

(20) [Urinary Tract Infection]

DOC: >How do you do.<
(0.9)
PAT: I got a "U" "T" "I",
(0.2)
PAT: I think,
DOC: Uhh huh ((laugh)) £Okay look. that makes
my job easy,£ y(h)ou've a(h)lr(h)ead(h)y
d(h)i(h)ag[n(h)osed (h)it.
PAT: [I know.
DOC: .hhh £Okay.£ .hh £have a seat over here.£

In this case the physician's response, though articulated through laughter and with good humor, nonetheless mildly sanctions the patient. Patients may also find that self-diagnoses attract questioning that, whether implicitly or explicitly, challenges their rights to know what they claim. This is most apparent in technical diagnoses:

[4] This volunteering is, of course, facilitated by the physician's use of acknowledgments (lines 3 and 6), which facilitate the patient's continuation of her presentation (see Beach 1993, 1995; Beckman and Frankel 1984; Robinson and Heritage 2003).

(21) [Bell's Palsy]

DOC: Tell me what's going o:n.
PAT: I got this Bell's Palsy and uhm I already
(.) I've had it from yesterday (0.3) I already:
DOC: -> Who diagnosed it.
PAT: Uh:: a doctor at UCLA: (0.3) right on campus.
DOC: Mm hm,

(22) [Torn Rotator Cuff]

DOC: .hh So: can you tell me:=uh what brings you
in today?
PAT: Uh=I got=uh- torn (roto cuff:.)
(.)
PAT: in my left shoulder.
(1.0)
DOC: -> (Ok[ay) who told you tha:t.
PAT: [An:'
PAT: Uh: family doctor,
(.)
PAT: I: did it about: nine months ago:=I really don't
even know how I did it.

And, in the following case, where the patient's previous experience with this medical problem would likely have been unforgettable, the physician pursues it as a means of evaluating the likely validity of the patient's proposal:

(23) [Kidney Stone]

DOC: ·hh u-What's been goin' o:n with ya.
(.)
PAT: -> Uh:m=hh I don' know if it's a (0.4) urinary
-> tract infection or a bladder infection b't (.)
feel like (ya) gotta (.) go=da thuh bathroom
all thuh time there's burning s- (0.4) and uh
(0.2) right before I (came/come) up I got a
real ba:d (.) sharp pai:n in (.) in my right
si:de. (wh-) (.) where my kidney's at.
(.)
DOC: Okay,
PAT: I mean it was- (0.2) mean I- my whole body went
numb, (.) thought (I would) pass out.

14 DOC: Really.
15 (0.6)
16 DOC: Oka:y,
17 PAT: -> I don' know if its kidney sto:nes, (0.3) er
18 -> what. b't (0.9)
19 DOC: -> Have you ever had kidney stones.

Another reason for caution in the presentation of diagnostic theories may be the anticipation of disagreement with the physician, a circumstance in which the lay opinion is unlikely to win the day. Moreover, where patients have come to believe that their symptoms imply a serious diagnosis, they may be reluctant to voice this conclusion. For if they are wrong, they may fear being perceived as the kind of person who tends, unnecessarily, to believe the worst. And, if they are right, they may believe that such a conclusion should be the outcome of an investigation that is not "primed" or "biased" in favor of their worst fears. All in all, patients may have good reasons for not presenting their diagnostic theories, and as Heath (1992) and Peräkylä (1998, 2002, this volume) have shown, overt diagnostic disagreements between patients and physicians mainly involve disputes about "no problem" diagnoses.

On the other hand, self-diagnosis can also be a trump card in claiming doctorability, and in expediting the move towards the physical examination and treatment (Stivers 2002b; Robinson 2003). Patients who are experienced with a particular medical problem can self-diagnose and cite a previous experience as the basis for their conclusion (see arrows 1 and 2 in [26]). In (24), the patient immediately cites an earlier diagnosis of skin cancer at his HMO:

(24) [Actinic Keratosis]

1 PAT: =Now look it here.
2 (0.2)
3 PAT: I got cancer here.
4 (.)
5 DOC: Uh hu[h,
6 PAT: [I know it's cancer because it=was told to me
7 from a doctor one time before [he said you have a
8 DOC: [Uh huh,
9 PAT: touch, .h I had some here an' they >cut it
10 out< over at [HMO name] ye[ars ago.

11 DOC: [Oka:y,
12 PAT: .hh But n:ow I think it's coming in here, here,
13 and over there.

In (25), the patient invites his wife to corroborate his cautiously framed (with "[I] don't know if it's . . .") candidate self-diagnosis (lines 3–6). At lines 9–11, he discloses that this is a regular problem, and he shortly afterwards describes hospitalization for the problem (data not shown):

(25) [Prostate]

1 DOC: .hhhh What's been goin' on with you:.
2 (0.2)
3 PAT: .hh h=I:- (.) -huh=huh=hh ((throat clear)) (0.7) don't
4 know if it's a flare up of that stinkin' infection I get or
5 not. I- couple years ago (I)='ad (2.0) pro:state infection.
6 wa'n't it.
7 (0.8)
8 WIF: Mm hm,
9 PAT: And about one once::- once a ye:ar I get- (0.5) (th')
10 symptoms and stuff. from it. an': (0.4) usually end up
11 gettin' an a:n'ibiotic for it.
12 DOC: Right.

In (26), the patient's slightly qualified self-diagnosis is supported at some distance with "See I get them all thuh ti:me" (line 13):

(26) [Kidney Infection]

1 DOC: W'l what brings ya in today.
2 PAT: 1-> I: (.) j's think I have a kidney infection.=
3 DOC: =Uh oh:,
4 (.)
5 DOC: When did this start.
6 (0.4)
7 PAT: ( ) but like- (0.2) beginning of july::,
8 DOC: Beginning of july::.
9 PAT: [#Yeah#
10 DOC: [Oh my:.
11 (.)
12 DOC: Okay,
13 PAT: 2-> e-=See I get them all thuh ti:me . . . . ((continues))

And in (27), a self-diagnosed "prognosis" is invoked to account for a visit in which the patient's current symptoms are mild:

(27) [Strep Throat]

DOC: .hh U:m: (2.0) what's been goin' o:n.
PAT: Ah just achiness sore throat, an' .h I jus' thought
-> rather than wait, um (0.2) I just have seen up a
-> predisposition t' pick up strep throat durin' the school
year.=I teach kindergarten.=
DOC: =Oh you do.=
PAT: =So but thuh ^school year hasn't [^started yet,
DOC: [eh heh heh heh heh heh
heh ((laughs)) [.hhh
PAT: [I jus' thought rather than wait, °I want
to stop in and check.°

Here the patient justifies her decision in terms of what her symptoms may come to, rather than what they are currently.

Yet self-diagnosis may need to be handled with caution. Absent the possibility of analogy to a previous, on-the-record diagnosis that can be retrieved from the patient's chart, patients may look for other ways to support a diagnostic proposal that would warrant the medical visit. Thus in (28), the patient is careful to attribute the diagnosis to a "girlfriend" to disavow any experience with the condition:

(28) [Sore Throat]

DOC: So you're having a bad sore throat huh.
PAT: Yes:: um (.) a- a girl friend of mine kinda made me
paranoid about it. =She said u:m (.) uh it could be
strep throat but I've never had it before
[so I have no idea what that is but um (.) I was just=
DOC: [Uh huh
PAT: =explaining to her that my throat's been hurtin' up.

In this case, the patient also describes her visit as a product of "paranoia" induced by the girlfriend's suggestion (see below).

In other cases, as an alternative to self-diagnoses, patients may offer optimistic versions of their symptoms. In (29) the patient (at line 2) may be beginning a version of "I don't know what it is but . . .," which she abandons in favor of the more optimistic "I'm hopin' it's nothin'."

(29) [Cyst]

DOC: .h u-What's been goin' on that I can help you with.
PAT: I: don't- (.) I':m hopin' it's nothin'. (0.4) °But I°

fou:nd a lump under my arm pit_
(0.4)
DOC: Okay,
PAT: That I don't think should be there.
DOC: ( ) Oka:y, when did you notice that.

While these offer "benign" troubles-resistant (see below) versions of symptoms, patient optimism is often belied, as in (29), by the fact that the optimism is presented without any basis. This contrasts with (12) above, in which the patient's evidentially grounded reservations allowed her to align with the physician's subsequent "no problem" diagnostic evaluation.

While diagnostic claims are not very frequent in patients' problem presentations, and are often cautiously managed and indirectly communicated, those that occur are clearly oriented to issues concerning the doctorability, and in many cases the treatability (Stivers 2002b), of the complaint. This suggests that, while patients are generally quite inhibited from making diagnostic claims, these inhibitions can be overridden by doctorability concerns, especially when the patient is able to make a connection to a medically validated prior diagnosis.

Invoking third parties

Patients' descriptions of the reason for the visit often embody accounts of a prior process of decision-making and action. These can include an account of the reasoning that led to the conclusion that the presenting problem was probably doctorable, and of the decision process in which the patient made an appointment and arrived for the consultation. In portraying this process, patients quite frequently present their conclusions and/or their decision-making as shared with third parties. This presentation can have two major benefits, which are clearly illustrated in (12) above. First, patients can present their conclusions about their problems as already shared and, to this extent, validated or "sanctioned" (Zola 1964, 1973) by another person. The judgment that they should seek medical assistance is no longer theirs alone. Thus, second, their own responsibility for making the appointment and attending the physician's office is reduced and attenuated, potentially reducing the reputational costs of a visit held to be inappropriate. Both of these effects are maximized when the third party involved is a referring professional but, as earlier examples have suggested, other nonprofessional third parties are quite commonly invoked in patients' case presentations.

A clear case where citing a referral is the first, and indeed the only, component of a volunteered problem presentation is (30). Here the patient reaches for his medical records at line 2, and transfers the records to the physician at line 4 as an initial and designedly comprehensive response to the physician's opening inquiry:

(30) [Referral from Planned Parenthood]

DOC: So can you tell me what brings you in today?=
PAT: =I'll: tell ya exactly what's bringin' me in [tuhd(h)ay.
DOC: [(huh huh huh,)
PAT: -> .hh This is what's bringing me in tuhday.=hh
DOC: O[kay.
PAT: -> [.hh I was referred, .hh tuh you by Planned Parenthood?
hhh ((sniff)) hh
(1.5)
PAT: An' that is why=hh.
DOC: Okay. So uhm what was thuh reason you were seen over
there?

As this kind of example makes clear, referral by other professionals is a "reason of first resort" for patients who are explaining the reason for the consultation.

Of course, medical professionals are not the only third parties invoked in patient's problem presentations. Family members (as in [12]) and other third parties can also be recruited to these accounts. In (31), a person who was initially described as a "friend," in the patient's conversation with the nurse, is described as a "pharmaceutical sales rep" to the physician when her role in persuading the patient to seek medical help is invoked:

(31) [Asthma-like Symptoms]

DOC: You went camping and now have some difficulty breathing,
since the camping or something else?
PAT: -> Yeah actually a friend of mine is a pharmaceutical sales rep,
-> and she noticed the way I've been talking?
DOC: Okay.
PAT: I've been like (.) (breathing in) and she thought maybe I was
having some kinds of symp[toms.

8 DOC: [Okay.
9 PAT: And I've noticed (.) just like at night, or in the morning
10 it seems more severe.
11 DOC: Okay.
12 DOC: [Uh
13 PAT: -> [So she thought I should take a breathing test.
14 DOC: Yes (.) um wheezing as you breathe in?

The practice of invoking third parties is also quite commonly associated with self-diagnosis. In (32), the patient invokes his wife ("Jill") as having recalled his sinus infection of a year previously as a means of indirectly self-diagnosing:

(32) [Sinus Infection]

1 DOC: e=Uh#::# Sounds like you haven't been feelin'=so spiffy?
2 PAT: No::.
3 (1.9)
4 PAT: Thought=it was goin' awa:y, an' it come back over
5 thuh wee:kend.
6 DOC: Uh huh_
7 (.)
8 PAT: Jill's like you got=a sinus infection a year
9 ago. (.) it's
10 got=a be:_=
11 DOC: = (Uhh/Oh). How's Jill doin' these days,

A similar case is the following, in which a potentially "worst-case" self-diagnosis is described as the patient's husband's idea. Note that the husband is portrayed as an experienced sufferer with skin cancer:

(33) [Seborrheic Keratosis]

1 DOC: What's up?
2 (4.0)
3 DOC: (Mm) (A growth's) on your ba:ck?=
4 PAT: Ye:s, uh huh.
5 DOC: On a:, [has it been-
6 PAT: [O::h, they've been there for a long time, and I just
7 didn't pay any attention to 'em, but my husband's upset about
8 it, .hhh and my:, I've been having back spasms, and .hh my (.)
9 -> daughter-in-law rubbed my back the other day, and she says,
10 -> "These don't look good." (.) And=uh, so he would like me to go

to Doctor [Name], (.) because she's been taking cancers off
-> of his hands=an' (.) face, and she thinks m- he thinks maybe
-> they're cancerous.
DOC: ( ) let's take a look.

What is common to all these cases is that the patients portray their presence in the physician's office as the product of a process in which they were not the sole agent or decision-maker.[5] By diffusing responsibility for initiating the consultation, patients reduce their own agency and accountability in the matter. Moreover, the recruitment of others in support of a decision to seek medical help shows that the decision was neither idiosyncratic nor unconsidered, but rather is socially supported by others. The invocation of medical professionals, third parties, or even the routine status of the visit itself as the partial or entire basis for their decision to consult a physician, diffuses responsibility for the decision to make the visit, and lowers the social and reputational costs for raising a concern which turns out to be unfounded.

Troubles resistance

Notwithstanding Parsons' (1951) argument that persons labor under the obligation to resist the "sick role," by the time that patients

[5] An inversion of this process can occur when another person, acting as an intermediary for a patient, invokes the patient's authority as the basis for a medical visit:

DOC: How can I help,
CLR: .hhh Well- (0.3) all of a sudden yesterday evening, having been
perfectly fit for (.) you know, ages, [.hh
DOC: [Ye:[s,
CLR: [My husband was taken
ill: (wi') th'most awful stomach pains, and sickness, .h[h
DOC: [Ye:s,
CLR: .hh An' it's gone on a:ll night. He has vomited once. hh!
.hh[h
DOC: [Righ[t,
CLR: [An' also had some diarrhea,hh!
DOC: Right,=
CLR: =Uh: a:nd hh! You know he seems >t'be< almost writhing in a:gony,
h·hhh eh-hhh! .h[h (He's had) 'is appendix ouhht! hhh=
DOC: [°(Ruoh,)
CLR: =.hhh!
DOC: Ye:s. ((smile voice?))
CLR: -> Uhm: (.) an:d (.) you know he just feels he ought to see a
-> doctor,

have arrived at the physicians' offices they have relaxed this resistance to the extent that they have become prima facie committed to the need for help. Nonetheless, many patient problem presentations incorporate elements of that obligation to resist. In this section we explore patient orientations towards describing troubles that have their origins in the world of everyday social relations, but which travel across the threshold of the physician's office and inform patients' problem presentations.

In a masterful analysis, Jefferson (1988) proposes that everyday "troubles talk" properly involves tellers in displays of "troubles resistance." In their descriptions, circumstances are depicted both as distressing and/or as disruptive of the routines of everyday life, and also as self-manageable or as something to be "coped with." In these presentations to friends, relatives or other appropriate troubles recipients, there is a continuous tension between attending to the trouble and attending to the normal routine requirements and proprieties of interaction, which Jefferson glosses as "business as usual."

The norms and dynamics of the physician–patient relationship are of course not identical with those that apply in everyday life: in ordinary troubles-telling, the troubles recipient's focus is on the person-with-their-troubles, while the physician, as a service supplier, tends to focus on the troubles-telling as involving a problem-to-be-solved (Jefferson and Lee 1992). However, the general "troubles resistance" that is normally required of persons in the social world as they engage and disengage the trouble does manifest itself in the medical visit. For example, consistent with Jefferson's (1980b) observations about troubles-resistant responses to "How are you?" inquiries by persons with troubles to impart, patients ordinarily respond with "Fine" – a "no problem" response (cf. Sacks 1975; Jefferson 1980b; Heritage 1998; Robinson this volume). This response is sometimes used by pediatricians to playfully confound their young patients with questions like "Then why are you here today?," and it is sometimes exploited to invite the patient's presenting concern with the single word "but?."

In this section we focus on two aspects of troubles resistance in patients' problem presentations:

1. Efforts by which patients show that they have (or ordinarily would have) attempted to cope with the problem on their own

prior to seeking medical assistance. Showing troubles resistance in this first sense can involve the patients indicating that they didn't "come running" to the physician at the first sign of trouble, and that they either tried, or ordinarily *would* try, to outlast their complaint, or take other steps to fix the problem. These accounts are occupied with descriptions of self-medication, and of the time elapsed between the initial recognition of symptoms and the decision to seek medical care.

2. Efforts to display that patients are currently coping with their problems with fortitude. Showing troubles resistance in the second sense tends to be expressed in an objective "just the facts" approach to illness, the avoidance of reports of pain (except as itself a symptom), fear, or sadness, or of volunteering "worst fears." Faced with the choice between describing a problem as a "fact" or as a "complainable," patients overwhelmingly focus on the "factual" features of the complaint.

Troubles-resistant elements in a problem presentation justify a medical visit by portraying it as a last resort. The patient has waited for the problem to resolve and has made efforts to treat the problem using a combination of common sense and over-the-counter resources. These troubles-resistant efforts are now at an end; the problem has not resolved but worsened, and the patient is at a loss to understand why the efforts at self-medication have failed. The time has come to receive expert intervention. For these reasons, troubles-resistance is generally not a procedure that is associated with presentations of recurrences. Moreover, it is manifested somewhat differently in "routine acute" as compared to "unknown" medical problems.

Troubles resistance in "routine acute" medical problems

As we have already noted, "routine acute" medical problems are most often mild, self-limiting, and of short duration. Many of them – colds and related upper respiratory tract infections, for example – are potentially only marginally doctorable, not least because conditions of viral origin can only be treated symptomatically. In such a context, patients who present with them often offer special or unusual features – the persistent nature of the problem, the suffering or disruption associated with their symptoms, or exceptional or disturbing developments – to justify their presence at the physician's office. For example, in the case below the patient justifies the visit both by reference to the persistence of the problem and – similar to the patient in (13) above, who "wouldn' normally come with a cold" – by reference to "green stuff," which patients commonly associated with bacterial infection and antimicrobial treatment (Stivers 2002b; Stivers et al. 2003):

(5) [Flu – Expanded]

DOC:		What's been goin' o:n?
PAT:		I just got (0.4) chest cold a:nd it's been uh
		goin' on for a week- I don't seem to be able to
		[shake it-
DOC:		[O:kay
PAT:	->	And uh what caused me to call is uh 'bout fourth
	->	or fifth day in a row in thuh morning- [I was
DOC:		[Mm hm
PAT:	->	tryin' to get the engine started-
DOC:		Mm hm
PAT:	->	Coughin' up a buncha green stuff.
DOC:		Oka:y.
PAT:		So,
DOC:		Oka:y .hh uh now have you had much in thuh way
		of fevers or chills with this?

Alternatively, a patient can acknowledge that the symptoms they are experiencing are typical of a recurrent and routine problem, but assert their unusual qualities – in the following case, duration:

(34) [Atypical Migraine]

DOC:		.hhhh What can I do for yah. hhh
		(.)
PAT:		tch! I been having some headaches¿
DOC:		[Mkay.
PAT:		[U::m, sinc:e (0.5) Sunday¿
DOC:		Okay?
PAT:		A::nd (0.5) I get migraines occasionally. But (.) in this ca:se,
	->	(2.2) it's- it's been off an' o::n for the last four
	->	da:ys An' I'm-
DOC:		Okay.
		(1.0)
PAT:	->	Usually they- they don- I don't have [this,

13 DOC: -> [This isn't typical.=
14 PAT: =[Right. Exactly.
15 DOC: =[(of your) migraines.

Here, having described the duration of his symptoms, the patient begins a sentence which appears aimed at formulating them as unusual. This is certainly the physician's conclusion, and she is quick to draw out this inference on his behalf. And a putatively overly long duration for a problem is hinted at (lines 2–3), in (38) below, with "I can't get rid of" (see also [18] above), which is then disclosed as "four weeks'" (line 7).

(35) [Congestion]

1 DOC: So how are you fee:ling.
2 PAT: Well, (.) I- (.) I feel good now but=I can't
3 get rid=of=this:=uh:m (.) conge:stion.
4 DOC: Okay,
5 PAT: I've had this co:ld, >in my head,< it was- started uh
6 with a sore throat (.) four weeks ago this
7 [coming Friday.
8 DOC: [Uh huh
9 PAT: .hh And uh I don't know (0.2) ha my daughter had
10 something wrong with her she thinks that I
11 caught you know germ from her I don't know
12 ((laughs))
13 DOC: 'Kay now tell me are you blowing anything out of . . .

In sum, patients' presentations of routine illnesses tend to formulate them as basically recognizable and familiar, but as warranting medical attention by virtue of some feature which the patient characterizes as out of the ordinary, unusually disruptive of everyday life routines, or with an adverse prognosis. These exceptional features make it appropriate to seek medical care, despite the fact that the illness is generally likely to be self-limiting and that a "troubles-resistant" stance of waiting out the condition might be more appropriate under other circumstances.

Troubles resistance in "unknown" medical problems

When we turn to currently unknown medical problems, both troubles resistance and claiming doctorability can become a more complex undertaking. As we have seen, the status of a condition as questionable may be sufficient to warrant a medical visit (see [7]–[10] above). However, questionable conditions may turn out to be benign and this possibility may motivate more extensive and elaborate presentations:

(10) [Ringworm – Expanded]

DOC: What happened.
(.)
PAT: Well I got (.) what I thought (.) in Ju:ne (.)
uh was an insect bite.=in thuh back of my neck here.
DOC: Okay,
PAT: An' I (0.2) you know became aware of it 'cause
it was itching an'=I (.) scratched at't,
(0.2)
PAT: An' it persisted fer a bit so I tried calamine
lotion,=
DOC: =Okay,
(0.2)
PAT: An' that didn't seem to make it go away
completely, an' it=s:tayed with me,=w'll its
still with me. Thuh long and thuh short of it.
DOC: [Okay.
PAT: [Cut to thuh chase is its- its still with
me, .hhh but (its) got a welt associated °with it.°
DOC: Okay,
(0.5)
PAT: Its got a welt that's (.) no:w increased in
size to about that big=it was very (.) small
[like a di:me initially you know, an' now
DOC: [Okay,
PAT: its (0.3) like a (.) bigger than a half do:llar
(I bet [it's like-) [( )-
DOC: [And you [said it's no: longer
itchy. Is that correct,

This medical visit took place in mid-August and the patient begins his account with "Well I got (.) what I thought (.) in Ju:ne (.) uh was an insect bite.=in thuh back of my neck here." (lines 3–4), thus simultaneously projecting a narrative and indicating the amount of time he has waited before going to the physician's office. It is clear from the patient's use of "I thought" that he no longer believes that his condition is the product of an insect bite. Rather, and in line with other, more dramatic, narratives (Sacks 1992a; Jefferson

2004a; Halkowski this volume), he reports as his "first thought" an utterly commonplace and quite benign version of his complaint. He is also notably cautious in explaining how he became aware of the condition, going out of his way to explain (lines 6–7) that it was "itching" (cf. Halkowski this volume). Subsequently, he recounts the failure of his effort at self-medication (using calamine lotion), asserting (lines 13–15) the continued presence of his symptoms. At this point, the patient encounters a standard dilemma for patients who are describing a sustained period of "living with" the problem. This is to account for the "turning point": the considerations which made his earlier way of dealing with the problem untenable. He handles this by describing the development of something distinct from the consequences of an insect bite; namely, a "welt," which he articulates with great emphasis, going on to describe its progression in size from a dime to "bigger than a half do:llar" (line 25).

Finally, consider the following case in which a middle-aged diabetic women presents with a "bad foot":

(36) [Bad Foot]

DOC: Whatcha up to:.=h
(0.2)
PAT: I've gotta bad foot that I can't: get well.
(0.2)
DOC: Which part.
PAT: >Okay.< About ↑five weeks ago I went to Disneyland
and I wore uh pair of sandals that weren't very
supportive.
(.)
PAT: .hh And after that I started tuh have trouble.
(.)
PAT: It hurts in here,
(.)
DOC: (°Mm hm.°)
(0.8)
PAT: (Now s)=it's uh lot better than it was because I've
been wearing an ace bandage.
PAT: .hh But it still swells,
(0.2)
PAT: #An'# I don't know (.) what's wrong.
PAT: .hhhh Every day I've been wearing an ace bandage.
(0.2)

23	PAT:	But what r:eally made me come in here is that
24		this morning (0.5) when I woke u:p- (0.5) it was
25		kind=of- reddish blue, right here?
26	PAT:	.hh An' it hurts terrible tuh walk on my toe: an'
27		this part here.
28	PAT:	.hh Now if I press it it don't hurt very much but
29		when I walk on it (h) (But) I don't walk on it. I
30		walk on (th') side uh my foot which is no good
31		for this:.
32		(1.5)
33	DOC:	Yeah:.=h
34		(0.2)
35	DOC:	#eh# I hope you didn't- may have uh s:mall fracture
36		there er something.

Here the woman's initial problem presentation at line 3 includes the clause "that I can't: get well.", which already suggests that this is a condition which she has tried to remedy on her own. Thus, from the very start of this account, there is an intimation of the troubles resistance which will subsequently appear in her account. When she is asked the first "history-taking" question at line 5 by her physician, she does not respond to that question's agenda (Boyd and Heritage this volume). Instead she begins a narrative which states that her problem began five weeks previously and suggests a theory of its origins (cf. Gill 1998a; Gill and Maynard this volume). Only having conveyed this does she respond (at line 12) to the physician's question. Subsequently she describes an improvement in the condition, which she attributes to her efforts at self-treatment ("an ace bandage" [line 17]), but describes that improvement as partial (line 18) and expresses puzzlement about the problem (line 20). Finally, she describes a specific discovery – a discoloration of the foot – as the "turning point": the factor that precipitated her decision to seek help (lines 23–25).

The patient's account also incorporates elements of the second type of troubles resistance described earlier – objective descriptions and the avoidance of complaints and "worst fears." Apart from a brief allusion to pain at line 12, used as a method of responding to the physician's question at line 5 by identifying the part of her foot which is giving problems, the patient defers any mention of pain or discomfort until lines 26–27; that is, *after* the conclusion of her entire account of the problem and the methods she has used to address it, and even here the mention is brief. This is despite the fact that pain could have been used as an index of the problem at almost any point in the account, and perhaps particularly at line 18. (The patient's involuntary conduct during the physical examination gives a clear indication that her foot is severely painful.)

Moreover, unstated in the patient's problem presentation, though emerging very much later in the consultation, is the patient's underlying concern that her foot problem is a manifestation of phlebitis and that it is diabetes-related. This concern is indexed, but not stated, in her observation that her decision to seek medical help arose because of the discoloration of her foot (line 25). It is significant that in this highly troubles-resistant description the patient still avoids disclosing what may be her most profound anxiety.

In this account, then, the patient's concern is presented as: of long duration, involving failed self-treatment, puzzlement about the condition, and an event that precipitated the visit. It also embodies a troubles-resistant form of delivery which avoids reference to the subjective experiences of pain, fear, or "worst-case" anxieties. In various combinations, these elements appear in other troubles-resistant accounts.

As a contrast case, an expansion of (11) above may prove instructive:

(11) [Breathless – Expanded]

DOC: =hhhhh So::. What's the problem.
hhh[hhhhhhhhhhhhhhhhh
PAT: [Well, me breathin's shockin'.
DOC: Ri:ght.
PAT: As I'm wa::lkin' [ah- (0.3) I 'av ta sto:p.
DOC: [Yeah, (.) Yeah,
DOC: Yeahs.
(.)
PAT: An' even when- >do you know when ya go< ta
shake the pillas up,
DOC: Yeah
(0.3)
PAT: I ga- I go out a bre:ath.
DOC: Mm
(0.5)
PAT: -> ·hhh An' I hav' 'ad a-=hh a cold over the
weekend.=cuz it got cold on saturday,

18	DOC:		Mm:m,
19			(0.8)
20	PAT:	->	An' I feel lo:usy,hh
21	DOC:		Mm
22			(.)
23	PAT:	->	I'm full of- (0.7) everything(k).
24			(1.0)
25	PAT:		·hhh So::=hhh can ya help me?
26	DOC:		°Sure.°
27	DOC:		·hhhhh (0.4) Th- this isn' something completely
28			new:: you've had it before . . . ((continues))

Here the patient begins with a relatively troubles-resistant description of her symptoms, describing the two practical manifestations of her breathlessness (lines 5, 9–10, and 13) in order of increasing severity, in an objective and "factual" fashion. As her presentation continues, however, she lapses into a more "troubles-attentive," subjective, or complaining focus (lines 20 and 23) before concluding her presentation with an overt request for help. It is precisely these latter elements that troubles-resistant problem presentations are at pains to avoid.

Concluding remarks

The problem presentation phase of the medical visit has been quite extensively studied in recent years, as have patient reasons for seeking medical care (Mechanic 1972; Zola 1973; Brody 1987; Stoeckle et al. 1963). Apart from the sheer expressive value for patients of being able to depict the nature of a medical problem in their own terms, including the description of anxieties and concerns and attempts to understand and explain symptoms (Roter and Hall 1992), the process of soliciting and presenting concerns is important because it can affect health outcomes:

1. Patients frequently have multiple concerns, which can be biomedical and/or psychosocial in nature (Barsky 1981; Lipkin, Frankel et al. 1995; Stoeckle and Barsky 1981; White et al. 1994; White et al. 1997);
2. Research suggests that soliciting the full spectrum of patients' concerns and illness explanations improves diagnosis and treatment (Arborelius et al. 1991; Cassell 1985a, 1985b; Fisher

> 1991; Korsch et al. 1968; Larsson et al. 1987; McWhinney 1981, 1989; Mishler 1984; Sankar 1986; Todd 1984, 1989) and, ultimately, medical outcomes (Brown et al. 2003; Greenfield et al. 1985; Kaplan et al. 1989; Orth et al. 1987). Yet patients may not overtly express their true concerns in up to 75 per cent of acute care visits (Lang et al. 2000).

This chapter has suggested a possible reason for this disconnection: arguing that patients' problem presentations are often primarily occupied with justifying the decision to seek medical help. Central to the need to justify this decision are general social norms that, at least in the Anglophone world, promote "troubles resistance" in the individual's interpersonal conduct, and resistance to the sick role in the specific context of medical care. We propose that the constraints on, and resources for, justification vary with the type of visit. Visits motivated by the patient's belief that a condition has recurred offer different justificatory affordances than visits for routine illnesses. Conditions that are outside patients' illness schemata, and whose symptoms are difficult to describe or interpret, tend to attract narratives of discovery and uncertainty which "lower the bar" of doctorability by providing that the physician's resolution of a concern as unproblematic is "good enough" as a motivation for a medical visit.

We have also described various practices which are commonly deployed by patients to justify the visit. Patients may claim to have already identified their complaint as one that required medical treatment in the past, thereby justifying the present visit. Patients may indicate that a range of others have urged or supported their decision to make the visit or contributed interpretations of aspects of their condition. Patients may wish to show that they have endured the condition for a while, and have attempted self-medication before a particular development in the condition became a "turning point" in their decision to seek medical help.

Underlying the dilemmas of this phase of the visit is the tension, first identified by Bloor and Horobin (1975), between lay and professional judgment. Prior to visiting physicians, patients must make a judgment that they have a legitimately doctorable concern. Yet this judgment will itself be judged over the course of the visit. From the patient's point of view, an initial manifestation of that judgment may seem to be the first history-taking question, which can be interpreted as a validation pro tem that the patient's concern is being taken seriously. This may account for the willingness of so many of the patients described by Beckman and Frankel (1984) to abandon the problem presentation role at the first significant physician intervention. The data presented in this chapter suggest that when, as in example (12), such interventions curtail significant components of the patient's justification for the visit, patients are prepared to override medical questioning and pursue an underlying agenda of self-justification.

Of course, the process of justifying the visit does not end with the problem presentation. As Halkowski (this volume) shows, similar concerns clearly manifest themselves during the history-taking process, and Heath (1992) and Peräkylä (1998) both have shown the (re-)emergence of these concerns during the process of diagnosis (see also Heritage 2005, forthcoming; Heritage and Stivers 1999). Nonetheless, the problem presentation phase is the first, and perhaps the most crucial, phase of the encounter for the credibility and legitimacy of patient concerns. It is for this reason, perhaps, that so many issues that bear on the legitimacy of the patient's presence in the physician's office are dealt with at this moment, and why the appropriate management of this phase of the visit by the physician is of such central importance.

4

Realizing the illness: patients' narratives of symptom discovery

Timothy Halkowski

It's not the story though,
not the friend leaning toward you,
saying "And then I realized—,"
which is the part of stories one never quite believes.

I had the idea that the world's so full of pain
it must sometimes make a kind of singing.

And that the sequence helps, as much as order helps –
First an ego, and then pain, and then the singing.[1]

Introduction

When people talk about a potential new health problem, they sometimes produce narratives of problem discovery (i.e., a story of *how* they realized that this problem might be serious).[2] Consider this letter from novelist Walker Percy MD to his friend Shelby Foote.

I gratefully acknowledge the support of my colleagues at the University of Wisconsin Medical School, and the Behavioral Science department of the University of Kentucky Medical School for the NIMH postdoctoral fellowship (Grant number MH15730) I held while initiating this project. I am especially grateful to the following for their advice, comments, and encouragement: Steve Clayman, Don Zimmerman, Tom Wilson, Doug Maynard, John Heritage, Emanuel Schegloff, Gail Jefferson, Mel Pollner, Rich Hilbert, Tanya Stivers, Virginia Gill, Elizabeth Boyd, and Susan Halkowski. Earlier versions of this chapter were presented at a UCLA EPOS colloquium (1996), and at the AILA conference in Jyvaskyla, Finland (1996).

1 "Faint Music" (Hass 1996).

2 Patients also report symptoms in a non-narrative format. This chapter will not address that topic, but we can note that non-narrative symptom reports may be a way for patients to claim a taken-for-granted "doctor relevance" of the problem (cf. Heritage and Robinson this volume; Zimmerman 1992).

(1) Dear Shelby—

Not such good news here.
a-> I've been having some abdominal and back pain for past few weeks.
b-> Thought it was my periodic diverticulitis.
c-> Went to hospital last week for exam. Colon was normal, but there were masses around the aorta and along spine. Don't yet know what it is, but presumably it's metastases from prostate carcinoma or pancreatic CA.
Will keep you informed. . . . (Tolson 1997:301)

Note three features of Percy's letter. First, he announces some pain that he has been experiencing (a). Second, he mentions his "first thought" (Sacks 1992b:215–21), or initial causal hypothesis for the pain (b). Then he describes the events that showed his first thought to have been wrong (c). These features appear to be common in reports of new health problems. Consider this excerpt from a sports article:

(2) "Dizzy spells send Cirillo to sideline"

a-> . . . Cirillo first began experiencing dizziness March 21, when he sat out an exhibition game against San Diego.
b-> At first, he thought he was suffering from withdrawals because he had quit chewing tobacco.
c-> But the problem has persisted off and on during the last month.
d-> "At first, I thought it was just me," he said.
e-> "But lately I've been missing pitches that I usually hit. There are pitches that, even when I'm struggling, I usually foul off.
f-> It's been going on a long time. I tried to play through it." (*Milwaukee Journal-Sentinel*, April 21, 1997, p. 7)

The article starts with a description of the initial problem – (a). Then Cirillo gives an initial attempt to account for the problem – (b) and (d). He also gives subsequent information, which is presented as rejecting the initial account – (c) and (e). Then, he formulates the duration of the problem, as well as his initial response to the problem – (f). Through this last bit of talk Cirillo presents himself as having made a good-faith effort to deal with the problem, rather than immediately treating it as "doctor-able" ("I tried to play through it").

In these two cases a person presents a narrative of symptom discovery regarding a potential health problem to a layperson.[3] Similar narratives can occur in patients' presentations to medical professionals. In this chapter we shall consider their structure and uses in some detail. Based on data from twenty-five videotaped medical visits in two primary care clinics, we will argue that, through these narratives of discovery patients display to the doctor accurate and appropriate witnessing and experiencing of their bodily states. They show that they are reasonable monitors of themselves (not overly observant, nor too lax). At the most general level, these narratives address what can be called "the patients' problem."

The "patients' problem"

Early work on the patients' role in the health care visit highlighted the notion that being sick entails certain rights and responsibilities. Parsons argued that the "sick role" provided exemption from one's normal role and task obligations, as well as from responsibility for one's incapacity. One also had the obligation to seek (and cooperate with) competent help to get well (1964:274–5).

But these issues, as Parsons lays them out, are sequelae of a more fundamental process: how one realizes that this is a doctor-able problem (i.e., one that should be brought to medical attention). Certainly there are situations in which one's illness seems to present itself unambiguously, but it is often the case that an illness is only realized over a period of time (cf. examples [1] and [2] above). Moreover, patients are also expected to be experts on their health problem and bodily experience *until* seated in the exam room. As Bloor and Horobin put it:

> . . . [D]octors tend to typify the ideal patient as someone who is able to assess symptomotology with sufficient expertise to know *which* conditions he should present, and *when* he should present them to the GP, but at the same time one who, having assessed his condition, will defer to the doctor's assessment on presentation. (1975:276)

[3] Since narratives of problem discovery also occur in calls to radio talk-show advice programs, calls to 911 emergency services (Zimmerman 1992; Whalen and Zimmerman 1990), and gossip (Bergmann 1993), they may be a generic device in social interaction. As such, examinations of their use in a particular activity environment may be informative for their use in other activities (e.g., Halkowski 1999).

Similarly, Strong presented the following assessment of child-patients' parents by medical staff.

> [A] key quality for which doctors searched was how far parents were "sensible". (1) Being "sensible" meant putting things in their proper context; not worrying without any cause; not letting one's emotions influence what one reported to doctors; accepting one's fate; and making hard decisions when these had to be made. In other words it meant an active and competent compliance with medical staff. While some mothers, "worriers", saw problems where there were none, and others tried to overcome the impossible, *the ideal patient had a nice balance of involvement and detachment*, subordination and concern. Here, for example, a therapist discusses the mother of a severely handicapped child:
> TE: She's marvelous. The best of them all. She's ever so detached and yet ever so loving and she genuinely wants to know what's best for her child. (Strong 1979:156; emphasis added)

Thus, when experiencing potential symptoms, one has to make several practical decisions. Is this a potential health problem, or part of the everyday sensations, aches, etc., that come with having a body?[4] Is this something I need to deal with, or something that will resolve itself? Should I consult a professional about this, or manage it myself? If I treat this, how should I? How long should I try to manage this before I go to a doctor, etc?[5] This set of practical issues can be grouped together as "the patients' problem" (see also Heritage and Robinson this volume).[6]

One way patients manage to present themselves as reasonably seeking care for an emergent (or *potential*) new health problem is via narratives of symptom discovery. Because these narratives routinely take the form of a report of "realization" ("How I became aware of 'X'"), it is tempting to think of these stories as parts of patients'

[4] This issue is nicely captured in the following quotation from a sports article regarding pitcher Jim Bruske ("Bruske hurts elbow," *Milwaukee Journal-Sentinel*, May 14, 2000, p. 6c): "Bruske . . . said his elbow had been bothering him off and on for the past few weeks. 'It's a fine line,' he said. 'You have to decide what is normal soreness and what is something more serious. It's been bugging me, but I just felt like I could pitch through it.'"

[5] If the above set of dilemmas can be considered "the patients' problem," there is a corresponding dilemma for medical practitioners, partially generated by the fact that most of the doctor's access to the health concern of the patient is via the patient's report (cf. Meehan 1989).

[6] This phrase originates with Freidson (1975a:288), who used it to mark the patients' dilemma of whether to trust their doctor or their own physical sensations. I use the phrase to capture a larger (but related) set of patients' problems, enumerated above.

psychological explanatory models. But if we recall that "realize" has a social sense as well ("to bring into concrete existence"), we can notice how these narratives are employed to do particular tasks.

In this chapter we will explore the occasioning of these narratives at particular moments in the outpatient visit, and the structure of these turns, in order to understand what these narratives are being used to do (Schegloff 1996b:12). We will give special attention to two features of these narratives: the "at first I thought 'X'" report, and the "sequence of noticings." Subsequently we will examine how patients' tellings of these narratives display the "doctor-relevance" of a candidate problem, and their "unmotivated, out-of-the-blue" discovery of it. Via this work, people show themselves to be "reasonable patients" properly monitoring their bodies, (i.e., neither too lax, nor hyper-vigilant).

Thus what this chapter will offer is a way to make visible (and thereby analyzable) some of the ways that reports about our bodily sensations (presumably the most private and interior of phenomena) are shaped by social interaction, i.e., a social epistemics of sensation (cf. Hilbert 1984, 1992; Wittgenstein 1953, 1964).

Teach us to care and not to care[7]*: the "balance of involvement and detachment"*

To get a sense of what these narratives might be designed to achieve (and avoid), we will consider how the following issues are managed in one clinical interaction: Did I bring this problem to the doctor at the right time?; Is this a reasonable problem to bring to the doctor?; and Am I monitoring my bodily sensations appropriately?

In this clinical example, a retired man comes to the primary care clinic for a scheduled follow-up of his hypertension, and a newly discovered swelling in his abdomen.

(3) [UKFP2: 2]

```
1  DOC1:        [and you-   ]
2     PAT:  ->  [(and       )] I do have one thing I want ((cough))
3               you folks to look at today that (0.4) that's
4               come up (0.5) ah (.) °real° (0.7) (tk) (0.8)
```

[7] "Teach us to care and not to care, teach us to sit still" ("Ash Wednesday," T. S. Eliot).

ahh since I (.) saw doctor lyons last =matter of
fact I only noticed it about ahh (0.7) I'm gonna
sa:y (0.5) two (.) weeks (.) [(or)] three weeks
DOC1: [okay]
PAT: ago.
PAT: -> (.hh) I have ah- ah little swelling here.
(0.3)
DOC1: Oka:y,
PAT: -> an:d ah (.hh) I don't know whether its ah (hh)
. ah hernia, (0.4) or (ah) (.) something inside
there causing it ((cough)) but ah ((cough)) it-
is- ah little lop sided (.) maybe I'm just
growing that way.
DOC1: Hm hmm,=
PAT: But I think maybe its something ought ah be
looked at.=
DOC1: -> =You just noticed it two weeks ago,
PAT: Yeah.
DOC1: Okay.=
PAT: = (Hey) it coulda been there for ah year. (.hh)
I don't look at myself very much.
(.)
PAT: [you know
DOC1: [I see.
PAT: -> But I was shaving or something an I (0.4) I do
some side to side exercises an I guess I was
doing it an kindah maybe in front of ah (0.3)
mirror or something [an I] just noticed that
DOC1: [hm hmm,]
PAT: this side is (1.0) extended
DOC1: Okay.
PAT: rather than this side. ((Pat. continues))

In lines 2–7 the patient introduces this (new) agenda item for the visit, and provides a temporal context for it, a context that accentuates the problem's sudden onset. Note how this sense is achieved. The problem has:

a. come up (0.5) ah (.) °real° (0.7) (tk) (0.8)
b. ahh since I (.) saw doctor lyons last
c. =matter of fact I only noticed it about ahh (0.7) I'm gonna sa:y (0.5) two (.) weeks
d. (.) (or) three weeks ago.

Part (a) of the patient's turn suggests that the problem has emerged quickly. Part (b) marks the problem as having occurred *after* his most recent doctor visit. Parts (c) and (d) highlight that he "only noticed" the problem two or three weeks ago, but he also marks this timing as approximate ("about ahh (0.7) I'm gonna sa:y (0.5) two (.) weeks (.) (or) three weeks ago."). The cumulative effect of this problem introduction is to demonstrate that, while the patient did not excessively delay bringing this possible problem to his doctor's attention (a and b), he was not paying excessive attention to this symptom (the approximation in c and d).

After receiving a "go-ahead" from the doctor (line 8), the patient names the problem (line 10), and then offers some candidate causes for it (cf. Gill 1995):

a. an:d ah (.hh) I don't know whether its ah (hh) ah hernia, (0.4)
b. or (ah) (.) something inside there causing it ((cough))
c. but ah ((cough)) it- is- ah little lop sided (.)
d. maybe I'm just growing that way.

Part of the work the patient achieves here is to convey the reasonableness of bringing this problem to the doctor. The patient shows himself as aware that this could be a "routine" problem ("hernia," "maybe I'm just growing that way."), but also as concerned that it might be something more serious ("something inside there causing it"). He marks this as his account for bringing this problem to the doctor in his very next turn: "But I think maybe its something ought ah be looked at." (lines 19–20).

The doctor responds by attempting to confirm the timing of the problem discovery (line 21) in a manner that displays possible surprise that the patient has only just noticed the swelling (thereby potentially sanctioning the patient for being insufficiently attentive to his bodily symptoms).

After confirming the timing (line 22), the patient continues his answer in a way that treats the doctor's question as having been possibly sanctioning (lines 24–25). His answer treats the doctor's question as asking not simply for confirmation, but also for elaboration – "(Hey) it coulda been there for ah year"–, and an account of how he might have missed this problem before – "I don't look at myself very much."

Subsequently, the patient begins a narrative of symptom discovery (discussed in more detail later in this chapter), accounting for the problem discovery, given that "I don't look at myself very much." This is nicely highlighted by the way the patient introduces his narrative ("But" line 29), treating this discovery as discontinuous with his prior stance of not monitoring his own body very much.

This narrative of discovery, while responding to the (potentially sanctioning) question about when the patient first noticed the problem, also does the quite elaborate work of demonstrating how the patient has an appropriate balance of involvement and detachment. His involvement is displayed by his expressed concerns (lines 13–17); his detachment by his report of an almost accidental discovery of this problem (lines 29–32, 34, and 36).

We can see the finely calibrated ways that the patient demonstrates appropriate awareness of his bodily sensations and symptoms. In addition, note the finely tuned ways he shows himself to be reasonable, seeking medical care when (but *only* when) he should.

Establishing the "reason for visit" vs. "taking a history"

In his research on everyday interactions, Harvey Sacks argued that *where* and *how* a place is made for stories has implications for *what* they are used to do (1992b:229–31). In primary care encounters the narrative of problem discovery can be occasioned by either the doctor or the patient, and can be occasioned either near the beginning of the encounter or later during the history-taking. In both phases of the encounter, patients display an orientation to what we have called "the patients' problem." Patients' orientation to this is more acute at the start of the visit, where there can be a palpable sense of wonder (for both parties) about whether there is a reasonable health concern for this primary care visit.

By contrast, narratives during the history-taking, while addressing the same "patients' problem" concerns, do so without the overhanging issue of "Why am I here at the clinic in the first place?" At this point, the doctor and patient are in the midst of the medical encounter, and thus (at least provisionally) doctors treat patients as *reasonably* seeking care. Thus patients' narratives treat the visit as having been (provisionally) validated, and now address the issue "I should be here, and here's *why* I should be here."

Magnifying the locational aspects of these narratives, patients may treat the problem as difficult to name or characterize, thereby raising questions of its doctor-ability (cf. Zimmerman 1992). Consider the following example, introduced in the opening moments of a primary care visit, wherein the patient stays open to the possibility that this problem may not be doctor-able.

(4) [SSMC 0.1]

DOC: How can I help you.
PAT: -> Oh ah (0.2) I'm not sure how you can help me
but ah hhh=
DOC: =You're not sure.
PAT: -> It's ah (.) about ah couple of days ago I
noticed that (0.3) (ah) I just started to hurt
-> on thuh side en I thought I was getting a cold.
[(0.8)]
DOC: -> [((1 nod))]
PAT: -> an I jest you know (0.5) laid down an (.) it
-> seemed like it went away again later.=This
morning (0.7) when I got up out of bed I noticed
I was walking with ah limp. (0.5) an I felt like
I had to ah (0.2) urinate.=But I didn't have to
urinate.
[(0.4)]
DOC: -> [((1 nod))]
PAT: and then I (.) filt my (.) side (here) an its
real painful.
[(.)]
DOC: -> [((1 nod))]
PAT: an when I started wa:lking fa:st (0.2) or if I
laugh hard then its really irritated I have to
stop- [(1.2)]
DOC: -> [((3 nods))]
PAT: it's almost like somebody jest (0.2) poking me
in my side with their fist when I (0.2) do
sneeze >you know like I say< if I move rapidly
(.) or laugh hard.
[(1.0)]
DOC: -> [((2 nods))]
PAT: -> an it's just been like this since today. (0.6)
-> But it's been like you know kind ah sore (.) all
weekend.
[(1.2)]
DOC: -> [((2 nods))]

PAT: So I thought I'd come (in) an get it checked
out.
[(1.8)]
DOC: -> [((4 quick nods))]
DOC: Any other problems.
PAT: N::o.=that's it.

With the very first part of his answer (lines 2–3), the patient gives the sense that he is uncertain about whether he has an appropriate problem to bring to the doctor. After this the patient gives a short course of action narrative about his first symptom (lines 5–7), and the initial sense he made of the pain (line 7: "I thought I was getting a cold."). He thereby indicates that initially he was treating the symptom as an ordinary phenomenon, not something that needs a doctor's attention.

Next, the patient pauses for 0.8 seconds, and the doctor encourages him to continue, via his head nod (lines 8–9). Thus the patient is given the sense (right at this early point in the interaction) that the doctor is treating this narrative as (at least possibly) leading up to a point at which a "doctor-relevant" problem will be evident.

The patient then reports how he attempted to treat this problem ("laid down"), and the result ("it seemed like it went away", lines 10–11). In lines 11–15, the patient reports some more recent symptoms, after which he pauses for 0.4 seconds, and receives another continuer nod from the doctor (line 17). The patient gives three more symptom reports (lines 18–19, 22–24, and 26–29), each followed by a pause, during which the doctor gives a continuer nod (lines 20–21, 24–25, and 30–31).

Next, the patient summarizes the time-course of the symptoms (lines 32–34). By saying that the symptoms have "just been like this since today." the patient marks how recent this amalgam of symptoms is, thereby giving his report a more tentative sense than if he had been experiencing and dealing with various pains for a longer period of time. He does this marking lexically ("just"), and intonationally ("this," "today"). The patient then contrasts this part of his report with the next part: "But it's been like you know kind ah sore (.) all weekend." (lines 33–34). Via this contrast marking, the patient is able to indicate that, while most of the above symptoms are quite recent, there is a symptom that he has been experiencing and dealing with for the whole weekend.

Thus the patient reports a cluster of symptoms in a manner that shows himself as appropriately concerned (not too worried, not too lax), while also open to the possibility that after all there might not be any serious medical problem here.

By contrast, consider the next data segment, wherein the patient does not give a narrative of problem discovery until she is well into the history-taking portion of the visit.

(5) [SSMC:MSE:96]

DOC:		(About the) pain is it [sharp,] or dull,
PAT:		[(Well I)]
PAT:	->	at first I thought it was some uhh cramps from
	->	my period. Because that was coming in like three
		days, an I had to go home an- an lay down
	->	because it- an I usually don't get cramps.
	->	an then when it lasted thuh next weekend it was
		over an I'm still getting these cramps y(h)ou
		kn(h)ow
	->	(h)an I thought this isn't period cramps.
DOC:		Okay,
PAT:	->	This is something else.
	->	an an then it(s) just (real) sharp. Its- its like
		ah dull throb that's kind of always there an- its
		aching.
DOC:		Okay,

This patient is asked a focused history-taking question (regarding the pain quality), but responds with her narrative of problem discovery (lines 2–12). Placed just before the patient's more direct pain description (lines 13–15), this narrative is a way for the patient to describe the pain quality (via talking about it as possible period cramps). But while one might be tempted to assume that these comparisons are *only* pain descriptors, we must note their use *within* this narrative. This patient's narrative builds a context within which her subsequent pain description can be heard. Specifically, the patient shows that she tried to treat this as a normal, nonmedically relevant pain (lines 3–5).

She then underscores for the doctor her almost heroic effort to treat this as a normal, nonmedical pain, by mentioning that this normalizing attribution was tenuous ("an I usually don't get cramps." line 6). After this, she describes the persistence of the symptom, which led her to reject her "first thought" that this might be period cramps (lines 7–12).

In this example (occurring in the midst of the history-taking), the patient's narrative of symptom discovery is used to highlight how she is a reasonable experiencer of her bodily sensations. Indeed, she was prepared to go out of her way to treat her symptom as normal. This makes her subsequent pain report more credible, because her narrative provides a calibration of her "sensitivity" to bodily sensations.[8]

The prior two data segments demonstrate that the portion of the outpatient encounter in which the narrative of problem discovery is initiated matters for what it is being used to do. In (4), the narrative is offered in response to the physician's question "How can I help you?" Occurring in this interactional "slot," the narrative is offered by the patient as the accountable reason for the visit.

At the start of a primary care visit, there is often a very real question (for both doctor and patient) about whether this is a medically relevant problem, or just a "normal" pain. By contrast, when these narratives occur in the midst of the history-taking, the doctor has typically already treated the problem as "possibly medically relevant." Hence these narratives are weighted more toward displaying the reasonable stance the patient took toward this *likely* medically relevant problem.

Features of problem-discovery narratives

In this section we will focus on two common features of these narratives: the "at first I thought 'X'" device and a "sequence of noticings."

"At first I thought 'X'"

People often report what they thought they saw (or heard, or believed to be true, etc.) as a prelude to introducing what actually was the case. Sacks (1984) and Jefferson (2004a) have analyzed

[8] "Sensitivity" here refers not just to physical awareness of bodily experiences, but also to what (if anything) one *makes* of them interactionally. That is to say, is one's sensation treated as an occasion for casual remarks on, say, the inevitable aches and pains of aging, or a "ticket" for seeking a physician's care?

how this "at first I thought 'X,' and then I realized 'W'" device is used in ordinary conversation. They show that this device allows one both to foreshadow that an initial assumption turned out to be incorrect, and to display an initial "good-faith" attempt to account for some phenomenon via less extraordinary means.[9]

This device, then, provides a method for displaying oneself as a reasonable, accountable witness to the world. Rather than having looked for the most dramatic or outrageous explanation for an event, we demonstrate ourselves to have looked for the most obvious and mundane account (Sacks 1984, 1992b; Jefferson 1986; Pollner 1987). Only if those fail do we broaden our search and include more dramatic hypotheses.

There is an important distinction to note here. In the examples analyzed by Sacks and Jefferson, the device goes, "At first I thought 'X,' and then I realized 'W'." Thus the teller offers a specific, defined subsequent realization. By contrast, in these data the device occurs as follows: "At first I thought 'X,' but the problem continued (or got worse), etc., so I decided it was time to see a doctor." Thus patients are not offering specific subsequent "realizations" (i.e., diagnoses of their own symptoms). Rather, the realization they regularly offer is that symptom persistence, worsening, or other failure of their "first thought" led them to treat this as a doctor-able problem. Via their "abstention" from offering candidate diagnoses as realizations, patients thereby display themselves to be proper patients, i.e., they are specifically not taking upon themselves the doctor's task of diagnosis (cf. Bloor and Horobin 1975; Strong 1979 – and especially Gill 1995; and Gill et al. 2001).

We can observe how this device is employed in the prior example, repeated here, where a woman arrived at a primary care clinic with acute abdominal pain.

(6) [SSMC:MSE:96]

DOC: (About the) pain is it [sharp, or dull,
PAT: [(Well I)
PAT: -> at first I thought it was some uhh cramps from
-> my period. Because that was coming in like three
days, an I had to go home an- an lay down
-> because it- an I usually don't get cramps.

[9] In his poem "The Gardener's Song," Lewis Carroll plays with this convention by inverting it.

7		->	an then when it lasted thuh next weekend it was
8			over an I'm still getting these cramps y(h)ou
9			kn(h)ow
10		->	(h)an I thought this isn't period cramps.
11	DOC:		Okay,
12	PAT:	->	This is something else.
13		->	an an then it(s) just (real) sharp. Its- its like
14			ah dull throb that's kind of always there an- its
15			aching.
16	DOC:		Okay,

After the physician's question regarding pain quality (line 1), the patient gives a "first thought" report (lines 3–4), which forecasts that this hypothesis turned out to be wrong (Sacks 1992b:181–2). She follows that with an account for the "first thought" hypothesis (lines 4–5). After her report of the pain's initial impact on her (lines 5–6), the patient adds "an I usually don't get cramps." (line 6). This utterance casts her previous account for her "first thought" hypothesis in a new light. If she doesn't "usually" get cramps, then by displaying that as her "first thought," she shows herself to have gone out of her way to try to make sense of the pain as a "normal" pain (i.e., not physician-relevant).

In her next bit of talk (lines 7–10 and 12), the patient reports the way that she rejected her "first thought" hypothesis. This marking of her first hypothesis rejection is also hearable as the reason for her visit. She states that this is "something else." (line 12), but she does not know what it is.

Consider another example of this format below, where a man has arrived at a primary care clinic with severe headaches.

(7) [UK1]

1	DOC:		Okay. (0.2) what about thuh headaches (now)
2	PAT:		(.hh) We::ll they've been (1.6) ahh (0.2) ah I
3			think there've been three: major (0.5) sieges of
4			these things over thuh last five years or so
5			(0.2) an they've lasted (1.0) oh several weeks I
6			guess each time.
7	DOC:		°hmhm°
8			(1.1)
9	PAT:		(.hh) A::n (hhh/((sigh)) they're kindof ah bad
10			type of headache you know
11		->	an I thought (0.2) thuh first time I had it I
12		->	thought it was:: (.) related to some dental

13		->	problems I was having (but) that- they didn't go
14		->	away after thuh dental problems
15		->	[were tak]en care of so
16	DOC:		[hm hmm,]
17	DOC:		hmhm,
18	PAT:		((continues account))

This narrative is initiated just after the patient gives his report of the headaches' history and duration (lines 2–6), and assesses them as "kind of a bad type" (lines 9–10). Looking at the patient's narrative initiation (lines 11–12) we can note that his introduction of a causal hypothesis is started, then stopped to produce a parenthetical insert, then redone ("an I thought (0.2) thuh first time I had it I thought"). This insertion (especially via the intonational stress on "first") underscores that he's had several "sieges" of these headaches before. It also more powerfully marks that this "first thought" causal hypothesis was subsequently dropped by the patient, perhaps quite a while ago.

Thus this patient demonstrates that he did not just assume that this was a new medical condition that needed treatment. Rather, he first tried to find a preexisting account (dental problems) for his pain. When that account failed, he brought the problem to the doctor, along with this report of his prior hypothesis. Via his introduction of his initial causal hypothesis (dental pain), the patient shows himself to be reasonable (literally reason-*able*: able to look for plausible reasons for this pain). In both (7) and (6), the "at first I thought" device is used to display one's initial attempt to reasonably and accountably understand what is happening, and thereby to show oneself as *reasonably* seeking care.

A "sequence of noticings"

The "sequence of noticings" format is similar to the "at first I thought 'X'" format. But this format, instead of starting with "at first I thought," starts with some version of "I noticed." That is, the patient does not include an initial account or hypothesis. Instead, the patient reports a "first noticing," followed by other noticings, symptom persistence, worsening, etc., concluding with arrival at the doctor's office (e.g., "so then I decided to come see the doctor").

A key feature of the "sequence of noticings" problem-discovery narratives is that they are often presented as part of a patient's "course of action." These formulations are regularly used in reports by witnesses to events (Sacks 1984, 1992b:231–7; Zimmerman 1992). They are a device that displays interactants as having discovered something in an "unmotivated" fashion. The event is portrayed as having obtruded ("out of the blue") into the person's field of experience.

Consider the following, in which a woman comes to a primary care clinic with acute abdominal pain.

(8) [SSMC 3.5]

DOC:	->	When did it initially start.
PAT:	->	ahhhh (.) it started two weeks before I saw
		Marion.
DOC:		mm hmm,
PAT:	->	I noticed I would have this pressured feeling in
		the bottom of my stomach.
DOC:		mm hmm
PAT:	->	and then one day I went to the bathroom and it
		just literally set me on fire to use the
		bathroom like I had bathed myself in antiseptic
		or something
DOC:		mm [hmm,
PAT:		[cause it was burning just that bad. (.hh) an
		it did that one day and then it didn't do it
	->	again (0.5) then thuh next thing I notice I go
		to thuh bathroom to use thuh bathroom to urinate
		and (0.2) I'm spotting blood.
		(1.2)
PAT:	->	so then I f:igured it was time to call (0.2) the
		doctor to get in to see an appoint- to have an
		appointment that's when I went to see her. (0.8)
		when I started spotting.
DOC:		Alright, (3.4) ((cough)) Now today (.) you are
		having symptoms of what now.

In the patient's answer to the first question, she formulates her answer as a function of when she went to see a doctor ("Marion") about her medical problem (lines 2–3). As discussed above, this formulation highlights the amount of time the patient sought to solve or make sense of the problem herself, before seeking medical attention. Note also how the issue of going to see the doctor, mentioned at the start of the patient's story, is recycled in the last part of the story (lines 2–3 and 19–22).[10] The whole narrative is thus framed as "How I came to realize that I needed to see the doctor about this." This formulation asserts the "doctor-relevance" of the problem, presenting it as a legitimate medical issue.

Next, consider the marking of noticings in the narrative (lines 5–6, 8–11, and 15–17). These noticing markers constitute the marked talk as "an event," a phenomenon which stands out from the background of ordinary, taken-for-granted flow of experiences (Sacks 1984). The patient employs these markers to assemble the events that she reports as having led her to seek advice.

In addition, observe the particular "perceptual verb" the patient uses in this report: "notice(d)" (line 5). Its use here conveys the sense that the patient is giving "just the facts" – she's not adding her interpretation to these physical sensations, but is showing herself to be a neutral, objective reporter of her bodily sensations. "Notice" also conveys the sense of a reporter who did not hunt or search for these observations or experiences, but rather incidentally came upon them.

The patient wraps up her narrative of discovery by marking the upshot ("so then", lines 19–22). These two devices (noticing markings and upshot markers) display the patient as conscientiously sifting through her experiences to decide when it would be appropriate to seek her physician's advice. The patient thereby presents herself as an appropriate reporter of bodily sensations and experiences. Through the use of this narrative format, she can show that she is not making more of the experience than she ought to (Sacks 1992b:246–7).

Having looked in some detail at the formats of these narratives, we are in a position to consider the uses to which these narratives are put.

Doing things with stories: uses of the narratives

In this section we will consider how people use these narratives of problem discovery to demonstrate a reasonable orientation toward

[10] See Schegloff (1990:65, fn. 10): "Work in progress is describing a practice by which 'extended' or multi-unit turn answers to questions, sometimes involving stories or story fragments, show that they are coming to an end by the reappearance in them of elements (e.g., words) from the question to which they are a response."

the "patients' dilemma": a balance between being sufficiently attentive to one's symptoms while not excessively concerned about them.

How people display themselves as accurate and appropriate witnesses to events *in the world* (i.e., external to one's body) has been studied by Sacks (1992b), Jefferson (1986), Pollner (1987), and Whalen and Zimmerman (1990), among others. Writing about calls to 911 emergency lines, Zimmerman (1992:439) observes that callers can "package their report in a way that exhibits their status as ordinary, disinterested, reasonable witnesses."

One method of this packaging is to "frame an event and its noticing so that the trouble is seen to have imposed itself on someone otherwise minding their own business" (Zimmerman 1992:439; cf. Bergmann 1993). The same can be said of patients talking with their doctors about emergent, possibly new health problems.

In the following example, a man reports to the primary care clinic for his regularly scheduled hypertension follow-up visit.

(9) [SSMC 23 B]

DOC: Uhm you're here just for kinda (.) kinda checkin
up to see how you're doing with your high blood
pressure?
PAT: Yeah.
DOC: basic'ly,
PAT: °Yeah.°
DOC: Okay.
How [you been feelin,]
PAT: [and another thing] I've got.
I made (ah) (.) couple notations here.
DOC: Okay,
PAT: Here (.) just (ih-) recently (.) (started this
-> week so) (0.5) I ah (0.3) got up in thuh
-> morning, an went to thuh bathroom, (1.2)
-> °(an I) noticed there was blood in my urine.°
(0.4)
DOC: °O[kay,°]
PAT: -> [°(just)] ah little bit.°
DOC: Just ah little bit,
PAT: -> °It was just (real light).° An then (0.2) thuh
-> next time (after) (.) cleared up.
DOC: Mm kay,=
PAT: =It was
DOC: An its just been in thuh last week?

In lines 1–7, the doctor reconfirms that this visit was originally scheduled as a follow-up of the patient's high blood pressure. Just as the doctor asks how the patient has been feeling, the patient announces that he has another agenda item (lines 8–9). Note that he starts this turn at the first point at which he can see that the physician's turn-in-progress is not going to elicit further agenda items for this medical visit.

At line 10 the patient states that he has a "couple notations here." as he unfolds a piece of paper. Via this turn the patient shows that the problem about to be introduced will not be simply *named*; rather it has features which will be reported. In this way the patient's utterance functions as a story preface, letting the physician know that the patient will use more than one turn constructional unit to report the candidate health problem, and seeking acknowledgment of this forthcoming story from the physician (Sacks 1974). This turn also allows the patient to display himself as a conscientious reporter of this potential problem.

In addition, this placement of the narrative displays the patient's stance toward it as one of concern, in his treating it as important enough to raise early in the visit, as a new, albeit unscheduled, reason for the visit (Sacks 1992b:247–8; Whalen et al. 1988; Zimmerman 1992).

The doctor acknowledges the patient's problem story preface, and gives him a go-ahead (line 11). In his next turn the patient marks the problem as recent (lines 12–13), thus highlighting the newsworthiness of this symptom report (Sacks 1992b:171–2). This turn also shows the patient to be treating this problem as urgent, through the relatively short period of time he waited before consulting a doctor.

The 0.5-second silence in line 13 shows that the physician is treating the patient as being engaged in a longer unit of talk (i.e., telling a story, not simply giving the name of a new problem). The patient's next turn constructional units (lines 13–14) are a "course of action" formulation (Sacks 1992b:231–3). Such formulations are used to indicate what one was in the midst of doing just before the "storyable" event occurred. In addition, this particular reported action (getting up in the morning and going to the bathroom) is hearable as a story initiation. Not only is it hearable as "not news" (a feature of "course of action" reports generally), it also is hearable as a typical way to start a day, thus a way that a story could be introduced (Sacks 1992a:255–8). The physician's orientation to this talk "as a story in progress" is evidenced by her silence at line 14. For this full 1.2 seconds the physician withholds possible talk, indicating that she is expecting more talk by the patient.

At line 15 the patient gives a noticing marker plus his discovery ("blood in my urine."). He marks this discovery as serious by lowering his voice for this announcement. In addition, the patient treats his report as a "just the facts" account by use of the verb "noticed." This particular form also helps to mark this discovery as "unintended," or "not searched for." After this discovery announcement, the patient withholds talk for 0.4 seconds (line 16), waiting for some uptake from the physician.

The physician receipts the discovery with the same "quiet voice" that the patient announced the problem (line 17). By using the same sort of "quiet voice," the doctor can both demonstrate that she recognizes the stance the patient is taking toward the problem and display a similar (albeit unexplicated) stance toward the problem.

As soon as the physician does this (indeed, in the midst of the physician's receipt), the patient mitigates the problem discovery in three ways. First he mitigates the amount of the symptom (line 18). Then he mitigates the quality of the symptom (line 20). Last, he announces that the problem has since "cleared up."

Even though this patient's health problem is straightforwardly nameable ("blood in [his] urine") he only names the problem at the conclusion of his narrative of discovery. This narrative (lines 13–15) allows the patient to present himself as engaged in his normal, everyday activities prior to the onset of the story-able event. He was not going out of his way or "hunting" for an experience; rather, it happened to him (Sacks 1984, 1992a, 1992b; Jefferson 1986).

In addition, the patient's narrative allows him to set up the telling such that the doctor has to pull out from it the health problem, thus showing that she acknowledges it *as* a health problem. Note the silence at line 16, where the patient waits for some sort of uptake by the doctor, and as soon as that occurs (line 17) the patient starts to mitigate the symptom (lines 18 and 20–21). The patient did not offer these mitigations earlier (e.g., as in the following hypothetical version: "I noticed there was [just a little bit of] [real light] blood in my urine"). Instead they are withheld until the physician acknowledges the patient's problem discovery. By introducing the problem discovery with a course of action narrative, and only *afterwards* mentioning the mitigating aspects of the symptom, the patient is able to:

(i) convey the seriousness with which he initially viewed (and presumably experienced) it;
(ii) elicit from the doctor acknowledgment of (and perhaps agreement with) his stance toward it; and also
(iii) display himself as aware of its potentially reassuring features.

Thus this patient's narrative is a vehicle through which he can show himself to be attentive to, and concerned about, his health, but not unreasonably so.

In the following extract, we will see that these narratives of discovery, while typically used to demonstrate an agnostic stance toward the possible causes of the problem, can also be used to stake a strong claim of knowledgeability and/or experience.

(10) [SSMC 6]

DOC: -> Ok. When you f:irst (.) were aware of it (.) was
(.) did (it anything) in particular that you
noticed about it then, (or)
PAT: -> no I was washing my neck. (0.5) and I felt it
-> and I said oh god i'm coming down with ah boil.
-> (.) that's how I found the one (on) the back.
(0.6) So I didn't yeah I was telling (ahhh)
at that time (0.5) I was joking around (with) I
got ah boil and she said oh you and your boils.
-> (0.6) So we thought nothing about it an then
she'd start- we'd start with thee onions (0.5)
((Patient describes two home-remedy attempts to
treat her boil; 19 lines deleted.))
-> We tried all kind ah stuff.
DOC: Ri:ght.
PAT: And I said (thuh) girl this ain't working,
-> (0.6) so then we forgot about it (0.4) and I was
telling her oh about ah month ago (0.8) I said I
got ah have my boil taken care of. (0.5) so she
took (out) insurance and that's how I got down
here.
DOC: °°Okay. Alright

In this excerpt, the patient starts her narrative of problem discovery with a course of action formulation, telling the physician what she was doing when she first discovered this problem (line 4). By indicating the mundane activity she was in the midst of when the discovery was made, the patient conveys the sense that this problem was "chanced upon," not "hunted for." Unlike most other narratives of problem discovery, the first thought this patient reports upon finding the problem turns out to be correct ("oh god I'm coming down with a boil.", line 5). She then provides an account for being able to name the problem immediately upon discovery ("that's how I found the one (on) the back.", line 6). Thus her turn functions as a strong claim of knowledge or experience about this kind of health problem.

Through her description of how she related this problem discovery to her friend ("I was joking around", line 8), and her friend's reaction ("she said oh you and your boils.", line 9), the patient highlights how she and her friend were not excessively concerned about it, but treated it as an mundane feature of her life ("So we thought nothing about it", line 10). At this point in her narrative the patient expands on a series of home remedies she and her friend tried (lines 12–30, not shown), cumulating in her decision to give up those attempts ("and I said (thuh) girl this ain't working," line 33). Then (as in line 10 above) the patient states that she and her friend simply dropped the task of trying to cure her boil (line 34), thus displaying a casual stance toward the health problem. Then the patient outlines how she again brought up the issue of her boil, and what arrangements were made to get her to the clinic (lines 34–38).

This patient is dealing with the issues we addressed earlier in this chapter, but the whole tenor is different from the prior data segments. Here, while the patient's narrative does show an orientation toward being a reasonable observer of her health, nowhere does she display a sense that this problem might not be appropriate to bring to the doctor (i.e., doctor-able). Indeed, this patient's narrative bends toward the other extreme, via her work to show herself as an expert regarding her boils (including detailed descriptions of her home remedy attempts). Thus this patient's narrative of discovery may tell one more about the patient's stance toward her health problem than about her boils themselves (indeed, it may well be designed to do just that).

Let us now reconsider the following data segment (see also [3]).

(11) [UKFP2: 2]

1	PAT:	->	(.hh) I have ah- ah little swelling here.
2			(0.3)
3	DOC1:		Oka:y,
4	PAT:	->	an:d ah (.hh) I don't know whether its ah (hh)
5			ah hernia, (0.4) or (ah) (.) something inside
6			there causing it ((cough)) but ah ((cough)) it-
7			is- ah little lop sided (.) maybe I'm just
8			growing that way.
9	DOC1:		Hm hmm,=
10	PAT:		But I think maybe its something ought ah be
11			looked at.=
12	DOC1:	->	=You just noticed it two weeks ago,
13	PAT:		Yeah.
14	DOC1:		Okay.=
15	PAT:		=(Hey) it coulda been there for ah year. (.hh)
16			I don't look at myself very much.
17			(.)
18	PAT:		[you know
19	DOC1:		[I see.
20	PAT:	->	But I was shaving or something an I (0.4) I do
21			some side to side exercises an I guess I was
22			doing it an kindah maybe in front of ah (0.3)
23			mirror or something [an I] just noticed that
24	DOC1:		[hm hmm,]
25	PAT:		this side is (1.0) extended
26	DOC1:		Okay.
27	PAT:		rather than this side.
28			(0.2) And ah I hope it doesn't have anything to
29			do with (.hh) liver or cancer or anything like
30			that or tumor but (0.2) (en) I think maybe (it)
31			oughta be (0.4)
32	DOC1:		checked out,
33	PAT:		Ye:ah I think s[o.
34	DOC1:		[Okay.
35			Well we'll (0.2) take ah look at that,

This narrative of discovery has several remarkable features. First, consider the "or somethings" in lines 20 and 23. They function as "approximators," ways of doing: "being approximate" ("I was shaving or something"). "Being approximate" is a way to display oneself as having discovered this problem without having hunted for it. Along with "course of action" formulations, these approximators allow for a display of oneself as having almost accidentally discovered the problem.

Second, in how he reports *where* he was doing his exercises when he discovered the symptom ("kindah maybe in front of ah (0.3) mirror or something"), this patient highlights how much work patients may do to avoid presenting themselves as having hunted for symptoms (lines 22–23). If it is problematic to present oneself as one who hunts for symptoms, then we can see the particular difficulties this patient has to overcome. Since he was in front of a mirror (normally a place specifically used to observe one's body), he needs to present himself as *incidentally* in front of a mirror. He does this via the approximator, as well as the mitigators in this spate of talk ("I guess," "kindah," "maybe").

Last, we can see that he uses the particular "passive observation" verb form ("just noticed") to announce his candidate symptom discovery (line 23).[11] Through this series of moves the patient displays himself as having "unmotivatedly" discovered this possible health problem.

This narrative's (almost excessive) work of displaying the patient as not excessively monitoring his body allows him to raise particular health concerns in a "safe" non-implicative context. The patient can (in effect) say, "I have these concerns, but I'm not the kind of person who *always* has these concerns."

This point is brought home quite nicely in a later segment from the same clinic visit. The intern (Doc1) brings in the attending physician (Doc2), who asks the patient a similar question about the timing of the patient's problem discovery, thus eliciting a reiteration of the narrative of discovery.

(12) [UKFP2: 3]

1	DOC2:		And you think that that- that it jis- you
2			noticed it all at once or did you- what do you
3			think.
4	PAT:		No I jist noticed it all at once. I- (.hhh) I
5			don't look at myself very much. (1.0)
6		->	But I was (0.2) in front of thuh mirror
7		->	for some reason shaving
8		->	or taking ah [(bath-)]
9	DOC2:		[So it] didn't hurt. You jist-
10	PAT:		Never hurt.

[11] See Chafe and Nichols (1986), on these and other "evidentials."

Again, the patient's narrative displays him to have passively come across the mirror, and thus noticed his problem. Observe especially line 7 ("for some reason"), and the following lines (7–8). Through this talk the patient explicitly treats being "in front of thuh mirror" as something he has to account for (Sacks 1992a:72–80). The patient does not even say that he was "looking" in the mirror, but rather "I was in front of thuh mirror," thus highlighting the utterly incidental nature of his location when he noticed the problem. In these ways, the patient makes passive and accidental his possible symptom discovery, thereby underscoring its unmotivated occurrence.

This powerful emphasis on the incidental discovery of this problem is helpful to the patient if he is going to tell his doctor about particular fears or concerns he has about this problem. And this patient has been quite explicit in his expression of possible causes of (and concerns about) this problem. He notes (in (11)) possible benign causes (and marks them as such): "hernia," (line 5), "maybe I'm just growing that way." (lines 7–8). But he also (by contrast) notes possible serious causes: "something inside there causing it" (lines 5–6); "liver or cancer or anything like that or tumor" (lines 29–30).

Given this explicit sharing of concerns, the patient needs a way to demonstrate that, while he has these concerns, he doesn't spend every day looking for medical problems to be worried about. The incidental discovery, and the apparent lack of self-observation, combine to create a context in which one can have particular medical concerns without seeming unreasonable.

Conclusion: a social epistemics of sensation

> The language game of reporting can be given such a turn that the report is not meant to inform the hearer about its subject matter, but about the person making the report. (Wittgenstein, 1953:190)

The features of these narratives allow patients both to display the "doctor-relevance" of a candidate problem (showing one not to be a "negligent" patient) and to display an "unmotivated," "out-of-the-blue" discovery of a candidate problem (thus showing one not to be excessively attentive to bodily sensations). Via these two tasks, a person can show oneself to be "a reasonable patient." Harvey Sacks' remarks on the entitlement to experiences *in the world* are also applicable to how we experience and report on our own bodily states:

> The rights to have an experience by virtue of encountering something like an accident are only the rights to have seen "another accident" . . . you can't make much more of it than what anybody would make of it. We can, then, think of the way that you're entitled to an experience as that you borrow for a while that experience that's available, as compared to that you now invent the experience that you might be entitled to. (Sacks 1992b:246–7)

In these data, patients orient toward an awkward dilemma, born of the "patients' problem." While they attend to the doctor's need for information, they also take pains not to seem too certain that this problem is definitely medically relevant.[12] Through this balancing of bodily experience and diagnostic uncertainty, patients display "accurate and appropriate" witnessing of their bodily states, thereby showing that they are responsible monitors of themselves, not overly observant nor too lax.

Patients' demonstrate a strong orientation to the "patients' problem," and their solutions to it suggest its power – a power rooted in its fundamentally social and moral character (Hilbert 1984, 1992; Wittgenstein 1953, 1964). The "patients' problem" is profoundly social because people treat the answers to these seemingly private questions (e.g., "What if I decide I'm not ill, and it turns out I really am?"; "What if I decide I am ill, seek medical attention, and it turns out I'm really healthy?") as having social, interactional implications.

Furthermore, these social, interactional implications are experienced by people as intrinsically moral ("What if I seek care, but the doctor says I'm healthy?," "What if I fail to seek care in a timely fashion?"). The factual question "Am I ill?" is indivisibly intertwined with the moral question "Should I consider myself ill (and therefore seek medical attention)?" Since "the patients' problem" is experienced as both fundamentally social and moral,

[12] This is similar to Jorg Bergmann's "dilemma of the gossiper." In short, the more detail one provides, the more one is shown to have sought out information. As Bergmann puts it, "detail is purchased at the price of reputation" (1993:107).

it may be powerful enough to prevent some patients from seeking medical care in a timely fashion.[13] Our focus on these narratives thus opens up for investigation (in a new way) what can be called a social epistemics of sensation.

Problem-discovery narratives as patients' models in situ

As discussed by Kleinman et al., patients' explanatory models include ideas about one or more of the following: "[1] etiology; [2] onset of symptoms; [3] pathophysiology; [4] course of illness . . . and severity of disorder; and [5] treatment" (1978:256). Both Percy and Cirillo (see (1) and (2) above), as well as the clinical data segments in this chapter, included explanatory model components as part of the narratives of problem discovery.

While patients sometimes offer this information, researchers and medical educators have increasingly argued that physicians should actively elicit it from patients. For example, Kleinman et al. (1978) is used as an assigned reading in many medical schools' interviewing courses. In such courses, strong emphasis is given to eliciting and using "the patient's perspective on the illness." Cassell (1985a:12–40) has argued for the usefulness of asking patients to "tell me the story of this illness, please." One thing this question seems to elicit from patients is narratives of problem discovery.

Hunt et al. offer an important critique of how the patients' explanatory model concept has been used in social science and medicine. They note that patients offered examples of how they *used* illness explanations as "resources" in their lives.[14]

[13] Consider the case of asthma patients who need to decide whether or not a given exacerbation is sufficiently problematic to seek emergency care. As Becker et al. put it, these patients "walk a tightrope between delaying formal medical intervention and seeking treatment too soon" (1993:305). Another example is that of a person choking in a restaurant, who goes to the restroom. Then, isolated from any help, the asphyxiation becomes a death "by embarrassment" (Mittleman and Wetli 1982).

[14] By depending exclusively on questionnaires and interviews, researchers have denied themselves access to this phenomenon as it is actually used, *in situ* (Wittgenstein 1953, 1964; Sacks 1992a, 1992b). As Hunt et al. note, "Interestingly, this kind of information tended not to appear in response to our interview questions but rather coincidentally, as a passing reference to a conversation with a mother, sister, or friend" (1989:953).

> Illness explanations were constructed in ways which were useful as resources in the lives of patients and were also sustained by the day to day situations in which they become what we might call "interactional objects"; that is to say, they become topics in familial and friendship-network discourse. (1989:953)

Similarly, through their narratives of discovery, we saw how patients employed realization both as a topic and as a resource (Zimmerman and Pollner 1971). Realization is an explicit topic of patients' narratives of discovery: they talk about how they came to realize that they had a problem that might need medical attention. But, while the narratives in this analysis regularly take the form of how a patient came to (psychologically) realize that they had a "doctor-able" problem, we have also seen how the patient's narrative is itself an interactional process, wherein a candidate health problem is *realized*.[15] The patient has started to see that this problem is possibly doctor-able, but it is through one's sheer telling of this realization to the doctor (wherein the doctor's moment-by-moment reactions help to shape that telling) that a candidate health problem emerges as an intersubjective phenomenon.

Seeing how Percy, Cirillo, and the patients quoted above included explanatory model components in their narratives of problem discovery, we might gain a more accurate picture of how such models work (or, rather, how patients put such models to work) by looking at their natural occurrences in clinical interactions.

Clinical implications: working at being a reasonable patient

When a patient brings a new, emergent health problem to his or her doctor, there is a particular issue that is palpably relevant: what we called "the patients' problem." As we have seen in this chapter, through narratives of problem discovery people show that they did not go looking for this problem, but had it thrust upon them, and that they did their best to normalize or handle the (emergent) health problem before they arrived at the doctor's office.

We have also seen that patients often take it as their task to formulate, through their talk, descriptions of their health concerns

[15] See Maynard (1996), and cf. Volosinov (1973:93–4).

as doctor-able in a manner that displays them as reasonable patients, reasonably seeking medical care.

Consequently, when patients talk about an illness via a narrative of problem discovery, physicians and other health professionals may want to hold in mind what the patient's "project" might be, what the patient is trying to do via this story. If we resist hearing these stories as faulty lay-models of illness, "hot air," or even literal truth, and focus instead on what the patient is trying to *achieve* by this talk, we may hear our patients more clearly.

5

Explaining illness: patients' proposals and physicians' responses

Virginia Teas Gill and Douglas W. Maynard

Introduction

Patients visit doctors for a variety of reasons, and a prominent one is to find out what is causing some health problem or symptom they are experiencing (Korsch et al. 1968; Novack 1995). However, during the course of medical interviews, patients often offer their own "lay" or "folk" explanations for what is causing their health difficulties. In the view of many researchers, doctors routinely ignore or dismiss patients' theories (Cicourel 1983; Fisher and Groce 1990; Kleinman et al. 1978; Mehan 1990; Mishler 1984; Stoeckle and Barsky 1981; Waitzkin 1979, 1991). Doctors, because of their power and authority, are said to impose a biomedical perspective upon patients.[1] They maintain an exclusive focus on only those symptoms and disease processes that are under the purview of the medical model, rather than considering or appreciating patients' social experiences and perspectives regarding their illnesses. Thus, the "voice of medicine" is said to regularly silence the "voice of the life world" (Fisher and Groce 1990; Mishler 1984).

Despite such pronouncements, investigators have not described or analyzed, in any detail, the interactional structure of patients' explanations and doctors' responses (explanation–response sequences) as they occur within the context of clinic visits. Nor has enough attention been given to how explanation–response sequences relate to ongoing courses of activity, such as the different phases of the

[1] See the review and critique of literature on the "asymmetry" in doctor–patient interaction, in Maynard (1991c); Robinson (2001a).

medical interview.[2] This chapter draws on audio- and videotaped data of patient visits to an outpatient medical clinic[3] to examine the interactional strategies patients use to offer explanations for their medical problems and the methods doctors use to respond to these explanations. Our focus is how patients design and place their explanations in the phase of the medical interview where doctors are gathering information about symptoms.

What has been portrayed as a struggle between the doctor's "biomedical" perspective and the patient's "lifeworld" concerns can be recharacterized in terms of interactional dilemmas that doctors and patients face. These dilemmas involve sequential organization within two ordered phases of the medical interview: (1) *the collection of medical data* through verbal and physical examination or Byrne and Long's (1976) phase III of the interview; and (2) *the "consideration" or analysis of this data* or Byrne and Long's (1976) phase IV. During clinic visits, patients show that they face this dilemma: How, within a course of action that primarily involves *collecting medical data* (facts about the nature of patients' symptoms and other aspects of their experiences) can patients offer their *analyses* of these facts (explanations) so that doctors may consider them, yet without requiring such consideration immediately, in the data-gathering context?[4] That is, when the doctor is gathering facts about a particular symptom, it provides an opportunity for the patient to offer

2 Conversation-analytic and ethnographic researchers have considered patients' or "lay" perspectives when investigating other topics in medical or clinical interactions (Drew 1991; Heath 1992; Heritage and Sefi 1992; Maynard 1991c, 1991d; Silverman 1987; Stivers 2002b; Strong 1979; ten Have 1991), but few have given primary attention to patients' actual explanatory practices and doctors' responses (see Gill 1995, 1998a, 1998b; Gill et al., 2001; Raevaara 1998, 2000).

3 Data were collected by the second author at an outpatient general internal medicine clinic associated with a teaching hospital in a medium-sized city in the Midwestern United States. The data corpus includes 15 audio- and videotapes of clinic visits (involving 15 patients and 5 physicians), and 2 audiotaped follow-up calls (involving 2 of the patients and 2 of the doctors).

4 A related dilemma is discussed in Gill (1998a): patients often have explanations for their illnesses, but treat as problematic any display of personal authority about these explanations. Patients handle the dilemma by displaying certainty about the explanations in contexts where they are not inviting doctors' assessments. Conversely, patients *downplay* their certainty when their explanations solicit evaluation from doctors. Thus, patients do manage to insert their explanations into the medical interview yet refrain from requiring doctors to recognize them as authoritative sources of this type of knowledge. See also ten Have (1991), who argues that appearing "uncertain" is a way for patients to put explanations on the table yet maintain a subordinate role vis-à-vis the doctor.

an explanation for this symptom. This will enable the physician to consider it as he or she generates and tests diagnostic hypotheses. If the patient does not take the opportunity then and there, it may not arise again, for the next phase of the interview involves the "flow of information from the physician to the patient" (Cohen-Cole and Bird 1991:28).[5] Yet giving an explanation in the data-collection phase may be premature, since not all the facts are in. For their part, doctors show that their dilemma, in hearing a patient's explanation, is how to stay on course in the overall interview, rather than jumping the track and moving back and forth between data collection and data analysis or prematurely moving to the phase wherein they educate the patient by delivering diagnostic or other information.

Patients handle their dilemma by constructing explanations that do not disrupt doctors' information-gathering activities. When patients present explanations, doctors address their own dilemma by strongly orienting to the canonical organization of the medical interview (where data collection precedes data analysis). Although in some cases doctors do evaluate patients' explanations immediately in information-gathering contexts, they typically stay on course when this option is provided and continue to collect data from patients without outwardly indicating that they heard patients insert their analyses into the conversation. Thus, as in previous research, we find that physicians may leave patients' explanations unassessed or even unacknowledged. However, this is at least partly due to both participants' orientation to the overall organization of the medical interview.

Design of patients' explanations for health problems

In this section, we outline three basic components of patients' explanations as well as other dimensions of their design. To begin, we observe that, during clinic visits, patients regularly produce complaints. That is, they make reference to and describe the symptoms and health problems they are experiencing or have experienced. For example:

[5] See also Lazare et al. (1995) on the "three function" model of the medical interview.

(1) [10:594]

1 Ms. N: While we're on my gut.
2 Dr. D: °Yes.°
3 Ms. N: → A couple a weeks ago: hh u:m (0.6) I had (.) tremendous
4 amount of rectal pai:n?

In addition to producing complaints, a patient may overtly or tacitly propose that something is causing the symptom they are experiencing; that is, the patient proposes a diagnosis, etiology, or site of origin for the symptom. To make these connections, patients use *linkage proposals*. Linkage proposals range from attributive, wherein patients *overtly* propose a causal relationship, to non-attributive, where patients only *tacitly* suggest such a causal relationship.

Overt explanations

When patients produce overt explanations,[6] they explicitly mark that they are *accounting for* their symptoms, not just producing *accounts of* (i.e., descriptions of) their symptoms.[7] Patients use attributive linkage proposals to produce overt explanations. For example, they may use the "because" form to causally connect a symptom to a reported fact, such as a life experience or circumstance. That reported fact then becomes a causal factor for the

[6] There are 63 overt and 22 tacit explanations in the data corpus, for a total of 85. We arrived at these figures by tallying participants' *activities* rather than the *content* of these activities. For example, there are cases where a patient offers the same explanation for a symptom at three different points in time; this was counted as three explanations, in order to keep track of how patients design each one – the opportunities they provide for physicians to respond, the degree to which they invite a response, etc. – and how physicians actually respond at each available opportunity. If the explanations were counted by content (i.e., if several different explanations that cite the same causal factor were counted as one explanation), we would lose this detail. Similarly, if a patient offers three different explanations for the same health problem (i.e., proposes three different causes) and offers each only one time, this was counted as three explanations. In these cases we always note when the content changes (when patients propose different causes in successive explanations).

[7] In conversation analysis, "accounting" is a broad category that encompasses activities such as "describing" as well as "explaining." However, in doctor–patient interaction, describing a problem and providing an explanation for a problem are treated as two distinct activities; that is, there is a member-generated distinction between these types of accounts (Gill 1998b).

symptom. In excerpt (2), Ms. O uses "because" to attribute her depression and upset feelings to lack of sleep.

(2) [2:1(

Ms. O: … ınd

Patients … 'was," as att … :ases is a hyp … N uses "was … l to the condi …

(3) [

Ms …
Dı …
Ms … endous

Ms … ɔt sur:e
… tried

Simi … condition "brc … Dr. A are discussing the patient's chest pain.

(4) [6:383]

Dr. A: An so tha:t (.) came on with the exerci:[se
Ms. A: [M hm?
Dr. A: An- with other activities that you've do[ne.
Ms. A: [M hm?
Dr. A: °Oka:y:°
(0.5)
Dr. A: .hh (2.5) An in addition sometimes you wake at nigh:(.)[t wi]th that.
Ms. A: [M hm]
(3.5)
Ms. A: → An I was wondering if: °you know° stress could a (.) brought that on too.

Patients may link a pain or other symptom to a specific site of origin, such as an organ in the body, by proposing that the symptom is "in" that organ. Below, Ms. B cites her "gall bladder" and then her "kidney" as the cause of the abdominal tenderness she is experiencing:

(5) [7:365]

1 Ms. B: .hhh An: : :d then I get a lot of tenderness: in this area hh.
2 And again:, it's probably: (1.0) [whether: it's] in the=
3 Dr. A: [In the front]
4 Ms. B: → =gall bladder? Kidney?

Thus, patients' overt explanations are based on a three-part turn structure, consisting of a *complaint* (reference to a symptom or other discomfiting health problem); an *attributive linkage proposal*; and a *causal factor* (a reported circumstance, hypothetical bodily condition, or site of origin). Patients put these elements together to account for the existence of their symptoms.

Tacit explanations

A patient can offer a tacit explanation by describing or referring to a symptom and then reporting a life circumstance or experience.[8] The patient connects these elements with a non-attributive linkage proposal such as "and" or "but."[9] The patient invites the doctor

[8] Reporting is a generic strategy that speakers can use to accomplish various types of tacit or implicit activities in conversation. For example, a speaker can avoid taking an official position in relation to a proposal, such as an invitation, by producing a report of an activity or circumstance in response (Drew 1984:134):

I: How about the following weekend.
(0.8)
C: → .hh Dats the vacation isn't it?
I: .hhhhh Oh:. ALright so:– no ha:ssle, ...

In this excerpt, I issues an invitation. C's subsequent report (arrowed) provides I with "the materials from which she can see for herself that it will not be possible to go then" (Drew 1984:134). However, C leaves it to I to determine the implication of his report. I takes the report as a rejection of her proposal.

[9] Whereas "and" projects that a forthcoming utterance is "additional" (in relation to a previous utterance) and thereby proposes a connection between the two, "but" can be used to propose a relationship between two utterances by *setting off* a forthcoming utterance against a prior utterance. A variation is for patients to use "since" to propose a temporal relationship between a symptom and another circumstance, and thus tacitly suggest a causal connection. See Drew and Heritage's (1992:31–2) example, taken from Mishler (1984:165):

Dr: How long have you been drinking that heavily?
Pt: Since I've been married
Dr: How long is that?
Pt: (giggle) Four years

to analyze the report's relationship to the complaint, while stopping short of overtly proposing that those circumstances or experiences are causal factors. The patient merely implies or hints at such a relationship and provides the *doctor* with the opportunity to display recognition of the "upshot" and to officially make a causal connection between the patient's report and the patient's symptom (see Drew 1984; Gill 1995, 1998b; Strong 1979).

For example, in excerpt (6) Ms. B offers a tacit explanation. She complains of a symptom (line 1) and then reports that she has a new car (lines 1 and 3). The doctor does not immediately display recognition of an upshot. After two more reports related to the emergence of her symptom (line 6) and time spent sitting in the car ("shifts," line 7), the patient herself goes on to propose (in a speculative manner) a causal connection between the car and the backache (line 9):

(6) [10:523]

Ms. B: .hhh I've been having this backache:KHH. .hhh A[n:d we] do=
Dr. A: [Do you:]
Ms. B: =have a new car:::,
(1.0)
Dr. A: °M [hm°
Ms. B: [An:::d (.) it- (.) didn't bother me the first two weeks.
But we did do: a couple of three hour:: shi[fts.
Dr. A: [Mm hm?
Ms. B: Whether that's it:thh?
(0.4)

In contrast, in excerpt (7) the patient issues a tacit explanation and the doctor's response does immediately display recognition of an upshot. That is, by proposing to look for "underlying causes" for the patient's fatigue (lines 8 and 11), he also shows his understanding that in lines 3–5 the patient was offering an *explanation* for her fatigue, and that the real cause may be more serious than "burning the candle at both ends":

(7) [16:1032]

Dr. C: You mention some easy bruising? An bleeding? Fatigue?
Ms. I: Yea::h. I- an the- an: that you know: has been (.) most recently
that I have the fatigue. But I guess: you know: you're just

4 not supposed ta (2.5) °keephh° (0.5) °burning the candle° at
5 both ends all the ti(h)me(h)(h)[(h)
6 Dr. C: [.hh Ah:: well-?
7 Ms. I: .HHH
8 Dr. C: We'll (0.7) look inta tha[t.=See if there's]
9 Ms. I: [Y' know::]
10 (.)
11 Dr. C: might be any underlying cau[ses for fatigue.]
12 Ms. I: [I have had some ch]est pains.

In other cases, neither the patient nor the doctor produce an upshot, and the complaint and report retain the ontological status of observations (i.e., accounts *of* facts and circumstances), never attaining the status of overt explanations. For example, in excerpt (8) Ms. B describes how often she experiences her symptom (lines 3–4), abdominal tenderness. She then reports monitoring her activities for "lifting something or doing something." (line 5), tacitly proposing that muscle strain from such activities could be a cause of the abdominal tenderness if, in fact, she were engaging in these activities. In a type of response that we will explore in detail later in the chapter, the doctor queries the patient about how long the tenderness lasts when she experiences it (line 7). The causal connection between lifting (or other physical activity) and the abdominal tenderness is never explicitly explored in this clinic visit.

(8) [7:365]

1 Ms. B: °.hhh° Ptch [A::nd, hhhh]
2 Dr. A: ['Bout how often does] that come.
3 Ms. B: Uh:: hhhh (1.0) This cn: (1.5) m- be like at least once or
4 twice a week. And I've been trying to see if I've been:::
5 >you know,< lifting something or doing something. °.hhhh°
6 (1.5)
7 Dr. A: How long does it last when you g[et it.]
8 Ms. B: [Ah::m](.) maybe a day or
9 two.

Thus, patients can offer tacit explanations via a three-part turn structure, consisting of (1) a *complaint* (reference to a symptom or other discomfiting health problem); (2) a *non-attributive linkage proposal*; and (3) a *reported circumstance*. However, they require an additional turn, which either provides or shows recognition of an upshot, in order to turn the reported circumstance officially into a *causal factor* for the symptom.

The relevance of doctors' confirming and disconfirming assessments

Explanation design and placement

Patients exhibit sensitivity to the activity context in which they are offering explanations. In the "investigative" phases of clinic visits where physicians are gathering empirical information (ten Have 1987, 1991; see also Byrne and Long 1976; Heath 1992; Waitzkin 1991), patients especially avoid compelling doctors to provide immediate confirming or disconfirming assessments. As Gill (1998a) shows, patients typically offer their explanations as "trial balloons" that suggest causal factors for doctors to investigate (or relevantly rule out), but which do not compel here-and-now assessments from doctors and thus do not propose to interfere with their collection of medical data. Patients design and place their explanations in ways that allow doctors to maintain a focus on fact-finding; i.e., to continue gathering information about patients' symptoms or other medically relevant experiences. In designing explanations that can accommodate empirically focused queries, patients orient to the structure of a typical medical interview, where data collection precedes data analysis. Patients provide for the possibility that doctors will refrain from evaluating their explanations before all the "facts" are in (Gill 1998a). Accordingly, patients' strategies at once make visible and deftly handle the dilemma of how to put explanations on the table so that doctors can take the suggested causal factors into consideration, yet avoid occasioning a situation where, if doctors choose to gather more information, patients' theories would achieve the status of having been "ignored."

In the following section, we briefly introduce the features of explanation design and placement which provide doctors with opportunities to focus on the activity of collecting data, rather than compelling them to evaluate their explanations. In the final section of the chapter, we show examples of doctors availing themselves of these features.

Explanations that do not strongly compel doctors' confirming or disconfirming assessments

By design, a tacit explanation – complaining about a symptom and then reporting a fact or circumstance – puts very little pressure on the doctor to respond with a confirming or disconfirming evaluation, as in excerpts (6)–(8); that is, this set of actions does not firmly initiate an explanation–assessment sequence. The patient gives the doctor the option to display recognition of an upshot, but also gives the doctor the option to hear the report as simply that – a report of circumstances. The doctor may relevantly treat the report as "information" or "data" and proceed with information-gathering activities by simply nodding, or otherwise indicating receipt of the report. To say that the physician can *relevantly* take this option does not mean that this is the best option. It simply means that the patient does not put the doctor in a position where he or she must respond, or else appear to be ignoring an explanation that the patient put on the table. Officially, there is no explanation on the table for the doctor to evaluate.

Even though they officially propose causal connections, the design of some overt explanations can also put little pressure on doctors to produce an assessment. Patients often pose their overt explanations as *speculations* or out-loud musings,[10] which not only display uncertainty, but are also relatively non-constraining in terms of the responses they require from doctors (Gill 1998a); see for example, excerpts (3)–(5) as well as line 9 in (6). Speculative explanations are not forthright questions, and therefore do not clearly constitute the first part of a question–answer adjacency pair. If such explanations did, then that would firmly establish the "conditional relevance" of a doctor's confirming or disconfirming assessment, such that it would be "noticeably absent" were it missing (Schegloff 1972:76–77; Gill 1998a; ten Have 1991). Instead, speculative explanations provide for the relevance of an array of responses.

Similarly, overt explanations designed as *qualified proposals*, as in excerpt (2), are also relatively non-constraining for the doctor. Like a "first assessment" (Pomerantz 1984a:61), a qualified proposal makes a confirming or disconfirming assessment *relevant* as a next-turn activity, but does not require such a response. A distinctive

[10] See Sacks (1992b:405) on "musing aloud."

feature of qualified proposals is that they display slightly more certainty than do speculative explanations (patients preface them with "I think" rather than "I'm wondering if" or "I don't know if"), but, as we will show, patients offset this certainty by using qualified proposals in comparatively low-risk contexts, where agreeing assessments are likely – for example, when patients are proposing an explanation that is in line with the doctor's own displayed view.

Patients' *positioning* of overt explanations within turns can also lessen the degree to which they compel doctors' assessments. Patients may place overt explanations within multiple-component turns that include both symptom-related and explanation-related components. This gives doctors the option to relevantly respond to either component (Gill 1998a). For example, a patient may construct a two-component turn (*reply + explanation*) wherein the patient replies to a doctor's symptom-related question (regarding when a symptom occurs, how long it lasts, etc.) and then offers an overt explanation for the symptom. As Frankel (1990:237) notes, this type of turn design provides the doctor with "an option rather than an obligation" to respond to the second turn component (the explanation). This design is evident in excerpt (9) below. Dr. C seeks a confirmation of a problem Ms. I had mentioned earlier in her clinic visit, that she experiences pain with intercourse (lines 1–2). (Several years before, Ms. I had a surgery that included both a hysterectomy and bladder repair.)

(9) [19:1259]

Dr. C: .hh Kay. An then the other- the other thing you mentioned
was (.) you have (.) pain with intercourse. Is that right?
Ms. I: Yeah. But that's just since I've had that hysterectomy. An I
don't know if that bladder tie up? Was part of that?
(0.8)
Dr. C: For th last six or ten years. Ever since that [surgery. So]
Ms. I: [M hm? M]
hm?

Ms. I replies ("Yeah," line 3), clarifies the date of the onset of the pain ("since I've had that hysterectomy." line 3), which may also tacitly suggest that the surgery is the cause of the pain, and then she adds a more overt, speculative explanation concerning a "bladder tie up" (line 4). This turn design presents Dr. C with the option of focusing on either the reported timing of the patient's pain, or her explanation. He responds in terms of the timing of the pain (line 6) and goes on to query about its frequency (not shown here).

Patients may also add other turn components to overt explanations, so that the explanations themselves become less assessment-relevant. For example, patients may append turn components that return the talk to the activity of *describing their symptoms*. Then the doctor may attend to the descriptive portion of the patient's turn. For example, in excerpt (10), Dr. B asks Ms. D whether she experiences shortness of breath (line 1). Ms. D replies to the query with "So:me" (line 3), then produces her explanation ("that-'s:cuz I should lose wei:ght."). She adds a tag component: a downgraded description of how much shortness of breath she experiences ("NOT much." line 6):

(10) [9:431]

1	Dr. B:	Shortness of brea:th?
2		(1.0)
3	Ms. D:	So:me: but that-'s:cuz I should lose wei:ght. I know
4		that.
5		(.)
6	Ms. D:	I think- NOT much.
7	Dr. B:	When do you get short of brea:th.

Dr. B's next query (line 7) is directed toward her temporal experience of the symptom, rather than her explanation.

Patients consistently use this turn design, which "envelops" the explanation within turn elements that describe a symptom or circumstance, when they offer *unmitigated overt explanations*, as in Ms. D's line 3 utterance above (Gill 1998a). Accordingly, the explanations that patients deliver with the most certainty do not actively solicit assessment. We shall return to this matter later, when we explore other kinds of work that unmitigated overt explanations can do.

Explanations that strongly compel doctors' confirming or disconfirming assessments

Patients may pose their overt explanations as *frank questions* that narrowly restrict doctors' response options, such that doctors are compelled to provide "answers" by evaluating the explanations. However, out of 85 total explanations in the data corpus there are only 3 cases where patients embed their explanations within such questioning formats,[11] and in these cases the patients place their explanations in locations in the medical interview where physicians are not engaged in gathering information (Gill 1998a). For example, in excerpt (11), Ms. N embeds an explanation in a frank question, soliciting Dr. D's assessment at a juncture in the visit where he has paused to write her a prescription.

(11) [11:716]
((Dr. is writing a prescription))

1 Ms. N: You know do you think I'm getting depressed at these times
2 because'v my period? A friend- er my health aide pointed
3 that out.
4 (1.0) ((Dr. puts down his pen))
((10 lines omitted where patient
further describes her depression
and not feeling well))
14 Dr. D: No Anna I've never had a very good- (1.2) feeling for what-
15 makes you go down in the dumps

The interrogative (questioning) format of Ms. N's explanation (lines 1–2) does strongly establish the relevance of the doctor's confirming or disconfirming assessment. As noted, however, this occurs at a place in the interview where the doctor is not gathering information. He listens to her description and then, at lines 14–15, rejects her explanation, claiming not to know what causes her depression.

Note also that Ms. N shifts "footing" (Goffman 1981) and attributes the explanation to her "health aide" (lines 2–3), thus proposing that her knowledge is "derivative" (Bergmann 1992:142) rather than hers alone. Third-party attributions occur in each of the three cases where patients embed their explanations within frank questions (see Gill 1998a). By using a third-party attribution the patient partially shifts to that third party the responsibility for asking

[11] This is consistent with Frankel's (1990) and West's (1983, 1984) findings that patients' questions are dispreferred in medical interviews. See also Pomerantz (1988) on embedding "candidate answers" within questions.

for an assessment, and marks this as a sensitive activity (Drew 1991; Pomerantz 1984b, 1988).

Explanations and their responses

We now turn to explanation-response sequences, focusing on cases where patients have offered overt explanations for their health problems. When a patient complains about a symptom and overtly proposes that a particular activity or condition is causing it, or that the problem may be emanating from a particular organ in the body, a physician may treat that explanation as a proposal for which a *confirming or disconfirming assessment* is a relevant response. That is to say, the doctor may handle the explanation as if it were the first part of an explanation-assessment "adjacency pair" (Schegloff and Sacks 1973) and respond accordingly. This pattern can be characterized as follows:

Response pattern 1

Turn 1: Patient's explanation

+

Turn 2: Doctor's confirming/disconfirming assessment

Although the assessment may be slightly delayed by tokens of hesitation, in this pattern the doctor orients relatively quickly to providing an assessment, rather than, for example, responding with a symptom-related query. Nevertheless, doctors' immediate assessments as responses to patients' explanations are relatively rare in our corpus. Out of 63 overt explanations, doctors disconfirm (5) or confirm (9) immediately in only 14 cases (or a little over 20 percent of the time).

Explanation–assessment sequences

Doctors' immediate disconfirming assessments

In our five disconfirmation cases, the pattern is for doctors to respond in a cautious, disengaged manner. An example is shown below. Just prior to this excerpt, Ms. A reported having a problem with dry skin on her face, and Dr. A examined her face.

Ms. A speculates whether the hypothetical condition, "hormone deficiencies," could cause dry skin (lines 1–4).

(12) [9:539]

Ms. A: The only thing I was wondering if dere is .hhhhh you kno:w
ah::n (2.0) ((doctor turns from desk to look at patient))
hormone deficiencies or something like this that it (0.6)
(>°you know°<) that dries your skin out too.
(0.5)
Dr. A: °Mm°
(0.5)
Dr. A: Tch .hhh ah:m
(0.8)
Ms. A: Or no[t too much
Dr. A: [tch There are some hormone problems like thyroid
p[roblems]=
Ms. A: [°Mm hm°] ((nodding))
Dr. A: =which can do tha:t. Um we've never found that (.) on you
before.
Ms. A: No= ((shakes head))
Dr. A: =(though) we could certainly think about- °about that.°
Ms. A: An- how did my cholesterol test turn out.
(.)
Ms. A: Blood tests I'm curious about tha:t.

At lines 5–9, Dr. A delays answering and produces tokens that may portend disagreement, whereupon Ms. A revises her explanation in a way that anticipates a negative answer (line 10).[12] In partial overlap with Ms. A's revision, the doctor offers a disconfirming assessment (lines 11–12 and 14–15). She claims that, in Ms. A's case, there is insufficient empirical evidence to support the explanation. Dr. A's offering is cautious, in ways that "dispreferred" responses are canonically performed (Pomerantz 1984a). In addition to her initial delays (lines 5–9), she confirms the theoretical possibility of such an explanation (lines 11–12 and 14). But then she "cites the evidence" (Maynard 2004) in a way that could rule out these hormone problems in Ms. A's case (lines 14–15). Note that by referring to evidence from *previous* lab tests ("Um we've never found that (.) on you before."), she displays still more caution in that she does not rule out the possibility that the patient may *currently* have such

[12] Ms. A is revising in a way that observes the preference for agreement (Sacks 1987).

hormone problems. Ms. A shakes her head and says, "No," displaying knowledge of these findings (line 16). Dr. A goes on to qualify her disconfirmation, portraying herself as still willing to consider the matter (line 17). However, Ms. A does not pursue it any further. She shifts the topic, inquiring about the results of her recent cholesterol and blood tests (lines 18 and 20).

Doctors' immediate confirming assessments

While it is more common in these data for doctors to provide confirming than disconfirming assessments in response to patients' explanations, confirming assessments also occur relatively infrequently. As mentioned, there are 9 cases out 63 overt explanations where, without first initiating an extended series of symptom-related queries and responses and/or a physical examination, doctors respond with confirming assessments after patients offer their overt explanations.

Not surprisingly, doctors tend to give confirming assessments in response to patients' explanations that have *exhibited alignment with doctors' displayed perspectives*. Even so, doctors' confirmations are cautious rather than forthright. Excerpt (13) shows a doctor giving a qualified confirming assessment in response to a patient's explanation. Mr. E has pain in his forearm that Dr. B has provisionally diagnosed as being caused by ulnar nerve entrapment syndrome (a pinched nerve in his elbow). This clinic visit is a follow-up visit; the doctor is evaluating the patient's condition since he began using an elbow pad and an anti-inflammatory drug. Dr. B first examines Mr. E to determine whether he is developing muscle weakness in the afflicted arm. He explains that activities that involve vibration, gripping tight, and holding the arms bent for an extended period will be irritating (lines 1–2, 4–5, and 7).

(13) [5:258]

1 Dr. B: It makes sense that things like mowin' thuh lawn cuz ya know
2 you're grippin' tight an' [your arms are bent] an' you're=
3 Mr. E: [(that's right]
4 Dr. B: =holdin that position for uh long time 'n there's vibration,
5 n' that's all [irritating. So it] makes sense that those
6 Mr. E: [(That's right)]
7 Dr. B: =kinds o' things're gonna bother it.
8 (.)

Dr. B: .h[h
Mr. E: [.hh tch .h I think that >what it is < um- (.) da:maging
wa:s:a- (.) I- I do:n't (.) remember whether I me:ntioned to
you or not:a- was years ago:, almost like a- (.) bout six,
se:ven years ago. .hhh I work in a workshop in this machin:e
jis those:a- those gu::ns? Needle sh:ape
Dr. B: Yeah=
Mr. E: =to- drill da h:ole ta-
Dr. B: Yea[h
Mr. E: [ta (glue).
Dr. B: Right.
Mr. E: And those one I probably work on em (.) constantly work on
one ti:me. I[for]go:t,
Dr. B: [Mhm]
Mr. E: I didn't (.) [pay] attention.
Dr. B: [Okay.]
Mr. E: And I cont:inuously (0.5) sh:ake it.
Dr. B: Righ[t
Mr. E: [>I feel< that's what's the damaging
Dr. B: Yeah=
Mr. E: =°Ya° [(cause for that)]
Dr. B: [It may ha:ve.]
Dr. B: Yeah.

Mr. E agrees (line 6) and further responds (lines 10–14, 16, and 18) by offering a qualified explanation for what may have initially caused the damage to his arm: he worked at a machine that "continuously" shook his arm. Dr. B marks that he is following the patient's narrative by offering continuers and other tokens of acknowledgment, including indications of agreement (lines 15, 17, 19, etc.), even as the narrative progresses (lines 20–21, 23, and 25). A summarizing turn (lines 27 and 29) refers back to the circumstances he reported in his story and the condition he experiences, more overtly proposing that the circumstances caused the damage. Dr. B offers an agreement token (line 28), and qualified confirming assessment, "It may ha:ve" (line 30). Thus, in a context where the doctor has already gathered information and made a candidate diagnosis (a pinched nerve), and where the patient's explanation for what caused the problem (shaking the arm) is in line with this diagnosis and the doctor's pronouncement of what could irritate the arm (vibration), the doctor produces guarded agreement. And Dr. B produces it quickly (line 28) – in the way that preferred responses are done – after Mr. E finishes his explanation.

Explanation–query sequences

In information-gathering phases of medical interviews, doctors also respond to patients' explanations by attending to their symptoms. Specifically, doctors' responses are often queries that ask patients to provide information about *what* they are physically experiencing – for example, the timing, location, or duration of the symptoms for which they are offering explanations (see Mishler 1984). This pattern is organized as follows:

Response pattern 2

Turn 1: Patient's explanation
+
Turn 2: Doctor's query
+
Turn 3: Patient's reply to query

Doctors may also query patients about other components of their explanation turns. For example, doctors may direct their attention to the activities, experiences, or hypothetical conditions that patients cite as *causal factors* in their explanations. When doctors query patients about the existence of these factors, it provides patients with an opportunity to discuss them. Finally, doctors may direct their attention to *evidence*. That is, if after offering an explanation a patient reports evidence that either lends support to the explanation or implies it should be ruled out or otherwise excluded from consideration, the doctor may query the patient about this evidence rather than attending to the explanation itself.

An important feature of these types of queries, also observed by Mishler (1984), is that doctors typically do not mark whether or how the queries – and the responses they seek – are related to exploring patients' explanations per se and determining whether they might be right. Doctors do not indicate whether or not these queries constitute "insertion sequences" (Schegloff 1972:78) that are being initiated in search of clarification or additional empirical information, which if provided would allow doctors eventually to confirm or disconfirm patients' explanations. On the face of it, these queries solicit more data. In some cases, doctors' queries represent the end of the line for patients' explanations, in that these explanations are never confirmed nor disconfirmed during the clinic visit.

As we will show, however, there are instances where these queries do end up amounting to insertion sequences between patients' explanations and doctors' assessments; that is, in five cases in the data, doctors eventually do assess patients' overt explanations after gathering additional symptom-related information through queries and physical examinations, and thus they retroactively display that this information-gathering was actually hypothesis testing (i.e., it was used either to rule out or confirm the patient's explanation).[13] This is consistent with Heath's (1992) and ten Have's (1991) findings that doctors may delay confirming or disconfirming responses until the completion of the physical examination or the medical interview. Such a pattern looks like this:

Response pattern 3

Turn 1: Patient's explanation
\+
Turn 2: Doctor's query ⎤

Turn 3: Patient's reply to query ⎥ *Insertion sequence*
.
.
.
\+ ⎦
Turn n: Doctor's confirming or disconfirming assessment of explanation[14]

Crucially, in the immediate sequential environment of the first two turns in Pattern 3, where patients offer their explanations and doctors respond with queries, it is not possible to distinguish this pattern from Pattern 2, where the patient's explanation receives no eventual assessment. The two patterns begin identically and *in neither case do doctors initially mark how and/or whether their queries are connected to exploring the patients' explanations.* As Mishler

[13] It is possible that there were actually more delayed confirming or disconfirming assessments than we have noted. In two of the interviews where patients offer overt explanations and receive no assessments, the recordings end just before the physical exams. In these two cases the doctors may have confirmed or disconfirmed the patients' explanations during or after the exams.

[14] In our data, these are all confirming assessments. However, in one case – see excerpt (17d) – the doctor's assessment overtly confirms the patient's first explanation (hemorrhoids) while also *tacitly disconfirming* her second explanation (obstruction).

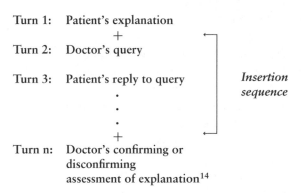

(1984:120) has observed, doctors do not show the reasoning that underlies their queries.[15]

However, this focus on gathering empirical data is not a unilateral accomplishment, nor is it simply a matter of the biomedical model suppressing "lifeworld" concerns. Although Mishler (1984:115) contends that patients may be "confused by shifts in the content of the physician's questions" and have "no clear idea of what [the physician] is trying to discover," our data show a more *bilateral* orientation toward the activity that predominates in the information-gathering phases of the interview: gathering medical data. Even if patients are unfamiliar with the exact diagnostic agenda physicians may be working to establish through their queries, this should not imply either naivety or passive acceptance of the biomedical model. *Instead, patients display an understanding of the interactional structure of the medical interview and the activities through which the biomedical model is realized.*

When patients place their own analyses within the data-gathering phase of the medical interview, they design and position these explanations in ways that accommodate continued investigation or fact-finding. That is, as we observed earlier, where doctors are collecting data about patients' physical states, patients' explanations are not sequentially restrictive; they do not constrain doctors to produce confirming or disconfirming assessments then and there. Patients' strategies for offering explanations thus adroitly handle the interactional dilemma noted in the introduction to this chapter: they allow patients to put explanations on the table for doctors' consideration, without being seen to request an assessment prematurely, before all the facts are in. For their part, doctors capitalize upon the non-restrictive design and placement of patients' explanations and respond in ways that focus on *what* patients are experiencing rather than on *why* they are experiencing it.

In addition, there are cases where patients' explanations invite rather than merely allow responses that focus on what they are experiencing. For example, patients may use explanation formats as vehicles to introduce and draw doctors' attention to additional concerns or complaints that may otherwise be difficult to put on

[15] Similarly, ten Have (1991:150) observes that in other positions (such as in the third turn position) physicians also "refrain from commentary, utterances displaying alignment, or any indication of their own information processing."

the table. In the next section, we show extended explanation–query sequences, highlighting how doctors delay or avoid producing immediate confirming or disconfirming assessments in information-gathering phases of medical visits, while pursuing their information-gathering activities. First, we show how doctors' focus on *what is occurring* (symptoms) rather than *why it is occurring* (explanations) can lead to patients' explanations being disattended for the entire interview. Subsequently, we examine how doctors may eventually confirm patients' explanations, after extended insertion sequences that deal with the nature of the patients' symptoms.

Query focuses on the patient's symptom, no assessment occurs

In the next excerpt, a patient offers an explanation that never receives a confirming or disconfirming assessment from the doctor. Dr. B has been taking Ms. D's health history.[16] At this point in the interview, he is gathering information about a variety of matters such as her family members' health, whether she smokes, and whether she experiences headaches or asthma. He then asks Ms. D if she experiences shortness of breath (line 1 below). She replies that she does have some shortness of breath, and then offers her weight as a cause for this condition (line 3). This reference ties back to the beginning of this medical visit, where they had discussed the fact that Ms. D had gained eleven pounds since her last appointment, despite the fact that she had said she was going to try to lose weight. In a laughing way, Ms. D displayed incredulity about this situation, and doctor and patient joked back and forth about what would have caused the weight gain. Her explanation at line 3 may be a way for her to display some authentic concern about this weight gain. However, Dr. B, at line 7, focuses away from the weight gain and on the shortness-of-breath symptom:

(14) [9:431]

1 Dr. B: Shortness of brea:th?
2 (1.0)
3 Ms. D: So::me, but that-'s: cuz I should lose wei:ght. I know
4 that.

[16] This interview, a portion of which is in excerpt (14), is explored in the chapter by Boyd and Heritage (this volume). Also see Gill's (1998a) analysis of the patient's portrayal of knowledge in this excerpt.

5		(.)
6	Ms. D:	I think- NOT much.
7	Dr. B:	When do you get short of brea:th.
8		(1.0)
9	Dr. B:	Stair:s? An: nat sort a thing? Er
10		(1.0)
11	Ms. D:	We:::h >after about-< (.) three fli:ght:s or four.
12		HIH huh huh huh.
13	.	(1.5)
14	Ms. D:	.h °Two.° N(h)o. Huh. .hhh
15		(1.5)
16	Ms. D:	Rea::lly not- not much. Uh uh.
17	Dr. B:	°Okay.°
18		(7.0)
19	Dr. B:	Are your bowel movements normal?

We noted earlier that Ms. D's response (lines 3–4 and 6) allows the doctor to focus on gathering information rather than requiring him to assess immediately whether her explanation is correct. At line 6, "NOT much." seems to characterize her shortness of breath rather than the weight she needs to lose; i.e., it appears to be a downgraded recharacterization of her initial reply ("So::me," line 3). Thus, her explanation by this point is effectively enveloped between two descriptions of her symptoms. Dr. B queries her about the shortness of breath, asking her to specify when she experiences this symptom (line 7). This query does not mark whether (or how) it is related to her explanation. After a silence (line 8), Dr. B produces a candidate answer (line 9) for the patient to confirm or disconfirm. Ms. D gives a characterization of how many flights of stairs it takes for her to become short of breath (lines 11–12), and appends a laugh. Next (line 14), she very softly upgrades this to "two" flights (i.e., she produces a characterization that displays the condition as more serious) and then quickly disclaims this upgrade ("N(h)o."), adding more laugh tokens and reasserting her line 6 recharacterization of her symptom: "Rea::lly not- not much. Uh uh." (line 16). As the laughter may be a display of "troubles resistance" (Jefferson 1984b:351), Dr. B (line 17) appears to accept it, and moves on (line 19) to another query related to Ms. D's health history.

Thus, when Ms. D inserts her explanation into an information-gathering phase of the medical visit, she provides for the doctor to take other avenues besides responding to and assessing this explanation. Not only does she use a turn design that envelops her explanation between characterizations of how much she experiences shortness of breath (thus allowing Dr. B to pursue additional information about this symptom), she also minimizes the problem by downgrading the extent to which she experiences the symptom, and by displaying a light attitude toward it. While Dr. B never does confirm or disconfirm Ms. D's explanation for the shortness of breath (being overweight), this reflects not just his unilateral actions and imposition of the biomedical model, but actions on his patient's part allowing for pursuit of symptom-related information during the information-gathering portion of the medical interview.

Query focuses on the causal factor, no assessment occurs

Doctors may also query patients about whether the causal factors they cited in their explanations do, in fact, exist. Such questioning offers patients an opportunity to discuss the causal factors, which suggests that when patients produce explanations they may be doing additional work – explanations may be an oblique or delicate way to get particular concerns on the floor when it might otherwise be difficult to do so.

Put differently, patients may use physicians' orientation to gathering data and evidence as a resource for achieving their own ends. When a doctor queries a patient about whether a causal factor exists (sidestepping the issue of whether the causal factor in question actually causes a problem to occur), this topicalizes a possible problem that the patient, by virtue of positioning it as ancillary to a more primary complaint, has shown hesitance in bringing up. For example, in excerpt (15) Dr. A and Ms. A are discussing chest pain that Ms. A has experienced during exercise. This is after Dr. A has given the patient good news about her cardiology tests, which disconfirmed "heart disease." They are now discussing a "symptom residue," the pain that Ms. A had that was therefore not explained by any such disease or condition.[17]

[17] See discussion of this case and the problem of "symptom residue" in the Maynard and Frankel chapter (this volume).

(15) [6:383]

Dr. A: An so tha:t (.) came on with the exerci:[se
Ms. A: [M hm?
Dr. A: An- with other activities that you've do[ne.
Ms. A: [M hm?
Dr. A: °Oka:y:°
(0.5)
Dr. A: .hh (2.5) An in addition sometimes you wake at
nigh:(.) [t wi]th that.
Ms. A: [Mm hm]
(3.5) ((Dr. is writing in file))
Ms. A: An I was wondering if: °you know stress could a (.) brought
that on too.°
(2.0) ((Dr. is writing in file))
Dr. A: °Are you feelin: stressed?°
(1.0) ((Dr. is writing in file))
Ms. A: U::m (.) I'm been going through some problems with my: (.)
so:n wh[o's now eighteen.]
Dr. A: [A::h yeah you mentioned that.]
Ms. A: Bu:t- I:'m pretty much (1.0) I think I cope pretty well.
(0.7) ((Dr. gazes at Ms. A, then writes in file))
Ms. A: Cause there's very little I can do:? n:d (1.0) I: (.) m: you
know made that decision on how I'm gonna handle the
situation with him an:d
Dr. A: °H:m°=
Ms. A: =I feel that I have to be firm and consistent.
(3.5) ((Dr. is writing in file))
Dr. A: Tch na- he's at home yet then.=
Ms. A: =N:o he: is: (0.8) staying with his girlfriend.=
Dr. A: =°Oh yeah°=
Ms. A: =°Mm hm?°
(0.7) ((Dr. is writing in file))
Ms. A: .hh But he has ta:- um (0.5) mo:ve (.) i-his things.
(24.0) ((Dr. is writing in file, then reading it))
Dr. A: .hhh Before I go on tuh just=uh: kinda go on generally over
your history again were the:re other things that you wanted
tuh: (0.3) talk about?
(.)
Dr. A: Ms. A?
Ms. A: Well- thu: thuh one thing I wanted tuh ask you about was
(1.5) skin,

In the context of Dr. A gathering information about when the chest pain occurs (lines 1–8), Ms. A speculates about whether "stress" could cause the chest pain to occur (lines 11–12). Dr. A queries her about this possible causal factor; she asks the patient if she is experiencing stress (line 14).

Ms. A takes the doctor's query as an invitation to describe the problems she is having with her teenage son (lines 16–17). Dr. A displays familiarity with these problems (line 18), at least insofar as they have been "mentioned" before.[18] However, her claim of prior knowledge does not invite explication of the trouble; that is, as Jefferson (1988:425) has argued, there are two types of responses to a troubles announcement:

> one which marks arrival [at a troubles telling point] and elicits further talk on the matter but does not necessarily align recipient as a troubles-recipient . . . and one which, by displaying "empathy," commits recipient as, now, a troubles recipient.

Ms. A treats Dr. A's claim of prior knowledge as less than empathetic. In her further talk on the matter, Ms. A plays down the problem's effect on her (line 19), shows a kind of resigned attitude (line 21), and claims that she has a remedy for the problem (lines 21–23 and 25). Ms. A thereby displays what Jefferson (1984b:351) calls "troubles resistance." Still, after writing in the patient's file (line 26), Dr. A re-topicalizes the problem by making a candidate assertion about where the son is living (line 27), which invites Ms. A to provide more information (line 28). Dr. A responds to the announcement that Ms. A's son is "<u>sta</u>ying with his girlfriend" with a kind of news receipt (line 29) that again discourages troubles-talk development (Heritage 1984b; Jefferson 1981a; Maynard 1997). At line 30, Ms. A confirms that receipt and then (line 32) offers a further aspect of the trouble, after which there is nearly a half-minute silence during which Dr. A is writing in and examining the patient's record. Subsequently, Dr. A invites Ms. A to bring up "other things" she may want to discuss (lines 34–36), whereupon Ms. A asks the doctor a question about her skin (lines 39–40), and they continue on that topic. The issue of whether stress could cause her chest pains does not get resolved here, nor later in the interview.

Turning to the issue of how Ms. A formulates her explanation in the first place, note that she offers "stress" as a causal factor

[18] There is no previous mention of the problems with her son in this interview and we take it that the physician is recalling something from a previous visit.

without also asserting that she is experiencing stress. This resembles a device Sacks (1992b:405) has described, wherein a speaker "muses aloud" using an abstract reference to elicit interest in what he or she "meant by that." By implying but not actually asserting that she is under stress, Ms. A may be inviting inquiry about whether she is, in fact, experiencing stress. As noted, the doctor's empirically focused response ("°Are you feelin: stressed?°", line 14) gives her an opportunity to talk about the stress she is under.

While Ms. A appears to make attempts at troubles talk and to discuss what the medical literature calls psychosocial issues (Engel 1997; Stoeckle 1995; Frankel et al. 2003), Dr. A does not respond further in a way that encourages such talk. Nevertheless, we can see how a patient may use the doctor's orientation toward gathering medical data to occasion the delivery of announcements about troubles, psychosocial issues, or other matters that would not otherwise easily fit within a context where the physician is gathering information about a particular symptom.

Query focuses on the patient's symptom, assessment occurs after a delay

As noted, the non-constraining design of patients' explanations allows doctors to focus away from the explanations and onto patients' symptoms. Eventually, doctors may assess patients' explanations. This happens in the following excerpts. After the patient offers an explanation for a symptom, in excerpt (16a), the doctor initiates an extended series of symptom-related queries and conducts a physical examination. She eventually confirms the patient's explanation in excerpt (16b). Thus, the queries, replies, and examination become an extended *insertion sequence* between the patient's explanation and the doctor's eventual assessment.[19]

In excerpt (16a), Dr. A and Ms. B are in the phase of the medical interview before the physical exam where the patient is introducing her physical symptoms. She is holding a piece of paper, which she looks at as she reports experiencing tenderness in her abdominal area (line 1). As she raises this symptom, she also indicates its location with a gesture, motioning under her right rib. Then

[19] Similarly, Whalen et al. (1988) discuss an "interrogative series" that operates like an insertion sequence between a caller's request for help and a call taker's announcement of dispatch in 911 calls.

Ms. B appears to start a relatively firm explanation ("It's probably:", line 2), which she abandons in favor of a speculation as to "whether" the discomfort is "in the gall bladder?" (lines 2 and 4). Ms. B thus produces an explanation for the doctor's consideration, yet she does not expose herself to disaffiliative treatment by compelling the doctor's immediate assessment. The first part of this explanation overlaps the doctor's immediate pursuit of a candidate location for the discomfort: "In the front?" (line 3). Ms. B then offers an alternate speculative explanation, "Kidney?" (line 4). Dr. A, in overlap with what appears to be the patient's continuation of her turn, asks again about the location of the pain (line 5), and points to her own right side. Now Ms. B confirms the location (line 6). In this segment, accordingly, the doctor strongly orients to gathering empirical information before engaging in analysis.

(16a) [7:365]

Ms. B: .hhh An:::d then I get a lot of tenderness: in this area hh.
And again:. It's probably: (1.0) [whether: it's] in the=
Dr. A: [In the front?]
Ms. B: =gall bladder? Kidney? [Er
Dr. A: [Up in here.
Ms. B: Yeah. Like under the r:ib. Where I can't get- >it'll get-<
(1.0) very sore.
(0.8)
Ms. B: °.hhh° Ptch [A::nd, hhhh]
Dr. A: ['Bout how often does] that come.
Ms. B: Uh:: hhhh (1.0) This cn: (1.5) m- be like at least once or
twice a week. And I've been trying to see if I've been:::
>you know,< lifting something or doing something. °.hhhh°
(1.5) ((Dr. A gazes at patient, then turns to record))
Dr. A: How long does it last when you g[et it.]
Ms. B: [Ah::m] (.) maybe a day or
two.

Furthermore, the doctor maintains her focus on the patient's experience of the tenderness, asking her how often it occurs (line 10).[20] After Ms. B replies (lines 11–12), she reports monitoring her activities for another potentially related event ([lines 12–13]; see excerpt 8). There is a silence, where the doctor initially looks at

[20] This query (line 10) overlaps with the patient's line 9 utterance, where she again consults her slip of paper and projects the introduction of a complaint about another (different) symptom.

the patient and then turns her head to write in the patient's medical record (line 14). While she is writing, she queries Ms. B about another aspect of her symptom experience – how long the tenderness lasts (line 15). This line of questioning continues after Ms. B's answer at lines 16–17 (not shown on transcript), until the patient introduces a different complaint about feeling "sick" and a "sort of gla::h" feeling, to which the doctor directs her attention (see Gill 1998a).

Approximately seven minutes later, while examining the patient's abdomen, the doctor demonstrates that she has not forgotten or otherwise permanently disattended the patient's explanation for her abdominal tenderness. Continuing her examination of Ms. B, Dr. A asks her how long she has been experiencing the "sore times," how often they occur, how suddenly they come on, and whether food ever brings them on. Then, in the excerpt shown below, she produces a response that invokes and tentatively confirms (via the stress on "could," line 2) Ms. B's original explanation:

(16b) [13:677]

Dr. A: .hh Thee um- (0.7) it- cuz the pain that yer telling me
about up in this: (.) area (1.2) you know could be::? (0.3)
from your gall bladder, an- what [we think] happens is that=
Ms. B: [(thats::)]
Dr. A: =little sto:nes are let out. .hh periodically=
Ms. B: =Yeah=
Dr. A: =Us[ually in] response to a me:al,
Ms. B: [An (that's:)]
Dr. A: An:d tha:t they may get cau:ght? trangently?.hh an it
causes this sudden pa:in.
(0.7)
Ms. B: That would make sense.

This confirmation (lines 1–3) recasts the doctor's prior line of questioning as not just information-gathering per se, but as related to investigating Ms. B's explanation that her gall bladder is the source of the pain. It thereby also (retroactively) recasts that explanation as the first component of an explanation–assessment sequence, whereas in its initial production it was merely marked as a speculation or "out-loud" musing which did not compel here-and-now assessment.

In sum, patients and doctors both strongly orient to the overall organization of the medical interview. Patients' explanations present doctors with *options* to relevantly go either one way or another (to focus on gathering information about symptoms or to focus on analyzing that information), and doctors consistently follow a particular course (gathering information). In sequential terms, because patients provide for confirming or disconfirming assessments to be *relevant* but not *required* in the next turn, those assessments cannot be said to be *noticeably* absent (Schegloff 1972:77) when not produced there. In other words, it is neither the case that patients naively set themselves up to be ignored, nor that doctors, because of their status-based authority, disregard patients' opinions. The next-turn attention to symptomatology is collaboratively – rather than coercively and unilaterally – achieved.

Query focuses on evidence the patient provides, assessment occurs after a delay

Patients, as we have seen, may follow their explanations with tag components, reporting additional aspects of their experience (such as additional symptoms) that either lend support to their explanations or suggest that a particular cause should be ruled out. That is, patients may report evidence that bolsters explanations that they are apparently advancing,[21] but they may also report evidence that would eliminate a particular explanation from consideration (as a preface to proposing a more serious explanation, for example). In either of these cases, doctors may focus on the tag component of the patient's turn and topicalize the evidence itself, asking the patient for more information about it. The focus then stays *on* what the patient is experiencing and *off* the issue of whether the patient's explanation is correct.

Excerpt (17a) occurs in the information-gathering phase of a medical interview, where the patient, Ms. N, is presenting various complaints. Ms. N reports experiencing a "tre<u>men</u>dous amount" of rectal pain (lines 3–4). Then she offers an explanation for this pain – a speculation about "<u>wh</u>ether it was <u>he</u>morrhoids or not"

[21] See Pomerantz (1984b:624) on reporting the bases of assertions.

(line 6) – and she claims she is "not sur:e" in light of the following evidence: she experienced pain when she "tried (0.2) pressin:g." (lines 6–8). She thus suggests that the evidence points to a more serious problem than hemorrhoids. After a silence (line 9), she begins a repeat of what she "tri:ed" and during a hesitation in this utterance Dr. D seeks clarification by offering a candidate characterization, "pressing with your hand?" (line 11). Dr. D thus focuses on the evidence that the patient has reported.

(17a) [10:594]

Ms. N:	While we're on my gut.
Dr. D:	°Yes.°
Ms. N:	A couple a weeks ago: hh u:m (0.6) I had (.) tremendous amount of rectal pai:n?
	(1.0)
Ms. N:	No:w- whether it was hemorrhoids or not I'm not sur:e because there was a lot of (0.8) .h pai::n when I tried (0.2) pressin:g.
	(0.8)
Ms. N:	tch When I tri:ed hh[a:h
Dr. D:	[(y'mean) pressing with your hand?
Ms. N:	No. When I tried ta have a bow:el movement. [(Just-)]
Dr. D:	[Pushing] down?=
Ms. N:	=Yea [h
Dr. D:	[>Yea<
Ms. N:	U:m (1.3) Plus there was pain on the outside too,

In line 12, Ms. N corrects Dr. D's candidate characterization by clarifying that "pressing" referred to her efforts to have a bowel movement. In overlap, Dr. D produces another candidate characterization (line 13). Ms. N confirms this (line 14). Accordingly, while Dr. D exhibits responsiveness to the evidence, this leads them away from assessment and keeps them in the mode of seeking and providing information. In line 16, after Dr. D has acknowledged (line 15) her confirmation of his candidate clarification (line 14), Ms. N returns to describing her symptom, now in terms of *where* the pain occurred.

In subsequent talk (seven lines of transcript not reproduced here), Ms. N describes applying a medication that took some of the "pain and itch" away. She then reintroduces her explanation (line 1 below), expressing a hope that "it wa:s just hemorrhoids".

(17b) [10:613]

1 Ms. N: An I'm hoping it wa:s just hemorrhoids
2 (0.4)
3 Ms. N: >because it< really did °°hurt a lo:t°°
4 (0.7)
5 Ms. N: It's not as bad now.

With this expression Ms. N implies its converse: that the problem may be more serious than hemorrhoids. Her next utterance, a reassertion of how painful the condition was (line 3), underscores her implied proposal. She then claims that the symptom has since abated (line 5). Then (not in excerpt here), Ms. N states that she bought a new medication (Anusol), and Dr. D queries further about the symptoms and their location. Reporting that the pain occurred not just externally but also "up some (0.7) in the re:ctum" (lines 1–3 below), Ms. N next proposes (in a qualified manner) that the pain could have been caused by an obstruction (lines 3–4). Again, Dr. D pursues more information about the location of the pain (line 7):

(17c) [10:630]

1 Ms. N: >I mean-< there wa:s some external (1.0) pain a:lso but
2 there was a- it felt like it was up some (0.7) in the
3 re:ctum. Um (.) that it was hurting- Almost like it was
4 obstructed there somewhat.
5 (0.5)
6 Ms. N: °.hhh ° [(N:::)]
7 Dr. D: [Could you touch] anything that was tender?

Many minutes later, during the physical exam, Dr. D assesses (line 1 below) Ms. N's original speculative explanation that the pain was caused by hemorrhoids:

(17d) [22:1435]

1 Dr. D: (You do have) a fresh hemorrhoid here An[na=
2 Ms. N: [I do,
3 Dr. D: =over on the right si:de.
4 (0.5)
5 Dr. D: (They) also all around the anus it's very re:d.=h
6 (0.4)
7 Ms. N: Well it has been sore the[re
8 Dr. D: [An I think that's (probably from

your diarrhea)
.
. ((11 lines omitted))
.

Dr. D: Al:right well we'll jus' stop right there Anna cuz I think
we know what's goin' on
Ms. N: What
Dr. D: You Have A: hemorrHOID [jis like you] said
Ms. N: [Oh °okay °]
Ms. N: I thought you were going to say something to °scare° me
Dr. D: °be ° a good DOCtor Anna we'll hire YA
Ms. N: ((laughs))

Note that Dr. D constructs this diagnosis as a confirming assessment ("You do have a fresh hemorrhoid", line 1, and . . . "jis like you said", line 23), suggesting that the patient's explanation was correct. In this way, he pitches the diagnosis as responsive to that explanation and also as strongly affiliative. However, in light of Ms. N having designed her explanation in a way that suggested the pain was too severe to reflect hemorrhoids and may represent an obstruction, the doctor's response is also an oblique disconfirmation of that alternate possibility. Ms. N's response (line 24) exhibits a "change of state" in her understanding (Heritage 1984b). At line 25, she also displays an "At first I thought '(X)'" orientation, implying relief at this disconfirmation and the realization it entails a less serious diagnosis (Sacks 1984:419; Halkowski this volume).

Conclusion

During the information-gathering phase of medical interviews, if the focus typically remains on patients' symptoms and medically defined ways of exploring them, this is not wholly doctor-induced, nor a matter of doctors imposing a biomedical agenda upon patients who have little agency or understanding of medicine or the medical interview. Previous studies have failed to appreciate patients' dilemma of needing to offer their explanations in a relevant sequential environment while not disrupting the information-gathering phase of the encounter. Nor has previous research appreciated the doctor's dilemma of how to receive such explanations before gathering all the data necessary for analysis. Accordingly, the apparent struggle between professional and lay orientations in medicine is at least partially a more local matter that is related to the overall organization of the medical interview and the conversational sequences through which participants assemble it.

In other words, a distinctive aspect of medical practice is that the data the professionals (doctors) are to analyze derive from laypeople (patients) who may have their own perspectives about what causes health problems. The question for patients is where to insert their own explanatory analyses, so that doctors may consider these explanations as they make determinations about what is going on medically. Patients appear sensitive to the pattern by which medical inquiry typically proceeds. They are wary of disrupting the gathering of information and avoid compelling an analysis (an official assessment) too soon, before all the data have been collected. However, if patients do not offer their explanations in the environment of data collection, the next phases of the interview may be even less propitious, for the immediate next activity, after verbal and physical examination, is the diagnostic informing when the doctor's task is to deliver the news and the patient aligns to receive it.

Through the details by which they construct their turns at talk, patients address this dilemma by producing explanations during the collection of medical data and providing doctors with sequential options other than immediately producing confirming or disconfirming assessments. When doctors take the option to continue assembling data rather than engaging in analysis of it, they are, like patients, strongly orienting to the organization of the interview and to completion of its data-collection phase. Practices on the part of both patient and physician account for what comes off as a kind of tenuous introduction of, and minimalistic appreciation for, patients' causal theories.

Our analysis suggests that there is the potential for conflict but that it does not derive from inherent tensions between physicians' positioning within biomedicine and patients' parallel embeddedness in the lifeworld. The conflict is between the local, sequential organization of talk and the organization of the medical interview. Even so, when patients offer overt explanations, in approximately 30 percent of these cases (19 out of 63), doctors do either assess them immediately or respond to them in a delayed fashion. Also needing appreciation is the resourcefulness of both parties. Patients do have a device (the three-part turn structure) for introducing their explanations into medical interviews. Furthermore, they sometimes may have health worries about whose medical status they are not confident. This device for explaining their more clearly defined symptoms allows them to put these worries on the floor with minimal interactional risk. Given that the exploration of psychosocial factors is central to improved communication and medical care (Frankel et al. 2003), it is important for doctors to pay attention to patients' explanations that introduce such factors.

More generally, our research has this implication: *Doctors can increase their sensitivity to patients' experiences by being aware of the patient's and doctor's dilemmas, and interactional resolutions thereof, that promote tenuousness and minimalistic talk directed toward patients' own explanations for illness.* For example, after hearing a patient's explanation for a symptom, doctors can signpost that their subsequent queries about the symptom are related to exploring a variety of candidate explanations, including the patient's. This strategy does not require the doctor to present a diagnosis prematurely (i.e., to immediately confirm or disconfirm the patient's explanation); rather, it simply provides additional orientation about the direction of the doctor's questions and may provide some reassurance to the patient that, indeed, the doctor has heard and is considering his or her explanation.

Another strategy doctors can use is to propose that they will consider the patient's explanation later in the interview, during the physical exam. This occurs in the excerpt below, where (near the beginning of the medical interview) the patient and doctor are discussing the patient's chest pain. The patient speculates whether the pain "could had (.) <u>any</u>thing to do:" with the "<u>bre</u>ast." (lines 1–3). After a silence, she reformulates the causal factor in a progressively more specific way (lines 5–7), indicating what it is about her breast that could be causing the pain: "tha:t (0.3) <u>sur</u>gery", and then having the "<u>tu</u>mor removed." The doctor initially queries the patient about the causal factor, asking whether she is experiencing tenderness in her breast (lines 9–10). After the patient confirms this, the doctor indicates that she will check the patient's breast and "see" (line 13). Thus, the doctor exhibits responsiveness to the patient's explanation by proposing to examine the breast later in the interview, during the physical exam. She then continues querying the patient about her chest pain; see excerpt (15).

(18) [5:271]

Ms. A: An' the only other thing I was thinking of about da:: (.) da
pai:ns is if- that could had (.) anything to do: too is with
the breast.
(2.2)
Ms. A: When I had u::m (0.5) °pt° (0.8) tha:t (0.3) surgery da
tumor removed. If dat could be anythin:g (.) connected with
that.
(1.2)
Dr. A: Ptch .hh (.) ah:: >are you hav<ing:: (.) tenderness in in
your brea[st it]self?
Ms. A: [Mm hm?]
Ms. A: Mm hm=
Dr. A: =°You are.° (.) °I'll check that breast again: an see.°

Finally, after collecting data in the medical interview and arriving at a diagnosis, doctors could attune themselves better to the patient's dilemma by following up with a response to the patient's explanation, such as a confirming or disconfirming assessment, as in excerpts (16b) and (17d).

Others have suggested strategies that enhance the patient's participation in the interview.[22] For example, Lipkin, Frankel, et al. (1995) recommend that the concluding tasks of the medical interview be reconceptualized so that, besides doctors delivering information to patients, patients themselves enter the analytic discussion with their perspectives and beliefs. Physicians should ask patients what they have understood about what the physician has told them. Lipkin, Frankel, et al. (1995:79–80) write:

> In the course of the patient's exposition of what he or she has understood, the patient will reveal his/her explanatory model of the illness process – that is, to what the patient attributes the problem. These so-called attributions, the patient's sense of the meaning or causality of the illness, must be acknowledged or some patients will reject the clinician's approach as not appropriate.

[22] See the discussion of cultural influences on patients' "explanatory models" in Johnson et al. (1995).

We agree that physicians should encourage patients' participation in medical interviews. Our analysis, however, shows that patients may reveal their explanatory theories well before the closing moments of these interviews. Patients orient to the process by which data is gathered and analyzed; in overt and tacit ways, they offer their explanations in information-gathering locations such that doctors can consider them as they generate diagnostic hypotheses. To suggest, as Lipkin, Frankel, et al. (1995) do, that doctors should elicit patients' participation in the analytic discussion at the end of the visit, is to assume that patients will believe that doctors can take their explanations into account as possible candidate diagnoses at this point, even though they have finished collecting data and have already delivered a diagnosis. It is perhaps more likely that patients may interpret the doctor's efforts to give them (what Lipkin, Frankel, et al. [1995] call) a "final shot" at determining the agenda of the visit, as a move designed to make the doctor *appear* responsive. In addition, with this strategy doctors miss the opportunity to take patients' explanations into account while considering and testing various diagnostic possibilities. We therefore suggest that if a patient does not volunteer a causal explanation within the data-collection phase of the medical interview, the doctor should solicit the patient's explanation in that location, rather than wait until the end of the visit.

6

Taking the history: questioning during comprehensive history-taking

Elizabeth Boyd and John Heritage

Introduction

One of the foundational elements of the physician–patient relationship is the patient's comprehensive medical history (Bates et al. 1995). Elicited through a verbal examination of the patient by the doctor, the history is one of the key components of medical diagnosis (Stoeckle and Billings 1987) and forms the foundation of the relationship between physician and patient in primary care settings (Cassell 1997). Recorded by the doctor in the patient's medical chart, the comprehensive history includes the details of the patient's present illness as well as past problems, procedures, and family and social background (Bates et al. 1995; Heath 1982b; Cassell 1985a; Stoeckle and Billings 1987; Frankel 1996).

The medical history, both as a written document and as an interactional component of the doctor–patient consultation, evolved into its present form during the latter part of the twentieth century amid growing recognition that illness was interwoven with the life experience of the patient (Stoeckle and Billings 1987). Thus, the history has come to include not only the patient's account of the current medical problem (or "reason for the visit"), but also the patient's preexisting medical conditions, current medications, family history, social and psychosocial circumstances. As Cassell (1985b:86) observes, there is much more to a history-taking than bringing to light the patient's current condition. The doctor must also find out

> who the patient is, and how the kind of person the patient is, along with how he or she behaves, interacts with the pathophysiology to produce this specific illness. Next must come an attempt to discover whether other factors, environmental, familial, social, occupational, or personal habits, have played a role in making the patient sick.

Thus, from the perspective of the physician, questions in the comprehensive history are asked in order to elicit necessary information about the medical and social background of the patient, providing a "historical" context in which to understand the patient's situation and/or make a diagnosis. From the perspective of the patient, these questions may (or may not) provide an opportunity to reveal any observations, problems, or facts that might have a bearing on his or her current (or other) medical condition(s) (Mishler 1984; Beckman and Frankel 1984; Stivers and Heritage 2001). Within medicine the importance of history-taking for the physician–patient relationship has been recognized, and there is a growing literature on this portion of the medical consultation. Detailed "how to" manuals and training courses are targeted at new residents, all of whom are increasingly held acountable for conducting sensitive, complete, and efficient medical interviews – interviews that encourage patients to reveal their observations, concerns, and fears and that do not consume inordinate amounts of the physician's time (Coulehan and Block 1987).

When viewed within the context of the medical consultation as a whole, the medical history is more than a simple chain of questions and answers; it represents a recognizable activity within the overall set of activities that comprises the consultation as a whole. As a discrete activity, the history is best viewed as a set of sequences of action, with each sequence accomplishing particular tasks within the activity (Frankel 1995b). Thus, not only are doctors' questions designed to elicit information about the patient, they are also designed for specific tasks within the overall activity of history-taking. Similarly, patients' responses not only provide information to the doctor, but they also display the patient's understanding of the task at hand and the opportunities and constraints it affords.

In this chapter, we examine some basic principles underlying the design of the questions physicians ask during past and personal history-taking in a primary care setting, and in this way supply the beginnings of the theory called for by Frankel (1995b:235–6) "that will link both questions and responses together over time and space." It is important to emphasize here that this chapter deals with what has been termed "the personal history" – the details of the patient's past medical history as well as personal and social circumstances (Cassell 1985b) – and not the history-taking commonly associated with differential diagnosis – asking questions about the current, presenting medical complaint in order to arrive at a diagnosis. There are very significant differences between the two activities whose consequences for question design remain to be systematically examined (though see Drew this volume; Stivers 2000). In particular, we focus on the expectations, presuppositions, and concerns that physicians' questions about the patient's personal history unavoidably embody. We also examine some of the constraints and opportunities that different questions present to the patient, and some of the practices through which patients address these constraints and opportunities. Finally we consider the normative pressures structuring the interaction through which physicians and patients conjointly produce the patient's history as a routine activity.

The data

This chapter centers on a single case analysis of a primary care consultation that occurred in 1989 in a Midwestern city in the United States, and is supported by data from additional US primary care settings. The physician specializes in internal medicine at a university teaching hospital. The patient is an observably overweight, middle-aged woman with a 29-year-old daughter. She is the owner/manager of a small restaurant in a rural township nearby the hospital location. She has seen this physician on one prior occasion, some months earlier.[1] Her ongoing medical condition is high blood pressure, for which she has been prescribed the antihypertensive diuretic, Dyazide. This visit is for a routine pap smear and checkup for her high blood pressure; the patient does not present a new medical problem on this occasion.[2] The doctor conducts a comprehensive medical history, including past and current medications, family and social history, and systems review.[3]

[1] The exact date of this prior visit is unknown, as is the extent of the doctor's participation in that visit. No past history was apparently taken during that visit. In this sense, this case is perhaps somewhat atypical – the lengthy history-taking seen here is most often done on a patient's first visit. However, we have no reason to suspect that this aberration is consequential for the design of questions and answers and the construction of the activity as a whole. Our observations are supported from data in other first-visit primary care settings.

[2] Patients taking Dyazide for high blood pressure require frequent checkups to monitor their serum potassium levels.

[3] Systems review refers to a series of questions related to diseases or problems in the various systems of the body: head, eyes, ears, respiratory, cardiovascular, gastrointestinal, etc.

Our primary focus on a single case history permits readers to develop a sense of the course of questioning that develops during history-taking, and the particular aspects of the patient's circumstances which may or may not be addressed. We also include some data from additional primary care settings for comparison. For this analysis, we examined all of the question-and-answer types occurring during the history-taking segment of the visit. In this interaction, the history-taking begins after the patient explains why she has postponed her return visit and describes her concerns about the mammogram she has scheduled for later in the day. The doctor begins taking the history, with an inquiry about her current medications.[4]

Question design: some basic preliminaries

We can observe that, at the minimum, physicians' questions have the following features: first, they establish particular agendas for patient response; second, they embody presuppositions about various aspects of the patient's health, bodily awareness and background knowledge of medicine, and third, they incorporate "preferences"; they are designed so as to invite or favor one type of answer over another.[5] Similarly, patients can formulate their responses in ways that accept or resist (or reject altogether) any or all of these. Thus patients' responses engage (or decline to engage) the agenda set by the doctor's question, confirm (or disconfirm) its presuppositions, and align (or disalign) with its preferences. These possibilities are displayed in Table 6.1.

These three dimensions of questions are fundamental and inexorably relevant characteristics of question design and production. Because it is not possible to avoid them, physicians' questions can

[4] The history is taken with the patient's chart open and actively consulted. As the doctor records the patient's verbal responses to his questions, the doctor's (and the patient's) orientation is dually focused: on the interaction itself and on the written record. There is also a larger sense in which the doctor addresses himself to two "versions" of the patient: "the patient *in situ*" and "the patient inscribed" in the written history (Robinson 1998). Recurrently in the interaction the doctor's attention oscillates between the two. The many contingencies which this oscillation introduces into the question–answer exchanges of this interaction are, unfortunately, beyond the scope of this chapter. See Robinson (1998) for a consideration of these issues.

[5] These dimensions are taken from Heritage (2002b).

Table 6.1 *Dimensions of questioning and answering*

Doctor questions:	Patient responses:
Set agendas: (i) Topical agendas (ii) Action agendas	Engage/Decline to engage: (i) Topical agendas (ii) Action agendas
Embody presuppositions	Confirm/Disconfirm presuppositions
Incorporate preferences	Align/Disalign with preferences

only select between different possibilities for agenda setting, presupposition and preference. These selections are crucial for the work that questions do, and the kind of physician–patient relations which are conveyed through that work. Below, we briefly review these dimensions, illustrating some alternative possibilities.

Medical questioning sets agendas

At their most basic, questions solicit information from a recipient by pointing to some information gap or deficit that the recipient is to remedy. In this elementary sense, questions set agendas. These agendas consist of two elements. First, as Mishler (1984) notes, questions establish particular issues as the topics of inquiry, and thus establish *topical agendas*. For example, in the following excerpt, the doctor pursues the patient's marital status as a topical agenda (lines 1 and 5) before shifting to a lifestyle topic (line 8):

(1) [Midwest 3.4.6]

1	DOC:	Are you married?
2		(.)
3	PAT:	No.
4		(.)
5	DOC:	You're divorced (°cur[rently,°??)
6	PAT:	[Mm hm,
7		(2.2)
8	DOC:	Tl You smoke?, h
9	PAT:	Hm mm.

Second, questions request that recipients perform particular actions, e.g., answering yes or no, giving substantive information, explaining, clarifying, justifying, etc. In short, questions establish *action agendas*. In addition to establishing a topical agenda, each of the three questions in (1) sets a restricted action agenda. In each case, responses that engage the physician's action agenda consist of "yes" or "no"; other responses represent departures by doing something other than what was "asked for" by the form of the question. In the above example, the patient engages with both the topic and the action set by the doctor's first two questions, providing no more than minimal positive and negative responses.

In the next case, the doctor's questions pursue issues connected to the patient's father's mortality as the topical agenda, and do so with questions that establish closely related action agendas for patient reponse.

(2) [Midwest 3.4.4]

DOC: Tlk=.hh hIs your father alive?
PAT: (.hh) No.
DOC: How old was he when he died.
PAT: .hh hhohh sixty three I think.=hh
DOC: What did he die from.=hh
(0.5)
PAT: He had:=uhm:: He had high blood pressure,

Here the doctor's first question establishes the patient's father's mortality as a new topical agenda. The second and third questions maintain the father as the topical focus, but solicit additional information contingent on the patient's first answer (that her father is dead). In this instance, the doctor's first two questions are relatively constraining in setting an action agenda, inviting first a Yes/No answer and next a one-word numerical response. The third question, however, invites a more discursive answer. In all three, the patient's response engages both the topic and the action agendas that the questions set.

This agenda-setting aspect of physician questions has previously been intensively examined. Thus "closed" questions, by posing a restricted action agenda (as above), have been argued to severely limit the contributions that patients may make to the interaction (Byrne and Long 1976; Beckman and Frankel 1984; Mishler 1984; Roter and Hall 1992; Lipkin, Putnam, and Lazare et al. 1995; Frankel 1995b). For instance, Roter and Hall (1992:83) found that closed-ended questions (formatted as Yes/No questions) were two or three times more common than open-ended questions, and greatly limited patient participation in the interaction. They concluded that a predominance of closed-ended questions indicated high physician control over the interaction and the patient. Similarly, Mishler (1984) argued that, through the use of closed-ended questions (as well as other forms), doctors typically establish the relevance of the "biomedical world" to the exclusion of the patient's "lifeworld" experiences. By contrast, open-ended questions are seen as encouraging patients to respond in their own terms and permitting the emergence of narratives based in lifeworld experience.

Less examined in this literature are the resources with which patients can resist question agendas (cf Raymond 2003; Clayman and Heritage 2002a: Chapters 6 and 7) and expand beyond them (Stivers and Heritage 2001). In particular, Raymond (2003) has shown that Yes/No questions appropriately receive "yes" or "no" as the first component of an answer. With this in mind, we can see ways in which the agendas of Yes/No questions can be resisted or subtly subverted. For example, in (3) there is the near-"standard" patient response to questions about drug allergies:

(3)

DOC: Do you have any drug aller:gies?
(0.7)
PAT: .hh hu=Not that I know of no.

Here the patient defers her "no" response until the end of the turn, transparently in the interest of qualifying her response. And in (4) the patient defers an answer to the physician's question about the restaurant she owns, and "leaks" a comment, which she then quickly retracts as humorous, that suggests how burdensome the work of a restaurateur in a small town can be – a "lifeworld" concern in Mishler's (1984) terms:

(4)

DOC: How long have you had that?,
(0.8)
PAT: hhhuhhh How long has it had me.=[hh<No: it-
DOC: [(Yeah.)
PAT: We had it aba- - We built thuh building #abou:t#:
ten years ago. [(I think.)
DOC: [Mm.

In (5) the patient transparently exploits the “where” component of a physician’s question to launch the beginning of a narrative about her mother’s death from cancer (Stivers and Heritage 2001).

(5)

DOC: Is your mother alive,
PAT: No:.
(1.0)
PAT: No: she died- in her: like late (.) fifties: or:
I’m not sure.
. . . . . .
DOC: -> Whe[re was her cancer.
PAT: [(-)
PAT: -> .hhh Well:- she lived in Arizona an:’- she::
wouldn’t go tuh doctor much. She only went
to uh chiropracter. (h[u-)
DOC: [Mm [hm,
PAT: => [An:d she had(:)/(’t)
=> like- in her stomach somewhere I guess but (.)
thuh- even- that guy had told her tuh go (into)
uh medical doctor.
DOC: [Mm hm,
PAT: [.hhh An:’ she had- Years before her- (.) m- uh
hh mother in law: had died from: waitin’ too-
or whatever ya know (on-) in surgery, .hh an’

Once the narrative is launched and acknowledged (“Mm hm,” line 12), the patient briefly and offhandedly answers the question (lines 13–14), before resuming the story.

Finally, in (6) and (7) two similar questions are asked by British community nurses (health visitors) of first-time mothers about a week after leaving the maternity ward (Heritage and Sefi 1992):

(6) [HV 5A1]

HV: How about your breast(s) have they settled
do:wn [no:w.
M: [Yeah they ’ave no:w yeah.

(7) [HV 1C1]

HV: Are your breasts alright.
(0.7)
M: They’re fi:ne no:w I’ve stopped leaking (.) so:

In (6) the question conveys that the health visitor is aware that there has been a problem. It is answered with an appropriate "type-conforming" "yeah" (Raymond 2003) and an expansion which (with the repeat of "now") renews the relevance of the earlier problem before being concluded with a final reconfirming "yes." In (7), by contrast, no prior difficulty is acknowledged in the question's design, and the mother, with "They're fi:ne now," goes out of her way to avoid a simple and confirming "yes" answer. Her subsequent expansion identifies the previous problem as "leaking." In this way the mother, while confirming the absence of problems, resists the terms of the question and the Yes/No agenda with which she would otherwise be confined (Mishler 1984).

As these examples suggest, patients have a variety of resources with which to engage or resist the agenda-setting function of questions, and there are many degrees of engagement and resistance.

Medical questioning embodies presuppositions

In addition to setting topical and action agendas, doctors' questions tend to embody presuppositions about aspects of the patient's life circumstances, health status, bodily awareness, and medical knowledge with varying degrees of explicitness. For example, a question such as "What type of diuretic are you currently taking?" presupposes that the patient is, in fact, on medication, knows what a diuretic is, and can provide basic information with regard to the drug. Any or all of these presuppositions can be disconfirmed. Cassell (1985b:101) includes the following example in his chapter on the personal history:

(8)

1 DOC: What kind of contraception do you use?
2 PAT: None, since my menopause.

In this instance, the doctor's question presupposes that the patient both needs and uses contraception. As the patient's answer displays, both presuppositions were inappropriate given her particular history. The patient thus rejects both presuppositions embodied in the question – she does not use contraception, and it is not necessary that she do so. Elided in this sequence is whether the patient is sexually active and whether she, hence, could have a use for contraception, even if she were premenopausal.

In general, *wh-* questions (questions using "what," "when," "why," how," etc. as question frames) tend to embody more presuppositions than Yes/No questions. In our datum, the physician approaches the topic of contraception more circumspectly:

(9) [Midwest 3.4:10]

1 DOC: Are you using any contraception? Is that
2 necessary [for you?
3 PAT: [Huh uh (not now.)
4 DOC: °(Okay.)°

Here the physician's initial Yes/No question ("Are you using any contraception?") is less presupposing of the patient's need and use for contraception, and he goes on to reduce any sense that he is presupposing her needs by explicitly asking, "Is that necessary for you?" This additional caution is rewarded by the patient's negative response, "Huh uh (not now.)", begun in overlap with the second of the physician's questions.

Medical questioning can "prefer" particular responses

Finally, doctors' questions may be structured to facilitate or "prefer" one response over another and, similarly, patients' responses are managed so as to be aligned or disaligned with those preferences (Sacks 1987). Preference is perhaps most prominent in Yes/No questions, and here it is accomplished through a combination of grammatical structure and lexical choices that are built to structurally favor "yes" or "no" answers. Most, if not all, Yes/No questions function by inviting agreement or disagreement to a "candidate answer" (Pomerantz 1988). The default preference is that the recipient should align to affirmatively framed Yes/No questions with "yes," and to negatively framed Yes/No questions with "no." Negative framing is often accomplished with what linguists term "polarity items" (Horn 1989).

There is a large conversation analytic literature on the design of preferred and dispreferred responses (Sacks 1987; Pomerantz 1984a; Levinson 1983; Heritage 1984a; Schegloff 1988). That literature has established that, while preferred responses tend to be produced in brief and simple fashion, and with little or no delay, dispreferred responses routinely embody one or more of the following features: (a) delays, such as a pause before delivery, the use of a preface, or displacement over a number of turns via the use of insertion sequences; (b) prefaces, such as markers like "uh" or "well," token agreements, appreciations and apologies, qualifiers, or hesitation; (c) accounts, in particular, explanations for why the relevant or proposed action is not being accepted or done; and (d) declining, which is normally mitigated, qualified or indirect (Heritage 1984a:266–7). Many of these features having to do with the role of preference in framing and responding to Yes/No questions are clearly visible in (10) below:

(10) [Midwest 3.4:8]

DOC: Tlk You don't have as:thma do you,
(.)
PAT: Hm mm.
(1.1)
DOC: (hhh) .hh Any chest type pain?
PAT: Mm mm.
(3.4)
DOC: Shortness of brea:th?
(1.0)
PAT: Some: but that's: cuz I should lose weight. I know
that,
(.)
I think- NOT much.

In this instance, the doctor's first question, "You don't have as:thma do you," is formed as a negative declarative statement, together with a tag question ("do you,") that seeks confirmation of the negative (i.e., no asthma). The declarative component formulates a "B-event," a matter to which the recipient has primary access (Labov and Fanshel 1977; Heritage and Roth 1995). Its negative formulation favors a confirmation of the negative state of "not having asthma." The patient's response is both aligned to the polarity preference expressed in the question, and produced in preferred format: it is designedly brief and produced without significant delay.[6] The

[6] Also notable is the patient's use of the vernacular, minimal form, "Hm mm." to indicate a "no" answer to the question.

doctor's second question, "Any chest type pain?" also prefers a negative response through the use of the negative polarity term "any." Once again, the patient's response is aligned to that preference, and is brief and immediate. Only in response to the third question (hearable as a third in a series of questions preferring a "no" response), does the patient break with the question's preference structure. Unable to confirm the negative, she produces a dispreferred positive response, which is delayed by a full second of silence (line 9), mitigated and accompanied by an explanation for her shortness of breath.

This sequence incorporates many of the features routinely present in the preference design of medical questioning. For example, fully formed Yes/No interrogatives which would ordinarily prefer a "yes" answer can have their preference reversed by the use of a negative polarity item such as as "any," "ever," or "at all," e.g., "Do you have any drug allergies?," "Have you ever lost consciousness?," "Do you exercise at all?" Declarative questions (with or without tag questions) can be strongly polarized in both positive and directions. Thus the question "You have your gall bladder?" is polarized in a positive direction (favoring a "yes" response); "No heart disease?" is polarized in a negative direction (favoring a "no" response).

It is clear that many routine history questions are designed to favor what we shall term "no problem" responses: they propose that the patient does not have any indications of illness and, if confirmed, permit the doctor to move on to the next domain of inquiry. In this context, aligned answers embody three features that are positively valued in the circumstances of medical history-taking:

(i) They are aligned to the state of affairs that the question was designed to favor.
(ii) They confirm a state of affairs that is favorable for the patient's overall health status.
(iii) They permit doctor and patient immediately to move on to the next domain of inquiry – in line with the tacit interactional objective of a "no problem" question.

In fully aligned answers, all three features combine to prompt the brief and immediate "no problem" response that the question invites, as in the first two responses to (10) above.

In this section, we have outlined and illustrated three basic dimensions of doctors' questions during personal history-taking. Far from being neutral or objective, doctors' questions – as do all questions – unavoidably establish agendas, and embody presuppositions and preferences. But questions and their answers obviously do not occur as isolated instances during medical history-taking. Rather they are part of larger *sequences* of questions and answers. Thus medical history-taking is an activity that spans individual question–answer sequences. We turn now to consider how the questions and answers that constitute personal history-taking are conjointly managed as matters of routine medical relevance.

Two principles of routine medical questioning

As Cassell (1985b) and other physicians describe it, the goal of the personal history is find out as much about the patient's habits, illnesses, family, occupation, sexual activity, etc. as possible and to do so as quickly and efficiently as possible (see also Reiser and Schroder 1980; Stoeckle and Billings 1987; Waitzkin 1991). To accomplish this, physicians employ a relatively standardized list of questions and become, as Cassell (1985b:89) puts it, "a fixed measuring instrument," a kind of living questionnaire, neutral and consistent across patients.

Notwithstanding Cassell's evocative metaphor, physicians do not question their patients by becoming a "fixed measuring instrument." This is a style of information-gathering that is most prominently found among social surveyors, who must stick to a script that formulates questions in highly decontextualized ways (Converse 1987). Even though they may be moving through just the kind of routine "face sheet" issues that social surveys almost always address, physicians' designs of these questions are strikingly different. For example, it is quite unlikely that a physician, even when dealing with a full medical history from a new patient, would ask about the patient's marital status using the standard social survey format: "What is your marital status: are you single, married, divorced, separated or widowed?" There are obvious reasons for this. The social survey question is designed to reduce response bias. It does so by minimizing communicated presuppositions and preferences. But in the process it establishes a particular kind of relationship with the subject that might be described as "essentially anonymous" (Heritage 2002a). No physician can afford to sacrifice rapport with patients by questioning them in this way. Instead, physicians ordinarily build their questions so as to convey a form of relatedness and concern for the welfare of the patient. One way in which they do this is to adapt their questions in ways that are oriented to the known or expected circumstances of the patient, and to the local contingencies of the interaction. Consequently, as Cassell (1985b:4) also notes:

> even when we physicians ask questions, the structure of the questions and their wording provides information about ourselves, our intent, our beliefs about patients and diseases, as well as eliciting such information about patients; "taking a history" is unavoidably and actually an *exchange* of information. (emphasis in original)

Thus, although the goal may be to ask questions of the patient in as neutral or objective a way possible (Coulehan and Block 1987), the wording, the ordering, and the placement of these questions also unavoidably embody the concerns and understandings of the physician, and contribute to the formation of a particular kind of social relationship with the patient.

Two fundamental principles of interaction, drawn from the normative framework of everyday life, underlie the management of routine history-taking questions. These are: the principle of optimization, and the principle of recipient design. Medical questioning that embodies these two principles will generally tend to be heard as sensitive, concerned, and caring.

The principle of optimization

Questions that embody the principle of optimization display a respect for what Maynard (2003) terms "the benign order of everyday life." They do so by incorporating presuppositions and preferences that are biased towards "best case" or "no problem" outcomes. To illustrate this optimization bias, one need only consider some of the most basic face-sheet questions a physician can ask. For example, questions about parental and/or sibling mortality can, in principle, be asked in several ways:

(i) Is your father alive?
(ii) Is your father dead?
(iii) Is your father alive or dead?[7]

Both the first and second forms of the question offer a "candidate answer" (Pomerantz 1988), and are designed to prefer its confirmation in next turn. However, it is clear then that, while the first question carries a preference for the *positive* affirmation that the father is alive, the second carries a preference for the *negative* affirmation that the father is dead. Self-evidently this can structure the physician's selection of a particular design. For example, if a physician uses the second formulation ("Is your father dead?"), a patient who can assert a "best case" scenario (that her father is alive) is perforce obliged to do this in an answer that is disaligned with the preference of the question, and this is generically avoided in the social world (Sacks 1987). Thus, when there is no evidence to suggest otherwise, doctors in the context of history-taking tend to structure their questions in an optimized or "no problem" direction, thereby conveying a "best case" stance toward the patient's situation. It is, of course, in this form that our middle-aged patient receives this question, both about her father (arrow 1) and her mother (arrow 2).

(11) [Midwest 3.4:4]

1	DOC:	1->	Tlk=.hh hIs your father alive?
2	PAT:		(.hh) No.
3	DOC:		How old was he when he died.
4	PAT:		.hh hhohh sixty three I think.=hh
5	DOC:		What did he die from.=hh
6			(0.5)
7	PAT:		He had:=uhm:: He had high blood pressure,
8			(.)
9	PAT:		An:d he 'ad- uh: heart attack.
10			(4.0)
11	DOC:	2->	Is your mother alive,

[7] There is, of course, a more neutral, though hardly specific, formulation which might run, "Tell me about your father." However, this utterly open-ended question sets a very broad agenda for the patient, who may be at a loss for an appropriate or relevant response (cf. Boyd 1998). Indeed, for this reason, the question may be heard as inappropriate for most contexts outside of psychotherapy, and therefore as specifically ill-fitted to the context of history-taking (cf. Maynard 1991c).

Best-case design pervades other aspects of routine history-taking. This is primarily done through preference features. As we have seen, fully formed Yes/No interrogatives which would ordinarily prefer a "yes" answer can have their preference reversed by the use of a negative polarity item such as as "any," "ever," or "at all." As illustrated in many of the sequences shown in this chapter – such as (12) and (14) below – physicians do not design their questions so as to consistently favor the same answer; for example, a positive or "yes" response. However, they do consistently favor optimized, "no problem" responses. Thus, in (12), both positive and negative polarity is deployed to this end:

(12) [Midwest 3.4.9]

DOC:	->	Are your bowel movements normal?
		(4.0) ((patient nods))
PAT:	.	°(Yeah.)°
		(7.0)
DOC:	->	Tlk Any ulcers?
		(0.5) ((patient shakes head))
PAT:		(Mh) no,
		(2.5)
DOC:	->	Tl You have your gall bladder?
		(2.0)
PAT:		I think so. uh huh=hh

In this instance, the doctor's first question asks the patient a question that "nominates" the normal state of affairs, favoring a confirming response.[8] The following question, "Any ulcers?" – with its negative polarity item "any" – prefers a "no" response, while the final declarative question once again prefers a "yes" response. All three questions are geared toward optimized outcomes.

The principle of recipient design

Our second principle, the principle of recipient design, refers to the "multitude of respects in which the talk by a party in a conversation is constructed or designed in ways which display an orientation and sensitivity to the particular other(s) who are the coparticipants"

[8] On the role of "normality" as an optimizing scenario, see Heritage and Sorjonen (1994), Heritage and Lindström (1998), and Bredmar and Linell (1999).

(Sacks et al. 1974:727). It is this principle that informs the physician's question "Are you using any contraception? Is that necessary for you?," discussed in (9) above. This question is asked of a patient who, we can recollect, is about 50 years old, and divorced. It also occurs less than a minute after the patient has mentioned an earlier tubal ligation procedure. In these ways, the question can be seen, by the patient and by the observer, and (not least) the physician, to be fitted to her likely circumstances.

The principle of recipient design may cut against the principle of optimization by making it "unrealistic" to ask a question designed for an best-case response. For example, after it has been determined that our overweight, hypertensive patient has gained eleven pounds and works at least a sixty-hour week in a restaurant, considerations of recipient design clearly impact the physician's negatively polarized question about exercise:

(13) [Midwest 3.4:7]

```
1  DOC:  Tlk Do you exercise at all?
2        (2.5)
3  PAT:  N::o, uh huh huh huh (.hh-[.hh) huh [huh (.hh huh huh)
4  DOC:                               [Hm      [£Not your thing
5        [ah:,]
6  PAT:  [.hh ] £Would you believe me if I sai(h)d y(h)e(h)s,=
```

Given the patient's weight and working hours that had been discussed just previously, the more positively formulated question – "Do you exercise?" – would risk being heard as at least ill-fitted, and perhaps as inattentive or insensitive. The addition of the words "at all" to the question, by reversing its polarity, work to obviate this risk, and the physician made his choice accordingly. It is significant that the patient's response, though aligned to the preference for a "no" answer embodied in the doctor's question (with "at all"), is nonetheless produced as a dispreferred action – with the delay, the stretched intonation on "no," and the accompanying laughter which treats her response as problematic (Haakana 2001). While aligned with the preference structure of the question's design, her answer, produced in dispreferred fashion, also aligns to the social and medical *undesirability* of her not exercising. Thus, though she responds to the doctor's question with the aligning answer that the question was designed for, the patient also manages to show that she recognizes the undesirability of her aligning response. The patient's remark at line 6 stands as implicit confirmation that the doctor took the correct "line" in designing his question about exercise.

At other times, the principle of recipient design may shape aspects of the *content* of a question in a "best case" direction. For example, relative to "What is your marital status?", "Are you married?" – in (1) above – may seem to the physician to be, conventionally speaking, a "best case" designed question for a middle-aged woman whose daughter was born around 1960.[9]

In summary, questioning during the medical history is informed by two fundamental principles – of optimization and recipient design. These principles are embodied especially in the presuppositions and preferences of physicians' questions, and they can shape the character of patients' answers. We stress that these principles cannot easily be departed from. The more that physicians design their questions so as to exclude presuppositions and preferences, the more their questioning will become drained of the concern for, and understanding of, the patient that medical questioning should properly convey, and come to embody the "essentially anonymous" relationship of the social survey and other forms of bureaucratic questioning. The paradox that physicians face is that, to enter into relationships with patients, they cannot avoid communicating assumptions and expectations about themselves, their patients, and the relationship between them – assumptions and expectations which can subtly shape patient responses. Physicians, like other human beings, are without a hiding place in this matter.

Having examined some basic characteristics of questions, and their implementation as principles of optimization and recipient design in the context of personal history-taking, we now turn to examine the deployment of these principles in sequences of questions and answers.

Medical history-taking: constructing routines and contingencies

As an activity within the medical consultation as a whole, medical history-taking typically involves moving through a set of routine,

[9] Here we emphasize that we are not making a moral judgment, but rather unpacking the likely moral judgment that informs the physician's design of this particular question.

standardized questions. These questions, as we have seen, are concerned with eliciting additional information about the patient and various aspects of her background. Unlike questioning toward differential diagnosis, the background history involves the effort of moving through a complete list of routinized questions. This task may be seen as regarded as relatively uninteresting:

> [Other] parts of the history, while tedious at first, are in a sense easier (than differential diagnosis), because they deal with structured data and are specific questions about predetermined topics . . . The trick is to emphasize the relevant features of past health and medical care experiences without getting too overwhelmed with a mass of detail. (Coulehan and Block 1987:55)

Thus, this aspect of history-taking involves the deployment of questions that recover baseline data from the patient. These "checklists" of questions may arise from record-keeping protocols, or from the routine experience of the doctor, or from explicit guidelines taught during residency. However, regardless of the motivation, it is not the face value of the questions that makes them "routine" or "unusual." Rather, they are *co-constructed* as routine (or not) through the actions of *both* doctors and patients. Doctors accomplish this by designing questions as items in a series, addressed to predetermined topics, and built to receive short answers. Here the principle of optimization is adapted to a particular medical function: gearing questions towards "no problem" outcomes can be a way of indicating that they are being asked on a routine "checklist" basis and without the expectation of problematic information. This type of questioning will be immensely familiar:

(14) [Torn Roto Cuff:3]

1	DOC:	->	An' do you have any other medical problems?
2	PAT:		Uh: no.
3			(7.0)
4	DOC:	->	No heart disease,
5	PAT:		#Hah:.# ((cough))
6	PAT:		No.
7			(1.3)
8	DOC:	->	Any lung disease as far as you know:,
9	PAT:		No.
10			(.)
11	PAT:		Not that I know of.
12			(.)

13 DOC: -> Any diabetes,
14 PAT: No.
15 DOC: -> Have you ever had (uh) surgery?
16 (0.5)
17 PAT: I've had four surgeries on my left knee:.

The five arrowed questions are constructed as a series of "checklist" questions in search of basic background information. As checklist questions, the order and topic of each question is normally predetermined, though sometimes departed from, and each question is designedly brief. Each incorporates a polarity marker that works to favor a "no problem" response from the patient. The brevity of the questions is achieved in part by a form of sequential parasitism in which, after the first question, the next several are managed through phrasal increments that offer some specifications of the "other medical problems" identified at line 1. These questions are Yes/No questions that are designed for one-word answers. With the exception of the last question, the patient's responses confirm or accept the "no problem" state of affairs that the questions prefer, and do so immediately and minimally. After the patient responds to each question, the doctor proceeds to the next, treating the preceding one-word answer as sufficient. The patient's responses contribute to this developing line – each response is minimal, exhibiting the patient's understanding of the "checklist" status of the questions and his preparedness to comply with that understanding (Heritage and Sorjonen 1994). By their very brevity, the patient tacitly shows an understanding of, and an engagement with, the function of these questions as "taking a routine history." In this sense, doctor and patient progressively co-construct and realize this sequence of questions as embodying a "checklist" of routine questions dealing with background or "face-sheet" data. Notably, the final non-aligned response to the last question is produced in delayed fashion, exhibiting a departure not only from the preference of the question (which preferred "no"), but also from the routine series of "no problem" answers which had become the established modus operandi of the sequence.

As we have already commented, in preferring "no problem" answers, the design of this string of questions embodies an optimized stance towards the patient's health status, while simultaneously facilitating a rapid movement through the sequence of question topics. It is just this design that is more broadly caught by Waitzkin when he remarks that this kind of questioning in "systems review" (SR) can be

> quite exhaustive, even more so if the patient happens to be a "yea-sayer." Then, doctor and patient enter potentially endless labyrinths of questions and answers . . . Gradual recognition of these pitfalls during a medical career accounts for the exhaustive efforts that medical students devote to the SR, while their supervising physicians often truncate the SR to a very brief series of questions, for which they do not expect to hear "yes" as an answer. (Waitzkin 1991:30)

Here it needs only to be added that the physician's negative "expectations" about "yes" answers, to which Waitzkin refers, can be thoroughly conveyed to the patient in and through the design and sequential placement of Yes/No questions.

In sum, routine questions are brief, checklist-style questions that expect brief, "no problem" responses from the patient. As is evident in their details, these questions are in search of possibly relevant background information that might inform the doctor's management of the patient's medical condition(s), but they are built to discourage movement beyond the immediate agenda set by each question. Thus, they facilitate movement through the list of questions, and achieve the activity of routine history-taking as a course of action having continuity and cohesion across the interaction as a whole.

Handling contingencies

Not all questions are designed as routine, predetermined, checklist questions. Doctors also use *contingent questions* during the course of history-taking. Contingent questions are questions that are produced in pursuit of some specification of a prior answer. As described by Heritage and Sorjonen (1994), these questions are built to deal, ad hoc, with some matter that emerges from the prior response. Often that contingent "matter" may emerge as a *break in the alignment of the patient's response*. For example, in (10), the doctor's initial question – to our middle-aged woman with a grown daughter – is designed for a "yes" answer. But, given that the question is clearly but one way of inquiring into her marital status, the patient might be expected to elaborate on her dispreferred "no" answer:

(15) [Midwest 3.4:6]

```
1  DOC:  Are you married?
2          (.)
3  PAT:  No.
4          (.)
5  DOC:  You're divorced (°cur[rently,°??)
6  PAT:                        [Mm hm,
```

The patient's unelaborated "no" response is less than cooperative in relation to the objective of the question. And the physician is left with the possibility that the woman is single, divorced, or separated. His follow-up question nominates a likely, and relatively "best case," alternative and is, once again, designed for a "yes" answer, which it receives, in fully preferred fashion.[10]

Another case in which a break in alignment triggers a contingent question is the following. Here the patient's response departs from the action agenda of the question in what might be described as an "overcooperative" way: she responds to a Yes/No question with more information than was requested. The question "Do you have brothers 'n sisters?" is offered as a Yes/No question. However, the patient's answer delivers an embedded "yes," while anticipating a follow-up question addressed to quantity and intimating, with the use of the past tense, that at least one of her siblings may have died:

(16) [Midwest 3.4:5]

```
1  DOC:  Do you have brothers 'n sisters?
2  PAT:  Ah there was eight in our family.   hh
3  DOC:  How many are there now:.
4        (.)
5  PAT:  Ah: seven.
```

Here, the doctor's use of the word "now:." in his contingent follow-up at line 3, references the patient's use of the past tense in line 2 and, with it, the implication that, while there were once eight siblings in her family, there are no longer that many. The doctor's question, then, embodies the presupposition that she now has fewer than eight

[10] Once again, no moral judgment by the authors is intended. It can be added that the physician's sotto voce addition of the word "currently" also embodies a "best case" element, by indicating that her marital situation is temporary rather than permanent. The patient's failure to elaborate on her "No." answer to the question "Are you married?" may be heard to comment unfavorably on her previous marriage.

siblings. This presupposition is contingently introduced in response to the patient's previous answer.

Contingent questions are not confined to situations in which non-aligned responses emerge. Medical questioning involves a variety of circumstances in which aligned answers may require a further question-driven course of elaboration. For example, in the following case, a patient's fully aligned minimal response to a declarative question leaves a residual ambiguity, as to whether the patient was confirming the "dyazide" medication and its dosage, or the "just thuh dyazide" query. The doctor's contingent question addresses this ambiguity.

(17) [Midwest 3.4:2]

1 DOC: .hh Let's ( ) thuh medicines you're taking now:.
2 Just thuh dyazide two uh da:y,
3 PAT: Mm hm,
4 (0.2)
5 DOC: -> That's the only medication?,
6 PAT: Mm hm,

In this instance, the doctor treats the patient's minimal response as ambiguous and in need of follow-up. In following up, the doctor poses a second question to the patient on the same matter that seeks clarification, reconfirmation, or elaboration. This question seeks reconfirmation of a prior answer, thereby formulating a residue of doubt or uncertainty about the patient's drug regimen. A similar case is the following:

(18) [Midwest 3.4:9]

1 DOC: Tl You have your gall bladder?
2 (2.0)
3 PAT: I think so. uh huh=hh
4 DOC: -> £Nobody took it out [that you know (of er hhh)
5 PAT: [.hh hah hah hah

Here the physician humorously topicalizes the patient's apparent uncertainty about her gall bladder. Other contingent inquiries address still more obvious gaps and difficulties. For example, in the following case the patient's response (arrowed), while evidently designed to be helpful, does not give the physician what he needs:

(19) [Midwest 3.4:6]

1	DOC:		tch D'you smoke?, h
2	PAT:		Hm mm.
3			(5.0)
4	DOC:		Alcohol use?
5			(1.0)
6	PAT:	->	Hm:: moderate I'd say.
7			(0.2)
8	DOC:		Can you define that, hhhehh ((laughing outbreath))

This response attracts a contingent follow-up question (line 8). Such contingent questions are quite common in a range of medical contexts, and consistently formulate and deal with ambiguities or problems with the patient's prior response.

Contingent questions strictly preserve the topic of the original question and represent brief "interruptions" in the parties' progression across the broad agenda of questions that form the basis of history-taking. Through contingent questions, physicians may pursue ancillary but related matters that may be directly relevant to the patient's medical condition(s). However, the patient need not necessarily acquiesce in these maneuvers. Subsequently, we will describe a more substantial excursion away from routine questioning. A careful examination of the features of both questions and answers, as well as their sequential positioning, reveals consistent effort by the patient to subtly resist the doctor's line of questioning, and establish an alternative project through which she is able to introduce personal information about herself and her lifestyle into the history.

Optimization and recipient design: clashes and resolutions

We are now in a position to examine more recalcitrant and complex dilemmas of question design. Some of these can concern clashes between the principles of optimization and recipient design: how to frame a question in a desirably "optimized" fashion given information one has just received. In the following case, the health visitor is following a checklist (for details, see Heritage 2002a), the format of which requires her to evaluate the mother's delivery by ringing the word "normal" or "abnormal." However, the parents have just volunteered an extensive description of difficulties with the baby's shoulders during the birth:

(20) [1A1:14]

HV: =So you had a- uh:
(1.0)
-> You didn't- Did you- You didn't have forceps you had a:
M: =Oh [no:: nothing.
F: [( )
HV: An- and did she cry straight awa:y.
M: Yes she did didn't sh[e.
F: [Mm hm,
(1.0) ((Wood cracking))
HV: Uhm (.) you didn't go to scboo: you know the
spe[cial care unit.
M: [Oh: no: no:.]

At line 1, the health visitor is on her way towards a declaratively formulated (and optimized) "So you had a [normal delivery]." However, as she reaches the point at which the word "normal" would be due, she checks herself and, after a one-second pause, restarts with "You didn't-". This appears to have been heading towards "You didn't [have forceps]." However, this question, though somewhat optimized, is problematic: the parents had not mentioned forceps in their previous account, yet forceps might be a possibility under the circumstances. Abandoning this tack, the health visitor shifts to the potentially less optimized "Did you [have forceps]," before reverting to her previous formulation, "You didn't have forceps you had a:" which, again, she abandons at the point where the word "normal" would be due. Here there is a difficulty over designing a question that would meet the terms of the checklist entry in the context of the parents' account.

A related case is the following. The health visitor's quite optimized question (line 1) is responded to only minimally and after a substantial silence. Perhaps oriented to the mother's hesitancy in responding affirmatively, the health visitor abandons a question frame in the same terms, "And you're-" (line 5), to begin a question about the possibility of stitches. As in (20), the health visitor is caught between an optimized and a non-optimized approach to the question:

(21) [4A1:19]

1 HV: And you're feeling well.
2 (0.7)
3 M: . Yeah.
4 (1.5)
5 HV: -> And you're- (.) You didn't ha- Did you have stitches?
6 (0.8)
7 M: Ye[:es
8 HV: -> [You did. [('N) are you so:[re=
9 M: [(nh hnhn) [I had a third degree tea:r=
10 HV: =O::::::h. ^Did you::?
11 M: Yeah. (0.2) It's uh (.) they think what happened 'is
12 chin must 'ave caught me.
13 (0.3)
14 M: .hhh as 'e w'[z coming ou:t.
15 HV: [O::::h,

As this datum indicates, the non-optimized approach turned out to be the one most closely attuned to what actually occurred.

In other circumstances, optimization and recipient design reinforce one another but not in a fashion which is ideal for the surfacing of patient questions and concerns. The following case is taken from the closing moments of a medical consultation (see West this volume, Robinson 2001b):

(22)

342 DOC: ·hhh Uh if the 'X' ray is shows anything ba::d, (0.5)
343 I: will ca:ll.
344 PAT: Okay.
345 DOC: If I can't reach you, (0.3) I'll write you a letter.
346 (.)
347 PAT: Great.
348 (10.5) ((physician writes prescription))
349 DOC: -> °Anything e:lse.°
350 (1.9)
351 PAT: -> ·hhhhhh No:: I don't think so.=hhhhhhhh I'm doing
352 pretty well otherwise.
353 (1.4)
354 DOC: ·mtch=·hh >By the way< if this bu:rns your stomach
355 you should take it with foo::d_ you can take an
356 anta:c[id,
357 PAT: [(Mm hm)=

358 DOC: =·hh [Something like] that.
359 PAT: [(What med is it)]
360 DOC: ·h Indomethacin, (.) Indacine,
361 (.)
362 PAT: Okay.
363 DOC: ·hhh (0.2) hhhh °'Ka:y°
364 PAT: ( )
365 (0.8)
366 DOC: -> Any other questions.
367 (0.3)
368 PAT: -> No::,=>I just< wait to hea:r about the physical
369 therapy?
370 DOC: >Mm hm,< w'=you and thuh nurse can arrange
371 that right now.
372 PAT: (Okay.)
373 (0.7)
374 PAT: Thanks for getting me in so f[a:st.]
375 DOC: [^O^kay.]
376 (0.8)
377 DOC: We:(ll) you know I had nothin' to do with it. Thanks
378 my nurses.
379 PAT: Hheh hah huh huh huh huh.
380 PA?: (They do good) work. ·hh huh=
381 DOC: =Okay.
382 (0.2)
383 PAT: Bye.

In these closing minutes, this physician – like many others in the same circumstances – uses question designs that are negatively polarized, i.e., in search of *no* further questions (line 366) or concerns (line 349). It would be easy to assume that this physician is eager to move on to his next patient and is using this question design to facilitate a quick exit from the examination room. Yet it is also the case that, since the patient has had an opportunity to express additional concerns and could have done so earlier in the visit, considerations of recipient design would mandate this negative polarity. Moreover, this negative polarity also embodies optimization: it is desirable from a health status perspective that the patient does not have other concerns, and this question embodies that stance.

Of course, we also know that up to 40 percent of patients bring more than one concern to their primary care visits, and that a substantial proportion of these only surface at the very end of the visit as so-called "doorknob" concerns (White et al. 1994). Since a number of these may be serious problems, and since physician–patient relations may be significantly enhanced by addressing them, it is instructive to register the difficulty which many physicians can feel in framing these questions in an alternative, more inviting form – e.g., "Are there other concerns you want to address today?" – largely because of the conjoined pressures of optimization and recipient design which, in this context at least, can militate against quality patient care.

"Alcohol use?": an excursion into lifestyle

In this section we examine a sequence of questions and answers addressing the topic of alcohol – one of the 'lifestyle' topics that frequently engender complex definitional and social maneuvers (Halkowski 1998). This datum will permit us to show a further range of variation in patients' answers, and to examine how these variations are deployed to achieve specific interactional objectives. The sequence dealing with the patient's alcohol use is set out below:

(23) [Midwest 3.4:6]

DOC:		Are you married?
		(.)
PAT:		No.
		(.)
DOC:		You're divorced (°cur[rently,°??)
PAT:		[Mm hm,
		(2.2)
DOC:		Tl D'you smoke?, h
PAT:		Hm mm.
		(5.0)
DOC:	1->	Alcohol use?
		(1.0)
PAT:	2->	Hm:: moderate I'd say.
		(0.2)
DOC:	3->	Can you define that, hhhehh ((laughing outbreath))
PAT:		Uh huh hah. hh I don't get off my- (0.2) outa
		thuh restaurant very much but [(awh:)
DOC:	4->	[Daily do you use
		alcohol or:=h
PAT:		Pardon?
DOC:	5->	Daily? or[:
PAT:		[Oh: huh uh. .hh No: uhm (3.0) probably::

23		I usually go out like <u>o</u>nce uh week.
24		(1.0)
25	DOC:	°Kay.°

Here the doctor's question "Alcohol use?" (arrow 1) is constructed as one in a line of routine questions. Its action agenda, however, is somewhat ambiguous. Specifically it can be heard to equivocate between two alternative types of "alcohol" question: "Do you use alcohol," and "How much alcohol do you use?"[11] In her affirmative response (arrow 2), the patient treats the question as requiring an estimation of quantity. After a substantial, one-second delay (Jefferson 1989), the patient produces a non-lexicalized "Hm::", an object often used to indicate "thinking" or a "mental search" for something, and then offers "m<u>o</u>derate I'd say." Her description "moderate" anticipates a question about quantity, which would be the likely follow-up to a simple "yes" response. It is also qualified with "I'd say." This qualification conveys both the sense of a general estimate as well the sense that the term was thoughtfully chosen from an array of measurement terms that are as yet unspecified.

The doctor's next question (arrow 3), evidently a contingent one, now pursues the definition of "moderate." While the doctor's laughter at the end of this turn acknowledges the topic as somewhat delicate (Jefferson 1985; Jefferson et al. 1987; Haakana 2001), it is treated by the patient as a request for more direct specification of the amount she drinks. She goes about this task by launching into a description of the constraints on her social life through which she implies, among other things, that she is essentially a "social drinker," and that her opportunities to drink are limited because she doesn't get out much. A number of observations can be made about her response: she defers engaging with the question's action agenda by her responsive laughter which treats the alcohol issue as a "taboo topic," and by describing a lifestyle constraint that is hearably prefatory to an estimation of the frequency of her social outings; she presents the constraints on her social life in "biographical" terms (Sacks 1989; Button 1990a; Halkowski 1998; Mishler 1984; Drew and Heritage 1992); and she projects (with "but") the production

[11] As Sorjonen et al. (this volume) note, this distinction is socially significant. While Finnish women are normally asked, "Do you use alcohol?," Finnish men are normally asked, "How much alcohol do you use?"

of an estimate that would be likely cast in similar terms. It is this projection which is interdicted by the doctor with a specification that renews his previous inquiry: "Daily do you use alcohol or:=h" (arrow 4).

This inquiry offers a candidate answer that manages two tasks: it specifies an estimate of her drinking, and it provides the terms in which, from the doctor's point of view, such an estimate would preferably be couched. Halkowski (1998) has observed that "lifestyle" questions are recurrent sites for a conflict between "biographical" and "calendar" (and, more generally, arithmetic) methods of formulating time and quantity. Here "Daily" specifies alcohol consumption in "calendar time" (Sacks 1989), and represents a first move towards terms that would facilitate arithmetic calculation in terms of "units per week." The doctor's calendar formulation is offered as a replacement for the patient's biographical formulation, and thus is in tension with it. While the doctor's question pursues the definition which he asked for at arrow 3, it also renews the question with which he initiated the sequence by its repetition of the words "alcohol" and "use." We can further observe that his selection of "Daily" is exemplary of the kind of answer he is looking for. However we can also observe that it is non-optimized: indeed, it permits the patient to acknowledge fairly extensive drinking via agreement with his formulation. In this way, it "biases" the patient's response in favor of disclosure of a possible drinking problem in a way that, for example, "Weekly" would not, while also permitting that patient to engage in "righteous rejection" of its formulation of quantity. Finally we can observe that the question ends with the word "or," with which the doctor attempts to mitigate (Lindström 1997) his reference to "Daily" in the event that, as it turns out to be, it is grossly inappropriate to the patient's circumstances.

The patient's response to this inquiry ("Pardon?", line 20) is a general question – an "open" repair initiator (Drew 1997) – that requests a redoing of the previous turn, and it is here found in its canonical location: a circumstance in which the recipient is experiencing difficulty in understanding how the previous turn came to be produced (Drew 1997). Here, as becomes evident, the patient does not immediately see how the candidate frequency estimate "daily" was constructed from her previous claim that she doesn't get "outa thuh restaurant very much". The doctor's response, "Daily? or:" (arrow 5) is a reduced repeat of his earlier question, which preserves the candidate frequency estimate and its mitigating turn final "or:".

The patient responds to this repeated inquiry with an *oh*-prefaced negative response ("Oh: huh uh"), where the *oh*-prefacing also treats the question as inapposite (Heritage 1998), and the "huh uh" is a minimized form of the negative that further dismisses the nominated measure ("Daily") embodied in the inquiry. In the subsequent expansion of this response, the patient renews her negative response and elaborates it with an estimate of the frequency of her social activities which, now couched in calendar time, replaces "Daily" with "once uh week." as the general metric in which her alcohol use is to be calculated. This is accepted by the doctor with a sotto voce "°Kay.°."

Three more general points can be made about this sequence. First, the patient's responses from lines 16 to 23 consistently resist the action agenda set by the physician's questions, and are often in outright non-engagement with it. They are also non-confirming of the presuppositions of his questions, and disaligned with those questions' preferences. Second, even when the patient is brought to a description of her alcohol use which explicitly employs units of "calendar" time (i.e., "once uh week." line 23), she specifically embeds this unit in a formulation which presents her alcohol consumption in "biographical" terms ("I usually go out") and, in particular, renews the implication that she only drinks socially. In this way, she continues her resistance to the arithmetical calendar formulation of her drinking, while also furnishing an answer that implies that her alcohol consumption is minimal and not in need of further estimation. The doctor finally acquiesces to this response with a sotto voce "°Kay.°" (line 25).

Third, it will be obvious that this "lifestyle" sequence embodies a kind of struggle between doctor and patient. The struggle has been made familiar to us by Mishler (1984) as a conflict between the "medical world" and the "lifeworld." We do not see that doctors and patients have any easy way around these struggles, which, as Halkowski (1998) notes, are commonplace in discussions of smoking and drinking. Physicians, after all, are mandated by the terms of their profession to explore conduct which may be harmful to the patient. In the first instance, this means establishing a measure of the conduct in question. The patient, on the other hand, may be preoccupied with presenting their drinking or smoking "in context," for example, as social or sociable in character. Vacillating over quantity by describing the contexts of consumption can be a vehicle to this end. And it may also address another difficulty: too prompt a description of the quantity one drinks or smokes may be taken as indexing a preoccupation with smoking or drinking as something that one is concerned about. Social norms may militate against the display of such a concern – at least at the beginning of a conversation on the topic. There is thus a sense in which the doctor and patient in this sequence act in terms of the normative requirements of their respective positions, which mandate the doctor to pursue the matter quantitatively, while mandating a corresponding reluctance to "go quantitative" on the part of the patient.

And yet, all is not lost. If, as Cassell (1997) notes, history-taking represents the most important opportunity for primary care doctors to learn about the entirety of their patients' concerns, both medical and personal, then this patient has provided her doctor with a range of lifestyle information, any or all of which is potentially relevant to her medical condition. Through a subtle but nonetheless resistant series of turns, the patient has revealed to the doctor something of her personal life, its constraints, its pressures, and its concerns.

Discussion

In this chapter, we have begun to specify some recurrent, analytically relevant dimensions of questioning and answering during personal history-taking. Where much previous research has focused on the open or closed character of doctors' questions, we have broadened our attention to include both topical and action agendas, and we have directed attention to the presuppositional content and preference structure of those questions. We have also examined the ways in which these features are mobilized into principles underlying question design in the personal history, and how these inform the co-construction of personal-history questions as involving routine matters or, alternatively, as non-routine, contingent issues to be pursued. In so doing, we have specified some of the practices through which doctors and patients conjointly constitute history-taking as a coherent medico-social course of action.

It is important to note that the features of questions and answers we describe are not unique to a history-taking context; indeed, these dimensions are ever present in all environments of questioning and answering, whether medical, legal, or educational, or in the context of news interviews or, most fundamentally, ordinary conversational interaction.[12] Thus, it is inevitable that any question necessarily sets an agenda for recipient response, and almost all questions incorporate presuppositions and, particularly in the case of Yes/No questions, preferences. Physicians, in designing questions for patients, are continually faced with selecting between alternative forms of the "same" question. Ideally, their choices will be responsive to and shaped by a variety of concerns, including the context of routine history-taking itself (which tends to favor "optimized" questions designed for "no problem" answers), and the particular patient to whom the question is addressed.

The fact that choices within these dimensions of questions and answers are unavoidable and are shaped by "recipient design" considerations can set the scene for recurrent tensions in the terms of doctors' questions and patients' answers. For example, returning to the "alcohol use" sequence discussed earlier, there is a tension between the doctor's search for a quantifiable measure of the patient's alcohol consumption and the patient's response in terms of qualitative biographical detail. Although this might look like a straightforward conflict between the outlooks of doctor and patient, it can be suggested that neither party is a completely free agent in their choice of terms. As we have suggested, the doctor is mandated by the terms of his profession to arrive at an assessable grasp of the patient's alcohol use, and is trained to use objective measures to arrive at an appropriate assessment. The patient, on the other hand, may act in terms of norms that mandate her to embed her estimates of alcohol use in a context of sociability. "Biographical"

[12] Amid a large literature, see Atkinson and Drew (1979) and Drew (1992) for legal questioning; Mehan (1985) and McHoul (1978) for educational questioning; Heritage and Greatbatch (1991), Heritage and Roth (1995), Roth (1998), and Clayman and Heritage (2002a, 2002b) for news interviews; and Sacks (1987) and Schegloff (in press) for ordinary conversation.

measures of alcohol use are a central resource for this. Moreover, their alternative – i.e., descriptions of drinking in terms of drinks per day, or units per week – may, by contrast, risk betraying a technical interest in alcohol consumption, which may be negatively construed.[13] Thus normative constraints may shape doctors' and patients' formulations in conflicting or incompatible directions.

Finally, our data suggest that, while doctors' questions in various ways prefer engagement, confirmation, and alignment in patient's answers, this outcome is by no means inevitable. As we have seen, patients can and frequently do break free of these constraints, and exert initiative and agency in proposing alternative agendas, challenging presuppositions, and maintaining contrary preferences. Even during history-taking – perhaps the phase of the doctor–patient consultation that is most completely under the doctor's control – question–answer sequences remain *co-constructions* in which the doctors' questions, although constraining, are not determinative of patient response. Indeed, the construction of history-taking as a routine matter necessarily involves complementary actions of doctors and patients which convey just that.

[13] See Halkowski's (this volume) parallel discussion on the balance which patients may have to sustain between too much and too little attention to their bodily condition.

7

Body work: the collaborative production of the clinical object

Christian Heath

Not merely do practitioners, by virtue of gaining admission to the charmed circle of colleagues, individually exercise the license to do things others do not do, but collectively they presume to tell society what is good and right for the individual and for society at large in some aspect of life. Indeed, they set the very terms in which people may think about this aspect of life. The medical profession, for instance, is not content merely to define the terms of medical practice. It also tries to define for all of us the very nature of health and disease. When the presumption of a group to a broad mandate of this kind is explicitly or implicitly granted as legitimate, a profession has come into being.

(Hughes 1958:79)

License my roving hands, and let them go,
Before, behind, between, above below.
(John Donne, *Elegies* 1633/1950:88)

Introduction

In general practice, the physical examination forms a pivotal part of the consultation. It follows the interview of the patient and discussion concerning the signs and symptoms of the illness, and foreshadows the diagnosis or professional assessment. The observations and findings which arise during the examination form the

I would like to thank all those patients and general practitioners who so generously agreed to cooperate with the fieldwork and allow their consultations to be video-recorded. I would also like to thank Dr. D. Nicholls of Great Ormond Street Hospital for her advice and help. I should add that, without the support of the late Professor P. S. Byrne, onetime President of the Royal College of General Practitioners, the research discussed here would not have taken place. The comments and observations received from Douglas Maynard, John Heritage, David Greatbatch, Paul Luff, Jon Hindmarsh, Dirk vom Lehn, Peter Campion, Hubert Knoblauch, David Silverman, Charles Goodwin, Rod Watson, and Susan Morris proved invaluable in the preparation of the chapter.

foundation to treatment and the management of illness. They have a critical bearing on whether the patient gains access to the "sick role" or, as in certain circumstances, the grounds for seeking medical help are called into question. The empirical contribution of the physical examination, the facts and findings which emerge, derive from the systematic application of technical, and medically warranted, procedures by personnel – in our case, general practitioners. The application of those procedures, and the facts and findings which emerge, rely upon patients transforming the body into a site for professional inspection and investigation. The clinical procedures which are deployed in the physical examination are applied to a material object, the human body, which is presented by a conscious and participating subject – namely, the patient.

As Hughes (1958) points out, clinical practice relies upon a license and mandate which both serve to legitimize professional conduct and circumscribe the ways in which we, the public, should behave with regard to clinical activity. In the case of the physical examination, doctors are granted a mandate to undertake activities reserved for the very few, and activities which demand forms of cooperation which are perhaps unique in our ordinary lives. As Hughes (1958) recognized, these sociological characteristics of professional conduct disregard the contingent and situated organization of clinical practice, and the ways in which medical practice is accomplished in and through interaction with the patient. For example, as Goffman (1961), Emerson (1970), and the rising litigation figures point out, the clinical examination is a highly complex and potentially problematic event, in which it takes little more than a slip of the hand or misguided glance to reconfigure how participants "define" or make sense of each others' conduct. Clinical procedures are deployed with regard to the situation and circumstances at hand, and tailored with respect to the patient and the illness, and yet the possibility of generating facts and findings relies upon the doctor's ability to apply these procedures in routine and methodic ways. The examination requires a compliant, cooperative, and competent patient (a patient who is able to place himself or herself in the hands of the doctor) and a doctor who can deploy routine and methodic procedures with regard to contingencies which inevitably arise during the course of the examination.

This chapter is concerned with ways in which patient and doctor constitute the body as a site for clinical activity. In particular, it explores how the patient, in and through interaction with the doctor, transforms himself or herself from an active subject into an object of inspection and investigation; an object which is manipulated with regard to the moment-by-moment demands of clinical practice and procedure. In exploring the ways in which patient and doctor orient to, and constitute, the body during the physical examination, we can discern how the threat of embarrassment and awkwardness is managed, and consider how pain and suffering is put to the service of clinical practice and investigation. The physical examination provides an opportunity, therefore, not only to address the interactional and contingent organization of medical practice, but to reflect upon the relationship between the body and social action, a relationship which has received growing sociological interest in recent years (see, for example, Turner 1984; Harre 1991). The observations discussed here are based upon extensive fieldwork and the analysis of a substantial corpus of video recordings of general practice consultations.

One of the long-standing themes which has informed studies of medical practice and communication from Henderson (1935) and Parsons (1951) onward is asymmetry, and in particular the distribution of knowledge and expertise between patient and doctor. The physical examination raises an interesting and relatively unexplored issue in this regard. Whereas the interview and prescriptive phases of the consultation are primarily accomplished through mutually available natural language, the examination involves the application of clinical procedures which may be unfamiliar to the patient. Moreover, in the case of certain clinical procedures, such as auscultation, what is heard and attended to by the doctor is inaudible or invisible to the patient. Yet the doctor has to gain the cooperation of the patient, and the patient has to present and adjust the presentation of the body in ways that allow the examination to proceed unproblematically, and as far as possible without interruption. The physical examination therefore provides an example of human activity where the participants have highly differentiated access both to each other's conduct and its procedural organization. In such circumstances doctors have to provide patients with a sense of the developing course of activity and its prospective implications for their conduct; and patients – while presenting their body as an object of investigation – have to remain sensitive to the shifting demands of clinical procedure.

In the general practice consultation, the physical examination can be initiated by either the patient or the doctor. For example, it is not unusual for patients, as they describe their symptoms, to show the doctor the area of difficulty, and invite him or her to inspect the details of the complaint. The doctor may respond by taking no more than a passing glance, but the revelation of the problem may lead to a more extensive clinical examination. More commonly, however, it is the doctor who asks the patient whether he can undertake an examination – the request encouraging the patient to undress and present the relevant part of the body to the doctor, and the removal of the necessary items of clothing occasioning the beginning of the examination. The doctor's request routinely marks the completion of the interview or history-taking phase of the consultation, and is designed to reflect or embody the patient's presenting complaint and the signs and symptoms which have been addressed in doctors' inquiries. The request is designed and legitimized with regard to its particular relevance to the patient's difficulty and rarely leads to question or query. The patient often accepts the request simply by beginning to remove his or her clothes. Due to economy and changing attitudes towards modesty, few health centers retain separate examination rooms. Patients undress in the consulting room and are often examined in the same chair, by the side of the doctor's desk, in which they have been seated throughout the consultation.

Following the doctor's request, both participants become engaged in distinct, but related activities, which prefigure the examination. Doctors take the opportunity to write up the medical records or prepare the necessary equipment, whilst the patient undresses. It is relatively unusual for either patient or doctor to talk, or even glance at each other, whilst these various preparations are made; the fragmentation of involvement providing the patient with a little privacy in which to undress. The request, coupled with the discussion of the complaint, provides the patient with the resources and time with which to initially present the relevant part of the body to the doctor. As the last item of clothing is removed, and the patient begins to position himself or herself for the examination, the doctor begins to orient towards the patient, his movements guiding the ways in which the relevant part of the body should be presented (cf. Heath 1986). The doctor's request foreshadows a strip of technical activity which demands a shift in the ways in which the patient participates in the consultation.

Constituting the body as an object

In the following consultation the patient informs the doctor that she is suffering from a bad cough and wheezing, especially, at night. He suggests listening to her chest, and as he does she stands and begins to remove her coat and blouse. He reaches for the stethoscope. The doctor's "Thankyou" is occasioned by the removal of the blouse. The examination involves auscultation; listening for "abnormal" croaking and creaking at different locations on the patient's chest and back using the stethoscope (see, for example, Toghill 1990).

Fragment 1, Transcript 1

Dr.: Well er::::: shall I have a listen to your chest
P: Yes::
(7.5)
Dr.: Thankyou
(11.5)
Dr.: Just listen to your back please
(8.7)
Dr.: Do you::: still feel a bit (.) cartarry:?
.
.
Dr.: I am sure the cigarette smoking is playing a part now.

As the patient removes her blouse, she sits down, and aligns her chest towards the doctor. He stretches forward, stethoscope in hand, and turns and looks at the chest. As he stretches forward, and the bowl of the stethoscope nears the chest, the patient turns away from the doctor, and looks to one side.

A simple transcript including aspects of the participants' visual conduct may help illustrate the action. Unlike conventional transcripts, descriptions of bodily conduct are laid across the page. Each series of dashes represents silence, and each dash equivalent to one tenth of a second. The doctor's visual conduct is described above the talk or silence; the patient's, below.

Fragment 1, Transcript 2

```
Dr.:  leans forward      places stethoscope and      replaces stethoscope
                         begins auscultation         on new site
                v        v                           v
      ----------------, -------------------,-------------, ---------,---------------,
Pat:  ^                  ^                                      ^
      presents chest     raises head, turns to one   retains orientation . . .
                         side, and lowers eyelids
```

The doctor places the stethoscope at a series of sites across the top of the patient's chest and then moves the stethoscope downwards around her breasts. The patient remains unmoved throughout the examination. She neither looks at the doctor nor the site of the examination, and she produces no response to successive actions that are performed on her body. Only when the doctor asks to look at her back does she alter her orientation. She momentarily glances at the stethoscope and then, leaning forward a little, she adjusts the position of her head as the doctor begins auscultation on her back. She turns away, both from the shifting site of the examination and the doctor, and, looking to one side, her head raised and eyelids lowered, appears disattentive to the proceedings. For convenience we might characterize the patient's alignment to the doctor's activity as a middle-distance orientation.

When taking a patient's blood pressure, the doctor wraps a cuff around the patient's arm and attaches a sphygmomanometer. He inflates and then progressively deflates the cuff. The sound of the deflating cuff is captured by "h."

Fragment 2, Transcript 1

```
Dr.:  inflates cuff                    releases air
          v  v  v  v  v                v
      --------------------,-----------  -------hh,hhhhhhhh-,-----hhhhhhh,hh
      ^                                ^
Pat:  turns to one side lowers         retains orientation . . .
      eyelids holds arm aloof
```

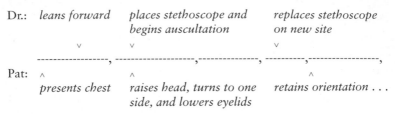

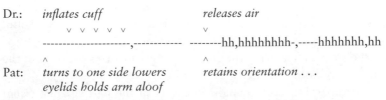

The patient raises his arm to allow the doctor to wrap the cuff. He turns to one side, raises his head, and lowers his eyelids. The doctor pumps air into the cuff, and then, after taking a reading from the sphygmomanometer, releases the air from the sock. Despite changes to the pressure on the patient's arm, the sound of the noise of air released under pressure from the cuff, and the doctor's accompanying activity, the patient preserves an orientation not unlike the patient in the first fragment.

Patients adopt the middle-distance orientation and withhold response to the examination even under quite disturbing and potentially embarrassing circumstances. The following fragment involves palpation, in which the patient's breasts are inspected for evidence of a growth. The doctor places the patient's legs between his own, reaches forward, and places the flat palm of the hand on the underside of the patient's left breast. As the patient begins to reply to his question, she turns away from the doctor and looks into the middle distance, lowering her eyelids and tightening her mouth. She maintains this orientation whilst the doctor presses his open hand at different locations on the left and then the right breast.

Fragment 3, Transcript 1

Dr. positions patient and places the back of his hand under her left breast

v v

Dr.: The pain was there wasn't it?

Pat: Yes err heh around there urm::

^

middle-distance orientation

The breast examination is followed by percussion, an investigation of the patient's respiratory system. Percussion involves laying the left hand flat on the chest wall, and striking the middle phalanx of the right middle finger smartly with the tip of the terminal phalanx of the middle finger. The note is assessed by a combination of pitch and vibration detected through the left middle finger. The doctor compares and contrasts the note by percussing in different locations on the patient's chest. The doctor arches the middle finger of his right hand and hammers the finger at different sites on the patient's chest, working his way up, across, and then down. As the doctor places his left hand flat on the chest, and lifts his right hand to hammer his finger for the first time, the patient once again turns away, raises her head, and lowers her eyelids. The patient largely maintains this middle-distance orientation, looking to one side and gritting her teeth, throughout the percussion. She responds neither to the doctor's glances at her chest and breasts, nor to the successive thuds on her chest. She is seemingly insensitive to the examination.

In each of the cases, the patient neither looks at the doctor, nor at the site of the examination. Rather, as the doctor begins the clinical examination, and focuses on the area of investigation, the patient turns "away" and looks into the middle distance. This orientation is often accompanied by a lowering of the eyelids and tightening of the mouth. The patient preserves this orientation throughout the duration of the examination, only returning their gaze to the doctor at the completion of the activity. This visual orientation is accompanied by a remarkable stillness of the body. The relevant area is presented to the doctor and held in the same position for some minutes whilst the examination proceeds.

The clinical examination is undertaken in accord with professional practice and procedure. Whilst the examination in general practice may – indeed, often does – involve truncated versions of particular procedures, which are tailored with respect to the problem "at hand," they are produced with regard to principles of clinical method. As we find within the few examples discussed above, the clinical procedures used in general practice involve a series of interrelated, or sequentially interdependent, actions performed by the doctor on the patient. These actions are accomplished in a relevant sequential order, which allows the doctor to systematically inspect the functioning of a particular bodily system. For example, the investigation of respiratory difficulties involves percussion. The pitch of the noise and the vibrations detected by the middle finger provide a means through which the doctor is able to detect any potential abnormalities. Percussion is properly performed on a series of specified sites on the chest and the back of the patient. Each action or series of actions is undertaken on a particular site and provides the resources with which to interpret subsequent noise and vibrations. For the doctor, the ordered sequence of actions not only allows him systematically to cover the necessary regions, but provides the resources through which he can compare and contrast the note from different areas of the chest and thereby determine what might constitute an "abnormality." Percussion, then, like other investigations, such as auscultation or palpation, involves a series of sequentially ordered actions, performed by the doctor; the interrelated actions forming a gestalt with which each contributes to the sense of the other and the understanding of the system as a whole.

In the cases mentioned above the patient adopts a middle-distance orientation and withholds response to a succession of actions, both visual and tactile, performed on their body by the doctor. In withholding response, and preserving a certain detachment, both from the actions of the other and the sensations which are inevitably experienced, the patient provides the doctor with the possibility of undertaking a series of actions on his or her body. The middle-distance orientation, coupled with the unflinching body, provides an undifferentiated opportunity to the doctor to undertake the clinical procedure. The patient's seeming absence of participation allows the doctor to coordinate his actions with regard to the principled organization of particular clinical procedures and practices rather than the in-course responses of the patient. The very possibility of undertaking particular investigations rests on the ability of the patient to temporarily suspend sequential commitment to the doctor's conduct; a sequential commitment that profoundly informs how they ordinarily organize their conduct with regard to the actions of others. In adopting the middle-distance orientation and withholding response to the actions of the doctor, the patient transforms himself or herself into an object which can become the subject of clinical procedure and practice. Patients become a suitable site for clinical examination – a site which, given the correct procedures, can serve to render certain physical functions clinically visible. By participating in the examination in this way, patients render their bodies visible, but leave untouched the organization of the activity in which the doctor is engaged – an activity which is guided by medical practice and convention rather than the momentary and shifting requirements of fully fledged interaction with a co-participant.

Patients cannot always be relied upon to conduct themselves in ways that render their body clinically visible. For example, some contemporary examinations are so disturbing or painful that a conscious patient will inevitably undermine the delicacy of the process by reacting to certain actions. In such cases anesthesia may be used to transform the patient into the object. More familiar, perhaps, are the difficulties that practitioners face in attempting to examine young children, who may wriggle, cry, or even scream in response to the coldness of the stethoscope, let alone the thuds of palpation. Parents or guardians, of course, attempt to lock the child in the correct position and render the small body as clinical object, and as the examination begins it is not unusual to find the parent adopting the middle-distance orientation as the child looks with fear at the doctor's work.

The physical examination consists of technical activities which are conducted with regard to the strictures of professional medical practice. It consists of highly specialized activities which are performed on the body, and the details of which may be unknown, if not invisible, to the patient. Through the ways in which the examination is initiated and legitimized with respect to the illness and the inquiries, the doctor secures permission to conduct the activity prior to its actual performance. In granting the doctor permission to undertake the activity, in providing a mandate (if only temporarily), the patient commits himself or herself to participate in ways that allow the examination to be undertaken and accomplished with regard to the strictures of professional medical practice. By adopting the characteristic middle-distance orientation and withholding response to a range of potentially disturbing actions, the patient provides the doctor with an uninterrupted opportunity with which to perform technical activities on the body. In this way, the patient provides the doctor with the possibility of coordinating a series of interrelated actions with regard to correct procedures of medical practices rather than the in-course responses of the "recipient." Even when encouraged to participate to illuminate a particular bodily function, the patient's participation largely precludes actively coordinating their conduct with the doctor. The patient's actions do not fashion the form and character of the activity undertaken by the doctor; they assist the examination rather than inform its procedural organization or trajectory. By participating in this examination in this way, patients render their bodies visible, but leave (untouched) the organization of the activity in which the doctor is engaged; an activity which is guided by medical practice and convention rather than momentary and shifting requirements of fully fledged interaction with a co-participant.

Configuring the site

If patients were simply required to make their bodies available and remain unresponsive throughout the examination, then one might find conduct other than the characteristic middle-distance orientation. Patients may, for example, watch the progress of the examination itself, turn well away from the doctor, or even close their eyes. In case after case, however, patients turn to one side, slightly raise their head, and lower their eyelids. While displaying some detachment from the proceedings, patients do not relinquish all participation in the practitioner's activity. Consider for example fragment 1. It will be recalled that the doctor listens to the patient's chest and then her back.

Fragment 1, Transcript 3

	withdraws stethoscope		*replaces stethoscope and continues auscultation*
	v		v
Dr.:	---------------------------------Just listen to your back please---------------------------		
	turns to doctor and then stethoscope	*begins to reorient*	*presents back and adopts a middle-distance orientation*

The patient, who has maintained a middle-distance orientation, remained unmoved for more than eleven seconds during the examination, turns to the doctor and then the bowl of the stethoscope. The change of orientation arises a few moments before the doctor asks to listen to the patient's back and anticipates the change in the organization of the examination. Indeed the doctor's utterance may well be responsive to the patient's shift in alignment. Even before the doctor speaks, the patient is sensitive to the upcoming change in the nature of the activity and its potential implications for the ways in which she should participate in the examination. The patient's shift in orientation, and her subsequent re-presentation of her body, is occasioned by the doctor's conduct. A second or so before his utterance, the doctor, still holding the stethoscope on the patient's chest, turns away from the site of auscultation. As he begins to look away, the patient abandons her middle-distance orientation and turns toward the doctor. He withdraws the stethoscope, she drops her gaze to the equipment and looks at the stethoscope.

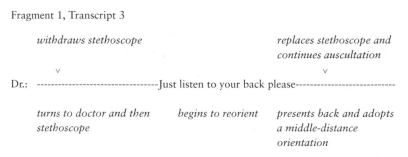

He does not, however, withdraw the stethoscope, as he might if the examination were over, but rather begins to move the equipment to one side of her torso. As the hand clasping the bowl of the stethoscope begins to move to one side of the patient, she adjusts her seating position and turns her back to align towards the doctor. The doctor's shift of orientation has the patient turning to the site of examination and the prospective path of the stethoscope as it leaves the body allows the patient to see that the examination will continue on her back. She is able to begin to position her body in the correct position for auscultation, even before being asked. Indeed, the doctor's request, "Just listen to your back please," appears sensitive to the patient's shifting alignment; more concerned with accounting for his conduct rather than providing instructions as to what she might should do next. As the doctor places the bowl of the stethoscope on her back, the patient once again adopts a middle-distance orientation. This time her orientation is a little different. The doctor is standing behind her and the patient aligns her head more in parallel with her shoulders.

Whilst seemingly inattentive to the proceedings, therefore, the patient is able to notice a shift in orientation away from the site of the examination, and to infer that the stethoscope is being removed from, rather than repositioned on, the chest. In turning and looking at the doctor's actions, the patient anticipates the prospective path of the artifact and the upcoming activity it suggests. In anticipating the upcoming activity, the patient is able to put her body in place, and provide the doctor with unhindered access to the relevant area to enable the examination to proceed. Consider a second example, taken as the doctor prepares to take the patient's blood pressure.

Fragment 2, Transcript 2

```
       reaches for pump        begins to
                               attach pump to cuff
           v                   v
Dr.:  ----------------,-------- ------------,----------------, ----------------,
                ^^                         ^^                  ^
       glances at              glances at hand raises   turns to middle
       pump turns to           arm                      distance
       middle distance
```

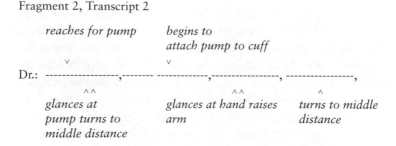

The patient adopts a middle-distance orientation as the doctor wraps his arm with the cuff. On a couple of occasions he turns and watches the doctor's hands. The shifts in orientation are responsive to the doctor's actions, even though they occur outside the direct line of the patient's regard. In the first case, the doctor reaches for the pump to inflate the cuff; in the second, he begins to attach the pump to the cuff. In the first, the patient resumes the middle-distance orientation as the doctor's hand returns to the arm. In the second, the patient follows the hand as it returns to the cuff and then raises his arm to allow the equipment to be attached. As the doctor removes his hand from the arm and begins to inflate the bag, the patient once again adopts a middle-distance orientation.

The patient's sensitivity to the shifting character of the doctor's activities also occurs during the examination itself. It will be recalled that in the following fragment the patient remains largely unmoved during the examination even though she is subject to potentially disturbing actions.

Fragment 3, Transcript 2

Dr.:	*releases grip and removes hand*	*repositions hand*		
	v v	v		
	--------------,--------------,--------------,--------------,--------------			
	^^^	^		
Pat:	*glances at hand and breast*	*reorients breast*		*turns to middle distance*

The patient preserves a middle-distance orientation as the doctor feels the patient's breasts and percusses various sites on the chest. At one point during the breast examination, the doctor begins to withdraw his hand in order to reposition his fingers. As the hand loosens its grip, but whilst the fingers are still clasping the breast, the patient abandons her middle-distance orientation and turns toward the site of the examination. As the doctor re-reaches for, and takes hold of the breast, the patient reorients her chest so that her breast neatly falls into the doctor's hand and the clasping fingers. The relaxation of the hand is treated by the patient as displaying a potential shift in the activity. By turning toward the site of the examination, she is able to see the hand's movement, and anticipate, in the course of its trajectory, its implications for the ways in which she should re-present her body.

The second example from this examination is more delicate still. We join the action as the doctor percusses the patient's chest. As the doctor's hands move progressively over the patient's chest, they near her right breast. At one point the hands move slightly to one side, a moment or so later, raising the breast on its back, as the doctor percusses the area below. The first movement appears to attract the patient's gaze – she abandons the middle-distance orientation and glances toward the site of the examination. As the right hand forms a bridge, the patient raises her arm, turns, and re-presents the breast to provide the doctor with easier access for percussion. Even as he begins to alter his position, she once again adopts the middle-distance orientation.

Fragment 3, Transcript 3

```
Dr.:  percusses        raises hand and forms     percusses
      chest            "bridge" for breast       chest...
              v v               v v          v v          v v
      --------------, -------------, -------------, -------------, -------------
      ^                          ^        ^        ^
Pat:  middle           glances         raises    readopts middle-
      distance         at hand         arm       distance orientation
```

Neither of these changes in the positions of the hands are accompanied by the doctor turning toward the face of the patient. The doctor maintains his gaze on the site of the examination, or occasionally, when shifting to a new position or "listening intently," turns to one side of the patient, almost mirroring the middle-distance look. For her own part, whilst repositioning her body to enable the doctor to gain access to the relevant part of the body, and momentarily glancing at the co-participant's hands, the patient does not look at the doctor's face. The participants do not once exchange mutual glances during the examination.

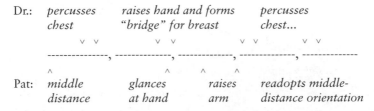

It should be said, however, that for many examinations there is no need for the doctor to look toward the patient's face. It may even be unnecessary to look at the actual site of the examination. For example, during percussion the doctor needs to listen carefully for the echo engendered by the hammering finger, but aside from deciding where to position the hands on the various sites around the chest and back there is no need for the doctor to look at the surface area of the body. Similarly, during auscultation the stethoscope needs to be guided and placed on particular areas of the chest, but listening to the patient does not require the doctor to look at the site of the examination. In the very ways in which the doctor undertakes the clinical examination, and in particular the ways in which the doctor organizes his visual attention with regard to the principal (shifting) area of activity, the doctor encourages the co-participant to disorient both from the activity and perhaps from the other. The doctor's own conduct, and the avoidance of actions that might serve to elicit the gaze of the other and thereby establish mutually oriented co-participation, encourage the patient to disattend the proceedings and to deliver their body as an object worthy of, and available for, clinical inspection and manipulation.

Other aspects of the doctor's bodily comportment also serve to encourage the patient to disattend the site of the examination. For example, consider the ways in which the doctor positions the patient's body with regard to his own. With the increasing use of the side-by-side arrangement where patient and doctor sit at a right angle across one corner of the desk, we find doctor and patient remaining seated during many examinations, the patient's legs being neatly tucked within the practitioner's. In establishing this position, which might appear a little intimate, the doctor is able to keep the patient at some distance during the examination. Palpation, auscultation, and even percussion, can be performed literally at arm's length, with the doctor's head tilted down toward the site of the activity. The arrangement allows the doctor to avoid a potentially more intimate arrangement, whereby the standing doctor leans over the seated patient, resulting in the close proximity of the participants' faces and making the middle-distance orientation more difficult both to adopt and maintain.

It should be added that doctors rarely talk during the types of examination that we have addressed so far, though some form of assessment often accompanies the completion of the physical examination or the conclusion of specific procedures. Where there are temporary shifts in the course of the activity, vocalizations are limited to task-related instructions and requests. The relative absence of talk during the examination may also derive, in part, from the interactional consequences of speaking, and in particular its implications for co-participation. The problem with talk is not simply that it might make it more difficult for the doctor to concentrate on the activity at hand, and certainly during some procedures such as auscultation it would be nigh impossible to talk and listen. It also avoids placing the patient under the obligation of looking at the speaker during the exchange of talk. The other's glance, and its ability to lead to mutual orientation, could inadvertently have the participants looking at each other whilst one touched the body of the other. In these and other ways, therefore, the doctor produces the examination to enable and encourage the patient to distance himself or herself from the activity. The middle-distance orientation therefore can be seen as a natural and suitable accompaniment to the standpoint adopted by the doctor to the body, and in particular to the ways in which the examination is accomplished by rendering specific sites relevant to particular activities.

Few clinical procedures in general practice require a patient to adopt a particular bodily orientation for the duration of the examination. Rather, the patient is required to remain sensitive to the developing progress of the activity and to shape how the body is presented with regard to the shifting demands of the procedure. Auscultation, palpation, percussion, and a number of other clinical procedures, involve a series of interrelated actions which are undertaken on successive locations on the body. The patient has to shape his or her participation within regard to the developing course of the activity. It is not enough simply to withhold response to a range of conduct performed on the body by the doctor. The patient has to discriminate the doctor's conduct with respect to its implications for the way in which the body should be presented to enable his actions to be properly accomplished. The patient has actively to withhold response to a range of actions performed on the body by the doctor, actions which may cause discomfort, embarrassment, even pain. However, the patient uses whatever can be discerned as a resource with which to configure the body so as to allow the activity to proceed. The patient transforms the body into an object, whilst simultaneously manipulating that object with regard to the emerging import of the examination itself. The patient actively constitutes himself or herself as a clinical object in and through interaction with the doctor.

On the one hand, therefore, the physical examination requires a patient to transform their self into an object of examination, to become a site for the application of clinical procedure. On the other hand, the patient has to remain sensitive to the accomplishment of clinical activity and, throughout its course, make changes to the ways in which the body is presented to the doctor. The middle-distance orientation is finely suited to solving these two, seemingly contradictory, demands. By not looking at the doctor, nor watching the activity, the patient can remain communicatively disengaged, and seemingly inattentive to the moment-by-moment accomplishment of the examination. The patient does not look at, at least in the direct line of his regard, the successive actions performed by the doctor on the body, and by not watching the actual activity is able to diminish his or her own desire to react. By adopting the middle-distance orientation, the patient can be seen not to be watching the activity, and by distancing himself or herself from the examination, provides the doctor with an uninterrupted opportunity to undertake clinical procedure and practice. Moreover, by turning to one side and adopting the middle-distance, the doctor is not placed under an obligation to return gaze to the patient; an exchange of looks which might not only serve to disrupt the performance of the examination, but also inadvertently lead to a moment of intimacy, even embarrassment. The middle-distance orientation provides patients with a way of dissociating themselves from the actions of the doctor, and being seen not to watch the examination within the developing course of its production. It displays a certain trust in the other, and provides the doctor with, as Hughes (1958) might suggest, the "elbow room with which to fulfil his or her professional obligations." The middle-distance orientation and the systematic transformation of the body into an object, is perhaps an embodiment par excellence of the sick role, and in particular the obligation of the sick to place themselves in the hands of the physician. As Parsons suggests,

> the fourth closely related element is the obligation – in proportion to the severity of the condition of course – to seek *technically competent* help, namely, in the most usual case, that of a physician and to *cooperate* with him in the process of trying to get well. It is here, of course, that the role of the sick person as patient becomes articulated with that of the physician in a complementary role structure. (Parsons 1951:437)

Patients do not relinquish themselves completely to the doctor. They actively transform themselves into an object. The middle-distance orientation provides patients with the ability to remain sensitive to the activity, "peripherally aware," whilst neither looking at, nor being seen to be looking at, the doctor and the site of the activity. In turning to one side and gazing into the middle distance, patients can appear inattentive, whilst able to monitor the actions of the doctor ongoingly. If patients were, for example, to close their eyes, or turn directly away from the site, they would no longer be able to discriminate the doctor's actions and would become insensitive to the ongoing demands of clinical procedures. The actual orientation adopted by patients during the examination is carefully shaped with regard to the location of the clinical activity, the visibility of its procedures, and the position and orientation of the doctor. Patients make small adjustments to their orientation during the developing course of the examination, so that they maintain their seeming distance from the activity and the doctor, whilst preserving their ability to remain sensitive to the accomplishment of the clinical procedure. The middle-distance orientation adopted during the examination, therefore, allows patients to remain sensitive to the examination, and in particular to notice and anticipate action which has implications for the ways in which the body should be presented to the doctor. It allows patients, if necessary, to momentarily glance at the actions of the doctor, and in this way determine just how the body should be presented to enable clinical activity to proceed, and proceed without interruption. The middle-distance orientation relies upon the ability of individuals to remain aware of, and discriminate, action outside the direct line of their regard and, where necessary, be drawn by changes in the production of the activity and the local environment of goings-on. During the physical examination our ability to remain peripherally aware, almost formalized in the middle-distance orientation, is put to the service of managing the almost contradictory demands of the physical examination.

Doctors encourage this remarkable detachment and stillness of being. As the patient aligns the relevant part of the body, and the examination begins, the doctor turns away from the other, and focuses on the site of the activity. Focal alignment on the shifting site of the examination is not infrequently preserved by the doctor throughout the course of the examination, even though it is neither necessary nor helpful to the procedure. Occasionally – for example, during auscultation – the doctors may turn away from the site, but in such cases, it is interesting to note, they look to one side and away from the patient, often adopting a display of intense concentration. We have mentioned, for example, how the doctor maintains his gaze on the site of the examination as it shifts to different areas of the body, even though many procedures do not necessarily require one to look. Moreover, the doctor does not respond to the patient's conduct, nor encourage response from the patient. So, for example, doctors do not acknowledge the patient's orientation, nor respond to their lack of response, or even remark upon the pacing of their breathing or the way in which the body is being held or presented. By organising their own conduct with regard to their own actions, and the properly ordered sequence of clinical procedure, they too disregard the other, and rid the other's conduct of sequential significance. The transformation of the body into a site for examination therefore is in a sense achieved by the participants ridding their conduct of interactional significance and the contingent and unpredictable course it inevitably entails.

In passing, it is worth mentioning, perhaps, that in both Fragment 1 and Fragment 3 the domain that forms the focal alignment of much of the examination is part of the body that is not ordinarily accessible to the gaze of others. In both cases, the doctor maintains his gaze either on the patient's breast or its surrounds. The alignment is legitimized by virtue of the ways in which it features in the examination, such that the doctor's gaze is constituted as a necessary feature of the activity itself. The activity, of which it forms part, renders the looking as a particular sort of alignment, not so much looking at the patient's body, but rather relying upon an orientation to enable the hands and instrument to be guided and positioned on relevant parts of the body. It is interesting to note that, freed from this embededness or connectedness, within the developing course of the examinations such glances, even when produced by doctors, can prove problematic for the patient and doctor. For example, in the following fragment, the doctor turns and glances at the chest of the patient, who is sitting undressed waiting for the examination to begin.

Fragment 4

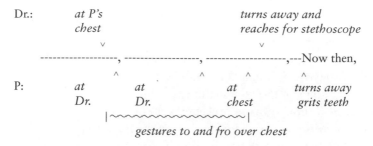

```
Dr.:      at P's                               turns away and
          chest                                reaches for stethoscope
              v                                     v
     ----------------, ----------------, -----------------,---Now then,
                   ^                  ^        ^           ^
P:        at          at                   at          turns away
          Dr.         Dr.                  chest       grits teeth
                 |~~~~~~~~~~~~~~~~~~~~~~~~~~~|
                     gestures to and fro over chest
```

The doctor's glance is not accompanied by the beginning of the examination. He does not lean forward to inspect the chest, as one might in palpation, nor does he take hold of a stethoscope to listen to the chest. Indeed, the examination, which does indeed involve auscultation, begins some moments later. Freed from the respectability of clinical activity, the doctor's glance engenders a series of gestures from the patient. The gestures consist of an open hand, which is passed to and fro over the surface of the chest. The gestures crisscross the line of regard of the doctor, partially concealing the chest from his gaze, and perhaps encouraging him to abandon his passing interest in her body. Indeed, as the doctor turns away, the patient immediately abandons her flustered gestural activity.

The patient's gestures, her accompanying glances, and gritted teeth, have many of the characteristics commonly associated with embarrassment (see, for example, Darwin 1979; Goffman 1956). The patient's moment of embarrassment is engendered by a glance, a glance freed from its embeddedness within a clinical activity. The patient's response, though seemingly haphazard, is perhaps sensitive to the practicalities of the moment. It serves in part to conceal the chest and discourage the doctor's gaze, and yet allows the patient to avoid the serious implications of covering the chest altogether. Not only would it inevitably cast aspersion on the conduct of the doctor, but it could undermine the participant's ability to proceed with the examination. As the doctor turns away, and the gesture subsides, the moment passes, and a few seconds later the doctor takes hold of the stethoscope and begins auscultation.

Revealing symptoms

The transformation of the subject into a clinical object does not necessarily rest on the ability to withhold response to a range of successive actions whilst making the body accessible for inspection and manipulation. A number of clinical procedures require patients to undertake particular actions so that certain signs, or the functioning of particular systems, become visible, at least to the professional eye. For example, consider how patients may be required to take slow, deep breaths, to enable the doctor to hear signs of consolidation in the lung, or cough, to reveal whether there may be infection. With other complaints, the patient may have to adopt a more active stance and, whilst presenting the body as a clinical object, will simultaneously (attempt to) reveal their subjective experience of the complaint. An interesting case in point is where the difficulty involves pain, and the examination explores its location and severity. The patient has to provide the doctor with access to the relevant part of the body, for inspection and in some cases manipulation, whilst both revealing, yet managing, the pain and suffering that the examination can cause.

Consider, for example, the following fragment. The patient has a painful ankle and has difficulty walking. We join the action as doctor places the patient's foot on his lap and begins to manipulate it back and forth. The doctor attempts to inflict pain in order to determine where the ankle hurts and thereby the source or cause of the difficulty.

Fragment 5, Transcript 1

```
  Dr.:  [Manipulates foot ]
        .
        .
• Pat:  Arghhh °hhh (°hm)=
  Dr.:  =Is that sore when I do that?
  Pat:                      mhm hhum
        (0.5)
  Dr.:  Where do you feel: it?
• Pat:  Here:agh:
        (0.4)
  Dr.:  °um
        (2.5)
  Dr.:  °hhh Just stand up Missus Delft will you?
```

The doctor bends the foot back and forth. As the foot is pulled back, the patient cries out, uttering, "Arghhh°hhh (°hm)." The cry consists of a conventional expression of pain, "argh," uttered through the teeth, followed by an out-breath and in-breath. As she cries out, the patient, who until then has adopted a middle-distance orientation, turns and glances at her foot. She then turns momentarily to the doctor, and once again adopts a middle-distance orientation. She retains this orientation as the doctor continues to manipulate the foot and largely abandons any further expression of her suffering. She participates by pointing to the location of the difficulty and answering the practitioner's questions, rather than expressing the pain she may be suffering.

The way in which the patient participates in the examination derives from the doctor's response to her cry of pain and his subsequent actions. In the following transcript, I have doubled-spaced dashes and letters in order show a little more of the action.

Fragment 5, Transcript 2

```
Dr.:  draws  pushes                                  turns from
      foot   foot                                    foot to
      back   forward                                 patient

      v      v                                       v
      - - - - -    A r g h h h  ° h h h (°h m)= I s t h  at sore when I
                   ^     ^        ^              ^
Pat:    turns to       turns      turns
        foot and       to Dr.     to middle distance
        grits teeth
      |~~~~~~~~~~~~~~~~~~~~~~~~~~~~~~~~~~~~~~~~~~~~~~~~~~~~~~~~~~~~~~~~~~|
                   retains foot in the hands of the Dr.
```

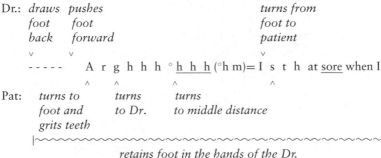

As the patient turns to the foot and cries out, the doctor provides no response. He continues to look at the ankle and manipulate the foot. The patient glances momentarily at the doctor, and then once again adopts a middle-distance orientation. As the cry subsides, and the patient adopts a middle-distance orientation, the doctor turns towards the patient, and produces a diagnostically relevant question, a question which attempts to identify the location of the difficulty within the continuing manipulation. The doctor neither responds to the patient's cry of pain nor provides sympathy or appreciation. By maintaining an orientation to the foot as the patient cries out, the doctor does not witness – and, critically, is not seen to witness – the patient's suffering. He establishes the foot, rather than the momentary suffering, as the focal area of attention. In continuing to grip and manipulate the foot, he demonstrates his commitment to continuing the examination. Finding the doctor continuing the manipulation, the patient curtails the cry of pain, tailoring her response to enable the doctor to continue the manipulation. By preserving a diagnostic stance toward the suffering, the practitioner encourages the patient to adopt an analytic standpoint toward her own pain; that is, to present the body as an object of clinical inquiry and to use her suffering as a resource to reveal when and where the pain occurs.

In this way, despite the pain she suffers, the patient cooperates with the examination. She does not withdraw her foot from the doctor's hands, nor is her suffering so severe that it undermines the progress of the investigation. The patient adopts an analytic standpoint toward her own suffering, presenting the object to the other, and answering questions concerning the location of the difficulty. She adopts this standpoint despite the suffering which continues to be inflicted by the doctor. For the examination, she transforms her body into an appropriate object of clinical inspection and object which relies upon the subject's ability to experience, and report on, pain.

Despite the patient's cooperation with the doctor's activity, she does not abandon all expression of suffering. In response to "where do you feel it" she points to an area of the ankle and utters the word "here."

The word "here" segments the gesture, marking the point at which the ankle hurts, or at least the surface position of the pain. The word "here" is spoken as "here:argh," and as the patient points to the ankle, her hand trembles. The patient's actions cooperate with the diagnostic inquiries of the doctor. They pinpoint the location of the pain, with regard to its location and the point within the manipulation in which it arises. In cooperating with the diagnostic stance of the doctor, the patient does not abandon all attempt to reveal, rather than describe, her complaint. The articulation of the word "here" embodies a cry of pain, "argh," a moment of suffering which is visibly revealed in the trembling hand that hovers over the ankle. In this way, the patient animates her symptoms, and renders them experientially visible to the doctor. He is not only informed where the pain is, and when it arises, but in that passing moment he sees and hears for himself the patient's suffering.

In animating signs and symptoms, patients systematically reveal difficulties which might otherwise remain invisible and unnoticed. In this and other cases, the patients' ability to reveal their suffering, and/or the functioning of a system, is put to the service of clinical practice. The examination relies upon the patients' ability to adopt an analytic or diagnostic standpoint to their body and their personal suffering. They adopt a middle-distance orientation, they withhold response to various actions performed by the doctor, and they present a particular part of their body to the doctor for inspection and manipulation. In rendering the body as an object, however, they have to manage their suffering and discomfort, their own subjective experience of the difficulty and the examination. Subjective experience is put to the service of clinical procedure. The patient is encouraged to present the body as an object, whilst simultaneously assessing, and reporting on, the suffering experienced through the object. The patient has to reveal, in the course of its presentation, characteristics of the object's functioning, characteristics, which themselves rely upon the patient's experience of the very object that is presented to the doctor.

Discussion: patient participation and professional assessment

The physical examination entails the application of technical procedures which are undertaken by doctors both on, and with, the patient's body. Whilst the application of these technical procedures is contingent on particulars of the patient's complaint and practicalities at hand – the amount of time for the consultation and the like – their accomplishment requires the production of a series of interrelated actions which are organized in accord with medical convention and practice. Unlike the material objects which form the subject of, say, the natural sciences, patients have to reflexively constitute themselves as a site for clinical activity. They present and manage their body to facilitate the application of these technical procedures and the actions they necessitate, and in particular transform themselves, or part of themselves, from an active experiential subject into an object of inspection, manipulation, and examination.

By presenting their body to the doctor, withholding response to a range of intrusive and potentially disturbing actions, visually orienting away from the site of clinical activity and the doctor, patients are able to transform themselves into an object of investigation and examination. Patients produce and manipulate this object with regard to the shifting demands of the clinical activity; its presentation tailored, moment by moment, to the examination and the implications of particular actions for the ways in which the body should be rendered visible with respect to the momentary requirements of the doctor's actions. This presentation may even demand that the patient, whilst presenting the body for investigation, exploit his or her personal suffering, for the practical purposes of rendering certain bodily functions visible. To corrupt Turner's (1984) theoretical critique of the ways in which the social sciences have disregarded the body, we find in the physical examination a rather different type of "separation practice," a practice in and through which patients actively render their body as object, whilst overseeing its manipulation and presentation.

The patient, as a self-constituting object of medical inquiry, has to manage the presentation of the body and his or her physical sensations during the examination. Many investigations, even relatively innocuous procedures such as percussion, involve physical experience, if only the sensation of a finger being tapped on successive locations around the chest and the back. The patient is required to withhold response to, and preserve an insensitivity toward, the sensations which he or she receives. Rendering the body as an object does not remove its sensuality. It is rather that the patient is required to act as if the actions of the doctor are of no effect, unfelt and unseen. Even in circumstances where the body's sensuality serves as a resource in the clinical examination, the patient is required to tailor his or her experience and its expression with regard to the ongoing requirements of the diagnostic activity. The patient does not simply give "voice" to his or her feeling; rather, the physical experience is animated, even experienced, with regard to the demands of the diagnostic activity at hand. The patient, for example, is required to experience and reveal pain, inflicted by the doctor, and to manage its expression in particular ways. In constituting the body as a site for examination, the patient constitutes himself or herself as an object, whilst preserving a relevant sensational arena with regard to that object and/or its operation. The patient is required to adopt an analytic standpoint towards his or her own body, to treat it as an object and express his or her bodily sensations in a clinically relevant way. With the cooperation of the patient, the subjective experience of bodily suffering is transformed into a resource for diagnostic inquiries; the object is re-embodied with relevant experience and expression.

The patient's ability to constitute the body as a site for clinical investigation and the systematic application of professionally warranted procedures and practices, provides practitioners with the resources with which to produce thoughts, facts, and findings concerning illness. Whilst it is widely recognized that the physical examination may well simply confirm an earlier hypothesis or idea, the findings it generates are often treated as the facts of the matter. The signs and the symptoms rendered visible during the course of the examination may stand in marked contrast to the "subjective" account presented by the patient during the interview phase of the consultation. Notwithstanding the recognition that the doctor's investigation is founded upon the patient's "verbal description of the problem" (Byrne and Long 1976), the examination and the procedures it entails provide the practitioner with direct and "objective" access to the functioning and malfunctioning of the body. It is not surprising, therefore, that the physical examination is routinely followed by the doctor delivering a diagnosis or professional assessment of the patient's illness (Heath 1992). The diagnosis or assessment gains its status by virtue of its immediate juxtaposition with the physical examination, and is designed to embody the findings which can be seen to have derived from direct technical observation of the patient's body. Whilst it may consist of no more than a single sentence which characterizes the illness or difficulty, its factual basis and its ability to form the foundation to the management of the complaint derive from the ways in which doctor and patient have, in collaboration, produced the body as a site of clinical activity. By actively transforming his or her body into a site for examination, the patient provides the opportunity for the doctor to generate clinical facts and findings, which form the basis of diagnosis or assessment. In turn, the diagnosis or assessment provides a foundation of, and grounds for, the management of the complaint.

Fragment 6

{*Dr. undertakes auscultation*}
Dr.: *hhhhh You've got erm: (0.8) bronchitis::.
*er:.
(4.5) {*Dr prepares to write a prescription*}
Dr.: *hhh (0.3) I'll give you antibiotics: to take for a week.

The diagnosis is delivered as the doctor withdraws the stethoscope from the patient's back. The "informing" is a simple monolithic statement which names the patient's difficulty. In this instance, as in many, it neither encourages nor demands response. It gains its character and status by virtue of its immediate juxtaposition with the examination; it is seen as the product of the doctor's clinical investigation of the patient's symptoms (namely, coughing and wheezing). The patient produces a downward intoned "er:.," which serves to pass the floor with dispatch back to the doctor. The doctor begins to prepare to write a prescription, and mentions the treatment he will give to the patient. The physical examination therefore forms the basis to the diagnosis, and in turn the management of the complaint.

A downward-intoned "er" or "yeh" is one amongst a variety of responses to post-examination diagnoses and assessments which can serve to encourage the doctor to progress directly to the "management phase" of the consultation. As discussed elsewhere, in producing a sequentially minimal response patients can orient to and preserve the professional, clinical status of the diagnosis and assessment, and in particular the ways in which it derives from the relevant application of medical procedure and convention by the doctor. Even in cases where patients attempt to challenge or disagree with the assessment, in our corpus of data they rarely question the relevance of procedures used by the doctor during the examination. Consider, for example, the following fragment, in which the patient has undergone a thorough investigation of the respiratory system. As the doctor finishes listening to the patient's back, he delivers the assessment.

Fragment 7 (simplified)

{*Dr. undertakes auscultation and palpation*}
Dr.: Well yer chest is (.) absolutely clear today::.
(1.0)

Dr.: Which is helpful:^ (0.4) and your pulse is (0.7) only eighty *thhh
which is er::: (1.2) not so bad.
(1.2)
P: Right it's:: there:: night time (.) it's:::ts
not clear then, I've got er::: (______). I've more or less gone to bed
when it <u>starts</u> : on us:^
(2.5)
P: I wake all the way through the night without getting any sleep
(un open).
(0.5)
Dr.: mm
P: I don't know what's fetching it up during the
nights (.) but it comes in at the nights.
(0.5)
Dr.: *thhhh. You've not had a history of asthma::
or er::: (0.3) *hh hay fever or anything like that?

The assessment details the outcome of the investigations and suggests that there is little evidence of the patient's presenting symptoms; namely, breathlessness, a persistent cough, and a racing heart. In reply, the patient produces an account of his condition. The account describes when the symptoms arise and underscores the severity of the difficulties and the discomfort they cause. The account does not question the physical examination nor the factualness nor accuracy of the findings that arose therein. Rather it describes the patient's subjective experience of the illness, and provides an explanation for the relative absence of signs and symptoms during the consultation. By reasserting his symptoms and suffering, the patient encourages the doctor to undertake further inquiries into the complaint, whilst preserving the integrity and reliability of the examination. The account underscores the patient's grounds for seeking medical help in the face of a physical examination that threatens the legitimacy of the patient's claims to being sick and his grounds for seeking professional help.

The ways in which the patient constitutes the body as a site of clinical activity, therefore, provides the practitioner with the ability to apply medically warranted procedures and practices and thereby generate empirically grounded observations and findings concerning the patient's illness. The examination and the findings it generates can help confirm the doctor's diagnosis, it can introduce a new issue or idea, and in some cases serve to question (even arbitrate) the patient's claims to being sick. The empirical findings of the examination, therefore, can serve to stand in marked contrast to the descriptions and reports found in the more discursive interview phase of the consultation. It provides a vehicle for the discovery and identification of empirically grounded observations concerning the illness, and in many cases forms the foundation to the assessment and diagnosis. It is hardly surprising, therefore, that diagnosis and assessment form a pivotal part of the consultation, retrospectively (re)formulating the patient's illness and the various signs and symptoms it may entail, and informing prognosis and management of the complaint. The ways in which the body is systematically made available to the doctor, and signs and symptoms rendered visible, serve to constitute the illness and provide access to treatment and the sick role.

8

Communicating and responding to diagnosis

Anssi Peräkylä

Introduction

In the literature on medical consultations, there are two strikingly different ways of thinking about the relation between doctors and patients. One emphasizes the doctor's authority, while the other, often programmatically, emphasizes the patient's knowledgeability and his or her participation in the diagnostic procedure and the decisions about the treatment. Writers who have emphasized the doctor's authority include, most notably, Talcott Parsons (1951), Eliot Freidson (1970b), and Andrew Abbott (1988). They point out that doctors possess technical and scientific knowledges that enable them to diagnose illnesses, and society has warranted them with the license to decide about medication and sick leave, and to perform surgical and other therapeutic procedures. The patient does not have such knowledge and licenses. Therefore, the relation between the doctor and the patient is necessarily characterized by the doctor's authority. However, there are other writers – for example, in medical anthropology (Stimson and Webb 1975; Kleinman 1980; Helman 1992) and on fields of research closely related to medical practice (e.g.; Pendleton 1983; Tuckett et al. 1985; Lipkin et al. 1995), who maintain that the patient, as well as the doctor, has ideas about the nature, the origin and the possible remedies of the patient's ailment. The consultation could and should be an encounter between two differently but equally resourceful agents where they negotiate diagnosis and treatment. In an ideal case, the parties' views will merge.

These two ways of understanding the doctor–patient relations appear as quite incompatible. Yet, at least for me, they both have some intuitive appeal. When I am a patient, I think that a good doctor is one that I can trust by virtue of the doctor's special knowledge and expertise. However, I also expect that a good doctor does not deal with me as if I knew or understood nothing about my illness, but instead respects my views about my ailment and guides me to an understanding of its diagnosis. Thus, to put it in terms coined by Billig and his colleagues (1988), the doctor's authority and the patient's knowledgeability in the medical consultation are in a "dilemmatic" relation: in spite of their incompatibility, both ideas seem to have some truth in them. Billig argues that many modern professions are characterized by similar kinds of "ideological dilemmas." These dilemmas cannot be resolved by the participants trying to subscribe exclusively to one or the other set of conflicting ideas, but instead by balancing them in their everyday practice.

In this chapter, I will examine the interactions between doctors and patients during a specific phase of medical consultation: at the delivery and reception of diagnosis. Through the examination of these interactions, I will show how doctors and patients simultaneously orient to the doctor's authority and still maintain a degree of mutual intelligibility of the diagnostic procedure. In other words, I will show how the participants in medical consultations find ways of accommodating the doctor's authority with his accountability and the patient's knowledgeability. The first half of the chapter deals with the doctor's utterances in which he or she tells the patient the diagnosis. The latter half focuses on the patients' responses. Before presenting the empirical results, however, I will briefly summarize some earlier research and give details of the data.

Earlier research on diagnosis

The delivery of diagnosis in primary care was first examined by Byrne and Long (1976) in their classic study of doctor–patient interaction in Britain in the early 1970s. According to their account, the doctors regularly adopt a highly authoritarian footing when telling (or, rather, failing to tell) patients about their disease. Most consultations, according to Byrne and Long, contain no real delivery of diagnostic information "of more than two seconds' duration" (1976:50). Doctors very seldom engage in activities such as "selling" their decisions to the patient. Thus the picture painted by Byrne and Long emphasized the doctor's authority and was very close to what one would expect on the basis of the theoretical writings of Parsons (1951), Freidson (1970b), and Abbott (1988): doctors interacted with patients in a way that implicated that diagnostic reasoning was their exclusive property.

More recently, Christian Heath (1992) found that in British general practice patients typically fail to respond with much more than minimal acknowledgment tokens to their doctors' diagnostic statements. He concludes:

> By withholding response to the medical assessment . . . patients relinquish or subordinate their knowledge and opinion concerning the illness . . . and render the co-participant's version as the objective, scientific, and factual assessment of the condition. (1992:264)

In emphasizing the knowledge gap between doctor and patient, Heath's interaction analysis also emphasizes the doctor's authority.

My analysis is grounded in the earlier analyses presented by Byrne and Long (1976) and Heath (1992); see also Heritage (2005). I add a new layer to the analytical depiction of the delivery of diagnosis: intertwined with the "authoritarian" elements, there are also features of interaction in the diagnostic sequences that maintain the doctor's accountability for the evidential basis of the diagnosis, and thereby preserve a degree of mutual intelligibility of the diagnostic process.

Data for the study

With a Finnish research team,[1] we video-recorded and transcribed more than 100 medical consultations. Four health centres were included in the data collection, and 14 doctors participated in the study. Each recorded consultation involved a different patient. Patients were not preselected according to their type of complaint or any other criteria.

[1] The team was led by Marja-Leena Sorjonen and myself, other members being Markku Haakana, Liisa Raevaara, Johanna Ruusuvuori, Tuukka Tammi, and Timo Vottonen.

From the recordings, I collected all diagnostic statements (n = 71). In them, the doctor named the patient's illness or asserted that the patient did not have a named illness.[2] The main analytical task was qualitative – it entailed developing a typology of the doctors' different practices of telling the patient the diagnosis, and of the patients' different practices of responding to the diagnosis. The qualitative analysis also involved an effort to describe the conditions, consequences and interrelations of these practices of the doctors and the patients. I also used quantitative analysis to assess the robustness of the qualitative conclusions.

The interactions presented here took place in primary health care environments. Interaction may be different in other medical contexts, such as specialized or hospital medicine.

How the doctors tell the patient about the diagnosis

As in any human interaction, the delivery of diagnosis can be performed in a number of ways. For example, the doctors have to choose which words they use and at which point of the consultation they deliver the diagnosis (cf. Drew and Heritage 1992). In this half of the chapter, I will focus on one central consideration of doctors when making these choices. (This consideration is not necessarily a conscious one, but by analysing tape-recorded data we can see that it is there.) It has to do with the ways in which the evidential grounds of the diagnosis are available for the patients to observe and to understand. I will argue that the doctors adapt their ways of delivering the diagnosis to the availability of evidence. Thereby, they maintain the mutual intelligibility of the diagnostic procedure. Through these actions, they indicate their accountability, vis-à-vis the patient, for the evidential basis of the diagnosis.

[2] Such statements were included only where the doctor named the illness for the first time, either after the examination of the patient or after the patient had rejected an earlier diagnosis. In other words, cases in which the doctors merely repeated diagnostic statements were not included in the analysis. I also excluded preliminary diagnostic statements: those in which the doctor reported diagnostic reflections during an ongoing examination, before the final diagnostic statement. It should also be noticed that, in professional medical discourse, "giving a diagnosis" is understood exclusively in terms of asserting the existence of a disease. By including the assertions of nonexistence of named diseases, I have adopted a broader definition of diagnosis.

Three types of diagnostic utterance

When doctors name a patient's disease, they can establish the relation between the diagnosis provided and the evidence used in medical reasoning in three different ways. In one type of diagnostic utterance, the doctor merely asserts the character of the condition without bringing out the reasoning on which the diagnosis is based. The second type of diagnostic utterance is designed so as to index a reference to an inferential process, but without explicating any details of that process. In the third type, the core diagnostic utterance is either preceded or followed by utterances with which the doctor, as an additional activity, details some features of the evidence on which his or her diagnostic conclusion is based. Below, I provide examples of each type of diagnostic utterance.[3]

Plain assertions. The following three extracts are examples of diagnostic utterances in which the doctor merely asserts the patient's disease.

(1) (Dgn 96 46B1)
Dr.: There's still an infection in the auditory canal

(2) (Dgn 20 11B1)
Dr.: Here's (.) luckily the bone quite intact,

(3) (Dgn 85 47A1)
Dr.: That's already proper bronchitis.

These utterances are presented as direct descriptions of reality. The doctors speak in a way that implicates their claim to knowledge as an unproblematic, taken-for-granted matter (see Pomerantz 1984b:609). This type of diagnostic utterance contains no verbal description of the reasons or the grounds for the diagnosis.

Diagnoses indexing inexplicit references to the evidence. Another type of diagnostic utterance in our data involves an inexplicit reference to the process by which the diagnosis was made. This reference is most often established by using verbs which formulate the diagnostic conclusion as based on sensory perception and inferences based on that. Extracts (4)–(6) are examples of this type of utterance.

[3] The original Finnish transcripts and word-by-word translations are available from the author.

(4) (Dgn 24 11B3)
Dr.: -> Now there appears to be an (1.0) infection at the contact point of the joint below it in the sac of mucus there in the hip.

(5) (Dgn 37 39B3)
Dr.: >Things like that but< no (0.5) bacterial infection
-> seems to be there.

(6) (Dgn 1 5A2)
Dr.: -> Otherwise the prostate feels really perfectly normal<

Instead of portraying their diagnoses as direct descriptions of reality, here the doctors point to the source of the diagnosis. By employing "evidential" verbs (Chafe and Nichols 1986) "to appear," "to seem," and "to feel," they allude to the sensory evidence on which their conclusions are based. Some of these evidential verbs indicate the general *type* of observation: "feels" in excerpt (6) indexes the observations made by the doctor during rectal examination; and "seems" in (5) indexes the observations made by the doctor while looking into the patient's throat. In (4), however, the construction "appears to be" does not single out any particular type of observation but indexes the doctor's more general observations. In sum, all the verbal constructions in extracts (4)–(6) index a reference to an observational and inferential process, marking the diagnosis as a conclusion that arises from the information that has been made available to the doctor. They do not, however, specify the details of this evidence. Simultaneously these constructions mark the diagnostic statement as tentative: extracts (4)–(6) do not claim the same level of certainty as do the plain assertions shown earlier.[4]

Explicating the evidence of the diagnostic conclusion. In the third type of diagnostic utterance, the doctors describe specific observations as evidence for their diagnostic statements. In some cases, the observations are formulated before the diagnosis; in others, the diagnosis is given first and the evidence formulated only after that. Extracts (7) and (8) are examples of the first type.[5]

[4] Uncertainty of diagnosis is discussed further below.
[5] For the other type, see extract (12).

(7) (Dgn 66 14A3; simplified)
((The doctor has just examined the patient's foot))

1	Dr.:		Okay:. .h fine do put on your,
2			(.)
3	Dr.:	=>	the pulse [can be felt there in your foot so,
4	P:		[↑Thank you.
5		->	.h there's no, in any case (.) no real circulation problem
			. . .
8	Dr.:	->	is <involved>.

(8) (Dgn 26–21A1)

1	Dr.:		(But but) I really can feel these with my fingers
2			here it is you see [( ) this way, a very tight=
3	P:		[Yes,
4	Dr.:		=muscle fiber,
5			(1.0)
6	P:		Yes a little th[ere<
7	Dr.:		[IT GOes here from the top but
8			it probably gives it (.) a bit further down then,
9			(1.0)
10			[((Dr. withdraws her hands from P's back))
11	Dr.:	=>	As [tapping on the vertebrae didn't cause any ↑pain
12		=>	and there aren't (yet) any actual reflection symptoms
13		->	in your legs it suggests a muscle h (h.hhhh)
14		->	complication so hhh it's [only whether hhh (0.4) you
15			[((Dr. lands on her chair.))
16			have been exposed to a draft or has it otherwise=
17			or has it otherwise=
17	P:		=Right,
18	Dr.:		.Hh got irritated,

Both extracts above contain a core diagnostic utterance in which the patient's problem is described by using a medical category (single arrows ->). These cases, however, differ from the others primarily because, in these, the doctor specifies some of his or her observations that form the basis of the diagnosis (double arrows =>). Thus, in extract (7), the doctor says, before delivering his diagnostic statement, that "the pulse can be felt there in your foot" (line 3). And in extract (8) the doctor reports two different observations: first, in line 11 (concerning the vertebrae), and second, in lines 12 and 13 (concerning the reflection symptoms). Using varying discourse

Table 8.1 *Frequency of types of diagnostic turns*

Turn design	Frequency	Percentage
Plain assertion	31	44
Evidence indexing	12	17
Explication of evidence	28	39
Total	71	100

markers, the doctors present their descriptions as reasons for, or evidence of, their diagnostic conclusions.

By explicating the evidence, the doctors make a part of their medical reasoning available to the patients, thus constructing them as *understanding recipients* of that reasoning.[6,7]

In numerical terms, plain assertions were the most frequent type of diagnostic turns in our database, representing well above 40 percent of the diagnostic utterances (see Table 8.1). Turns in which evidence was explicated were also quite frequent, whereas turns indexing inexplicit references to the inferential process were produced least often.

When we consider the verbal form of diagnostic turns, plain assertions seem to conform to the ideas that emphasize the authoritative relation between the doctor and the patient. The fact that diagnosis is delivered in the plain assertion format in not much less than half of the cases could be viewed as indicating the doctor's authority in relation to the patient, at least in these cases: these doctors seem to rest on their authority, without needing to resort to presentation of evidence in order to make the patients accept their diagnoses (see Freidson 1970b:120–1). In what follows, however, I argue that this is not the case. The doctors give plain assertions in activity contexts where the evidence is concretely present; thereby the evidential

6 In research independent of that reported on in this chapter, Maynard (1991d) identified a similar practice in delivering diagnostic news in a developmental disabilities clinic and in HIV-testing clinics. In those contexts, however, "citing of evidence" often accomplished the entire delivery of the diagnostic news: it was left to the patient to infer the conclusion. Heritage and Stivers (1999), on the other hand, described a practice in which the doctor describes the physical examination as it is happening "online." Through this practice, doctors can, for example, resist patient pressure to prescribe medications inappropriately.

7 This, of course, does not necessarily mean that the evidence presented by the doctor to the patient is always the evidence used by the doctor in his or her own reasoning.

grounds of the diagnosis are available for the patients to observe and to understand, and a degree of mutual intelligibility of the diagnostic procedure is maintained. In these actions, the doctors show their accountability for the evidential basis of the diagnosis.

Presence of evidence in plain assertions

When the diagnosis is given in the plain assertion format, the diagnostic statements are regularly positioned so as to allow for the observability of the evidential basis of the diagnosis. By giving the diagnosis at the completion of an examination or immediately thereafter, doctors establish an observable and inferable link between the examination, which the patient participates in or witnesses, and the doctor's diagnostic statement. For example, the doctor may look into the patient's ear, and immediately after doing so may assert that there is an infection in the ear; or he or she may examine a medical document (such as an X-ray) and state the diagnosis directly thereafter. By positioning the diagnostic statement next to the examination, the doctor minimizes what could be called the *inferential distance* between the diagnosis and its grounds: the activity context provides for the observability and the intelligibility of the evidence. In other words, even when giving their diagnoses in the plain assertion format, the doctors couch their actions in such a way that allows the patient to "keep on track" regarding the course of the diagnostic reasoning.

In (9), the patient has a damaged finger. This is his second visit for this complaint; an X-ray was taken between the two visits. (In lines 2–4, the patient talks about the circumstances of the accident.)

(9) (Expansion of [2])

```
1          (5.5)  ((The doctor is examining the X-ray picture
                    against the illuminated screen))
2     P:   It's probably a bit the water as well because,
3          hhh .hhh (0.5) as on the ground you couldn't but roll
4          it but, ,hh there you could lift it a bit.
5          (6.2)  ((Dr. switches off the illuminated screen and
                    returns to his seat. He holds up the X-ray
                    picture between himself and the patient.))
6     Dr.: Here's (.) luckily the bone quite intact,
7     P:   Yeah,
8     Dr.: So within a week it should get better ↑with that splint.
```

When producing his diagnostic statement in line 6, the doctor holds the X-ray in his hand so that it is between himself and the patient. In this context, the referent of the pronoun *here* (line 6) is clear: "here" refers to the X-ray. Therefore the diagnostic statement is hearable as a characterization of the X-ray. Thus the evidence of the diagnostic conclusion – the X-ray picture – is observably present in the activity context.

In the above excerpt, the observably present evidence took the form of a medical document. After a physical examination as well, however, doctors can assert the diagnosis without referring verbally to any evidence. In these cases, too, the positioning of diagnostic statements is critical: because no actions intervene between the examination and the diagnosis, the physical examination is understood as providing the basis for the diagnosis. (For the generic ways in which previous actions form a backdrop for interpreting subsequent actions, see Heritage [1984:254–60]; Schegloff and Sacks [1973:295–8]).

Extract (10) is an example of this situation. The patient has complained about a persistent cold.

(10) (Expansion of [3])
((Dr. has listened to the patient's chest))

Dr.:		Let's listen from the back.
		(0.3)
P:		.nff
	=>	(9.0) ((P breathes in and out, Dr. listens.))
Dr.:	->	That's already proper bronchitis.
P:		Is it [hh
Dr.:		[It is.

Because the doctor utters his diagnostic statement immediately after a single, recognizable act of examination, it becomes apparent that he gathered the information for the diagnosis through this examination. The inferential distance is short because the link between the examination and the diagnosis is transparently accountable for the patient.

Yet the fact that the grounds of the diagnosis are observable and intelligible does not mean that the patient perceives, interprets, or uses the evidence in the same fashion as the doctor. In extract (9), when the doctor examined the X-rays against the illuminated screen (line 1), the patient turned around and glanced briefly at the picture, which was behind him; when the doctor continued the examination (lines 2–4), the patient initiated talk that was not related to the X-ray; and when the doctor held the picture in his hand (line 6), the patient made no effort to look at it more closely. In (10), the patient was unable to observe the parts of her body that the doctor was observing, and the doctor did not describe what he actually perceived during the examination. Thus the participants do not coordinate their actions so as to make the evidence available for the *use* of the patients. The doctors, however, design their actions so as to preserve the observability and intelligibility of the bodily or documentary direction from which the evidence comes.

In summary, when doctors deliver diagnoses using the plain assertion format, they design and locate their diagnostic statements in a way that preserves a specific balance between the doctor's authority on one hand, and the patient's access to the diagnostic procedure on the other. By locating their plain assertions immediately next to relevant and recognizable examinations (as they always do), the doctors make the evidential basis of the diagnosis as transparently present. They design their actions with respect to their accountability for the evidential basis of the diagnosis. Yet, because the patients do not directly topicalize the evidence that is accessible, they orient themselves to the evidence as available to and grounded in expert knowledge and in the cultural authority (Starr 1982) of medicine.

In my database, this pattern – whereby a diagnosis, designed as plain assertion, follows immediately after a relevant, recognizable examination – is the most common format for delivering a diagnosis. Let us consider it as the default pattern of the delivery of diagnosis: "default" not only because it is most common, but also because it is the simplest and most straightforward way to deliver the diagnosis. In this pattern, the direction where the evidence for the diagnosis comes from is made observable for the patient, but the evidence is not verbally addressed, not put into words.

Departures from the default pattern

In some cases, the doctors depart from the default pattern. They move away from the tacit and incarnate accountability (Garfinkel 1967; Heritage 1984a) of diagnosis, and they refer to or discuss the evidence of the diagnosis. That move is made regularly in response to two kinds of contingencies related to the context in which the diagnosis is delivered. First, in some contexts the inferential distance between examination and diagnosis is long, either because the diagnostic statement is detached from the examination or the examination is relatively opaque. In such circumstances, the connection between the examination and its conclusion is jeopardized, and the doctors regularly adopt turn designs other than plain assertions. In this way, they re-establish the observability of the evidence.

In another kind of context, observability per se is not at issue, but rather the routine assumptions concerning the doctor's expertise are challenged, either because the diagnosis is uncertain or because there are manifestly discrepant views concerning it. The doctors manage these situations by using diagnostic turn designs other than plain assertion.

Problems arising from extended inferential distance

Detachment of examination and diagnosis. Temporal separation of examination and diagnosis is often accompanied with modification in the shape of the diagnostic utterance. When other events take place between the examination and the delivery of the diagnosis, the observability of the evidential grounds for the diagnosis is less apparent than when the diagnosis follows immediately after examination. In these circumstances, the doctors often take special measures to make the grounds of the diagnosis observable, referring inexplicitly to these grounds in their diagnostic utterance or by explicating them. In (11), for example, the patient is an elderly lady undergoing a regular checkup, who has reported difficulties in her bowel movements. The doctor examined her stomach by palpation; thereafter, on her own initiative, she examined the patient's breasts. During the breast examination, the doctor recommends that the patient regularly examine her own breasts.

(11) (Dgn U24 41A3)

1 Dr.: . . . it's the best of °all° examinations
2 what #you#,
3 (0.6)
4 Dr.: what you do yourself and then if you would ↑find something
5 from here then you could,

6 (1.1)
7 Dr.: come here and show it >but this is< ↑very smooth the breast
8 gland tis[sue.]
9 P: [° #Y] eah#° I have had in my breasts a very
10 VERy bad milk infection.
11 (1.3)
12 Dr.: How many children you #ha#ve,
13 P: I have one ↑chi°ld° and °I ha-° I [ha- I'm a bit > like a <
14 Dr.: [( )
15 P: risk #mo#th↓er: #ha-# °.hhhh° had difficult de[liver]ies
16 Dr.: [Yeah,]
17 P: or °(l[ike)°,]
18 Dr.: [>F:ine<] now you can pull,
19 (1.2)
20 Dr.: <do↓wn>?
21 (0.7)
((11 lines of discussion on children omitted.))
33 P: . . . God's blessing in that
34 iss(h)ue [t(h)oo (he]h) if you were not able to deliver them
35 [$Yeah:$,]
36 $then you get other ones$,
37 (2.2) ((P is dressing, Dr. takes away paper that covered the examination table))
38 P?: °Hmm°
39 (11.0) ((P dresses and sits down; Dr. takes the paper to trash container and washes her hands.))
40 Dr.: –> ((While returning to her seat:)) Nothing malignant
41 >really< (°.hhh°) #and no#
42 nothing ex[tra] can be felt as being there, (.) n[either the]re
43 P: [hh] [.nfff]
44 Dr.: in your bowels nor there in your <↓brea[°sts°>.]
45 P: [Yeah:]:

Towards the end of the breast examination, in line 12, the doctor asks about the patient's children. In lines 18 and 20, she instructs the patient to rearrange her dress, thereby indicating the completion of the examination. In lines 25–36, more talk about children and grandchildren ensues. While the patient is dressing, the doctor removes the paper cover from the examination table and takes it to the trash container. Thus, when the doctor gives her diagnostic statement in lines 40–44, other activities (discussion of family, patient dressing, and doctor arranging the examination table) have been inserted between the examination and the diagnosis. Moreover,

Table 8.2 *Turn design and positioning of the diagnostic utterance*

Turn design	Positioning relative to examination		
	Adjacent	Detached	Total
Plain assertion	31	0	31
Evidence indexing	6	6	12
Explication of evidence	20	8	28
Total	57	14	71

Chi-square = 15.9515 $p < .001$

the breast examination took place between the examination of the patient's bowels and the diagnosis.

Thus, when the doctor initiates her diagnostic statement in line 40, she is speaking in an environment that is sequentially detached from the relevant events and objects that could serve as grounds for the diagnosis. Unlike the cases in which the doctors used "plain assertions," the basis of the diagnosis is no longer prominent here. In this context, the doctor chooses to refer indirectly to the inferential process by using the construction "nothing extra can be felt as being there." Through this turn design, which suggests that what she says is based on the sensory data that she has gathered, the doctor *retrieves the examination of the patient* as a context for her talk (see Drew and Heritage 1992:18–19). In other words, the construction "can be felt" reinvokes the palpation of the patient's body as the basis for the diagnostic conclusion.

Quantitative analysis confirms the relation between turn design and the positioning of the diagnostic utterance in relation to the examination of the patient or relevant documents (see Table 8.2).

The plain assertion design is used exclusively in cases where the diagnostic statement follows immediately after the examination.[8] There are not many cases where the diagnosis is detached from the relevant examination, but when the diagnosis is delivered in such circumstances the doctors systematically choose more complex turn designs. By thus reinvoking the examination, they re-establish

[8] The results are not derived from a random sample, and the chi-square is used in this and the following tables only heuristically, to show the magnitude of the patterns discussed.

the mutual intelligibility of the evidential basis of the diagnosis. Thereby, they orient to their accountability, vis-à-vis the patient, for the evidential basis of the diagnosis. If the doctors did not reinvoke the examination, they would be heard as taking a more authoritarian stance than they actually take.

Opacity of examination. Another context where the balance between authority and accountability is achieved by modifying diagnostic turn design is one where the relevant events in the examination are opaque. For example, the examination of the patient may include a number of different actions, and it may be unclear to the patient which of these, if any, provide evidence for the doctor's diagnosis. By explicating some features of the evidence, the doctor may make the grounds of the diagnosis observable for the patient.

The plain assertion design is used, first and foremost, in cases where the relevant events in examination are transparent to a lay participant. After an opaque examination, on the other hand, the doctors are most likely to choose the design of the diagnostic turn in which they explicate the evidence (for a more detailed discussion, see Peräkylä 1998:311–12). If the examination is not transparent, the doctors, rather than "resting on the authority of their professional status" (Freidson 1970b:120), are likely to explicate the evidence for the patient.

In summary, in some cases the inferential distance between examination and diagnosis is long, either because the examination is opaque from the lay perspective or because it is temporally detached from the diagnosis. In these two types of case, the observability of the evidence is jeopardized; the doctors, as we saw, rather than trading on their authority alone, designed their diagnostic utterances so that these utterances inexplicitly incorporated references to the evidence for the diagnostic conclusion or explicated that evidence.

Problems arising from challenges to medical expertise

In the cases I will now discuss, observability per se is not at stake. Rather, in these cases the doctor's expertise becomes problematic because of uncertainty or disagreement. In such circumstances, a display of evidence is a way to retain a claim to knowledge.

Uncertainty of diagnosis. One type of context in which the doctor's expertise is potentially undermined involves uncertainty of diagnosis. In most cases involving uncertainty the doctors use turn designs other than plain assertion. Through these designs they can indicate their reasons for the proposed diagnosis. Thereby, the doctors orient themselves, in a special way, to their accountability for the evidential basis of an uncertain diagnosis. If the doctor does not know definitely what the patient's disorder is, he or she treats it as relevant to indicate verbally to the patient the basis of what he or she does know. Accountability and authority are closely intertwined here. Uncertainty undermines the doctor's authority as an expert; thus, when delivering an uncertain diagnosis, the doctor cannot rest on authority alone. By displaying evidence, the doctor earns his or her claim to knowledge. (For a more detailed discussion on uncertainty of diagnosis, see Peräkylä 1998:312–14.)

Discrepant views concerning the diagnosis. The doctor's authority is also potentially undermined in a diagnostic sequence where a discrepancy between the patient's and the doctor's views is manifest. In such circumstances, the doctors most often select a diagnostic turn design that involves explication of evidence.

Doctors often resort to explication of evidence when the delivery of the diagnosis involves explicit disconfirmation of candidate explanations expressed by the patient during the examination (see Gill 1998a; Gill and Maynard this volume; Raevaara 1996a), or when the doctor reasserts or corrects a diagnosis which he or she previously spelled out but which thereafter was questioned by the patient. Typically (but not exclusively) the discrepancy between the patient's and the doctor's views concerns the seriousness of the ailment: the doctor's diagnosis is less serious than the one proposed by the patient (cf. Heritage and Robinson's and Halkowski's discussions on "doctorability" in this volume).[9]

In the following extract, the doctor explicitly disconfirms the diagnostic suggestion offered by the patient. The patient suffered from intense pain in her leg and was making a follow-up visit after a sick leave. Early in the medical interview, the patient suggested that the pain in her thigh might have been caused by exertion or by "something either coming or going" in the thigh. The doctor

[9] Because the overwhelming majority of the consultations in our data set involve ordinary health problems rather than serious conditions or life-threatening situations, the management of serious diagnoses cannot be addressed properly here. See Lutfey and Maynard (1998) and Maynard and Frankel (this volume) for relevant discussions.

treats this comment as if the patient was referring to "thrombosis," a suggestion that the doctor explicitly disconfirms in her diagnostic utterance toward the end of the consultation:

(12) (Dgn 3 1B2)

1	Dr.:		Well (.) we'll have to follow up how this thigh of
2			yours, (0.6) .hh begins to respond and, (0.8) it has
3			indeed now clearly improved from °what
4			it is [and,°
5	P:		[It has at least in terms of pain th[e:n.
6	Dr.:		[Yeah:.
7			(0.4)
8	Dr.:		Yes:. .h >Did you have laboratory tests< now: sti[ll
9	P:		[NO:.
			((10 lines omitted))
20	Dr.:		Yes:.
21			(2.0)
22	Dr.:	->	.hh Well (0.8) I haven:'t (0.2) I I (1.0) haven't
23		->	(0.3) considered it as a (0.2) thrombosis.
24	P:		Mm hm,
25	Dr.:	=>	I think it isn't, (0.5) it would have,=if there would
26		=>	have been a beginning of a thrombosis then it would
27		=>	have been much more pain↑ful.
28	P:		Yes right.
29	Dr.:		So certainly there are the VARICOSE veins.
30			(0.8)
31	P:		Somethi- yeah I can feel the very lumps there
32			in a certain position ((continues))

The disconfirmation takes place for the first time in lines 22–23. Then, in line 25, after an acknowledgment by the patient, the doctor "elaborates" her view (cf. Maynard 1997). She first renews the disconfirmation and, thereafter, she explicates evidence that supports her conclusion. She explains what the symptoms for thrombosis would have been. The patient's agreeing receipt (line 28) is followed immediately by the doctor's substitute diagnosis in line 29. This, however, is presented as one that does not exhaustively explain the patient's problems. The patient aligns with the doctor's suggestion and herself refers to evidence for that (lines 31–32).

In extract (12), the discrepancy between the patient's candidate explanation and the doctor's rejection constitutes the controversial character of the diagnosis. In some other cases, the discrepancy arises at a later stage, through the patient's response to the doctor's initial diagnosis. In such cases, the doctor may resort to explication of evidence in pursuing the diagnosis.

In (13), for example, the patient has come to see the doctor because of a persistent cough. She has made an earlier visit because of the same complaint, but in spite of the medication the cough has not been cured. The doctor orders new examinations (chest X-ray and blood tests) for the patient. At the beginning of the extract below, the participants have already been finalizing the arrangements for the examinations and a new appointment. While the doctor is dealing with a paper, the patient asks a question concerning pneumonia vaccination in lines 1–3.

(13) (Dgn133 27A1)

1 P: How is it there, is it possible for me to have the,
2 the erm:: eh- which vaccinations are there, (.) >the
3 pneumonia vaccination<,
4 Dr.: Yes, but it cannot be given to you now as you have
5 this,(.) this disease?, kind of (.) [on, [so
6 [be- [Yes,
7 Dr.: this mu[st be cured] before, .hh[hh
8 P: [So later it,] [Quite right,
9 Dr.: before we can give [( ),
10 P: [Yes yes,
11 Dr.: Krhm krhm .hh
12 P: Was it pneumonia then really [as,
13 Dr.: [Well it has been pneumonia
14 because, #m:# there is, (0.8) #erm::# in the, (0.5) X-ray
15 of lungs it could be seen< seen and ↑the
16 se[dimentation rate was also so hig]h that, .hh that<
17 P: [Yes right,]
18 Dr.: really it is °but now for some,° (0.2) some reason it
19 has not got cured I'll eh- (.) I'll prescribe
20 for you still another medication ((continues))

The doctor tells the patient that she cannot be vaccinated before her current disease has been cured (lines 4–5, 7, and 9). It is notable that the doctor refers to the disease with the expression "this disease," thus not specifying the diagnosis but treating it as a known-in-common object. Thereafter, the patient inquires about the diagnosis in line 12. The question implies that the patient's disease has been considered as pneumonia; but on the other hand the question

Table 8.3 *Turn design and controversiality of diagnosis*

	Controversiality of diagnosis		
Turn design	Noncontroversial	Controversial	Total
Plain assertion	29	2	31
Evidence indexing	10	2	12
Explication of evidence	11	17	28
Total	50	21	71

Chi-square = 21.9525 $p < .001$

also incorporates a degree of doubt concerning this diagnosis. In line 13, the doctor reasserts the diagnosis of pneumonia initially made during an earlier visit. The reassertion is supported by the explication of the evidence in lines 13–16. In the final part of the doctor's diagnostic utterance (lines 18–19) it also transpires that the pneumonia has not been cured yet.

In the two cases discussed above, the doctors resorted to explication of the evidence when discrepant views concerning the diagnosis had been made manifest in the interaction. Discrepancy, like uncertainty, potentially undermines the doctor's expert role. The doctors responded by explaining the evidence; they pursued the diagnosis by accounting for it. Thus, when delivering a diagnosis in a context of discrepant views, they considered themselves as accountable for the grounds of their diagnostic statements. They justified their diagnostic conclusions by giving explicit reasons for those conclusions.

Quantitative analysis supports the qualitative results described above. All the diagnostic statements were coded in terms of their controversiality; the results are shown in Table 8.3.

When the diagnosis is controversial, the doctors seldom choose the plain assertion or the turn design in which they refer indirectly to the evidence. Instead they choose explication of the evidence.

Yet we could not observe open manifestations of the controversial status of the diagnosis in every case in which the doctor explicated the evidence for the diagnosis. In more than one third of these cases, the diagnosis was not presented overtly as involving a controversy between the patient's and the doctor's views. In some of these cases, however, a more subtle misalignment was observable between the doctor's and the patient's position: the doctor's diagnosis was hearable as suggesting that no major problem existed, whereas the patient had presented the condition as a serious trouble. Extract (8), for example, contains no open discrepancy between the participants' views. Throughout the description of the problem, however, the patient portrays the pain in the back as exceptionally intense and puzzling for her. She does not present any candidate explanations (see Gill and Maynard this volume) before the doctor gives the diagnosis, but the doctor's explication of evidence nevertheless may be a response to the patient's unarticulated worry. By explicating the evidence (which takes the form of symptoms that are not present), she demonstrates the grounds for excluding some other, more severe (but unnamed) diagnostic possibilities.

Telling the diagnosis: a summary

In the empirical analyses presented thus far, we have seen that doctors in Finnish primary care adapt their diagnostic utterances to considerations that concern the visibility and the intelligibility (for the patient) of the evidential basis of the diagnosis. In their actions, they orient to their accountability, vis-à-vis the patient, for the evidential basis of the diagnosis. In the "default pattern," the doctor does not verbally refer to evidence, but locates the diagnostic utterance immediately after a transparent examination, thereby making it possible for the patient to see the link between the examination and the diagnosis. I have also argued that there are four kinds of circumstances where the doctors resort to implicit references to evidence or outright explication of evidence. This happens when the diagnostic utterance is temporally detached from the relevant examinations, when the examination is opaque for the patient, when there is uncertainty, or where there are discrepant views concerning the diagnosis. In other words, in those circumstances the doctors take extra measures to secure the visibility and the intelligibility of the evidence.

The patients' responses to the doctors' diagnostic utterances

In the remaining parts of this chapter, I will explore the ways in which the patients' responses to the doctors' diagnostic statements incorporate the patients' claim of knowledgeability concerning the diagnostic reasoning, and an expectation of the doctors' ultimate authority. My main focus will be on cases in which the patients respond more than minimally to the diagnoses, and it is in these extended responses that the patients display their knowledgeability. The patients talk more than minimally after about one third of diagnostic statements. First, I will show that the extended responses occur most likely after diagnostic statements in which the doctor displays his or her own diagnostic reasoning through the design of the diagnostic utterance. Thereafter, I will explore some types of extended responses, showing how the participants cooperatively maintain a balance between an orientation to the patient's knowledgeability concerning the diagnosis and an orientation to the doctor's authority.

When do the patients talk after hearing the diagnosis?

The patients' ways of receiving the doctors' diagnostic statements can be divided into three broad classes: silence, minimal acknowledgment tokens such as "yeah," "yes," and "ahem,"[10] and extended responses. Some of the minimal acknowledgment tokens are designed to encourage further elaboration of the diagnostic statement or its implications in terms of treatment, while others do not overtly have such characteristics. Silences may also operate as elicitation of elaboration (cf. Maynard 1997). Further research is evidently needed regarding the work that the minimal responses and silences do after the diagnostic statements (see Robinson [2003] for a discussion on "progressivity" between the diagnostic sequence and the talk about diagnosis).

The third class of responses includes all responses where the patients do something more than just minimally acknowledge the diagnosis, e.g., cases where they (for example) show that the diagnosis is unexpected from their point of view, or verbally indicate agreement or disagreement, or describe symptoms that may be discrepant with the diagnosis. These responses entail that the progression of talk from diagnosis to other business (usually treatment) be postponed, at least for the time that the patient produces his or her

[10] These are English representations of Finnish response tokens used in the consultations. The original Finnish tokens include, e.g., "Joo.," "Juu.," "Nii.," "Jaa::," "Mm:," and "Aha," (cf. Sorjonen 1997, 2001).

Table 8.4 *Controversiality of diagnosis and the patient's response*

	Patient's response		
Controversiality of diagnosis	None or minimal	Extended	Total
No explicit controversy	37	13	50
Explicit controversy	11	10	21
Total	48	23	71

Pearson chi 2 (1) = 3.1561 p = .076

response. Moreover, the extended responses often incorporate the patient's claim to knowledge concerning the diagnosis.

In our sample of 71 diagnostic statements, these three types of responses are almost evenly distributed: no response was given by the patient in 23 cases, minimal acknowledgment in 25 cases, and an extended response in 23 cases. Thus, the Finnish patients actively took part in the diagnostic sequence in almost one third of cases. At least one extended response was produced in consultations of all except two doctors.

What, then, encourages the patients to talk, and thereby to adopt the role of a knowledgeable agent? According to Heath (1992:246–60), active patient responses typically follow diagnoses that are formatted as questions, presented as uncertain, or show implicitly or explicitly that the doctor's view of the condition differs from what the patient expected. In the Finnish data, there were no diagnoses formulated as questions. However, there were diagnoses that were presented as uncertain and those that showed discrepancy between the doctor's view and the patient's expectations. These features of diagnostic utterances are associated with the type of patient response that also occurred in the Finnish data; see Tables 8.4 and 8.5.

Table 8.4 indicates the relation between conflict in diagnosis and the patient's response. As in Table 8.3 shown at an earlier part of this chapter, the diagnosis here was also regarded as one involving conflict when the delivery of the diagnosis involves explicit rejection or correction of diagnostic suggestions expressed by the patient during the examination, or when the doctor reasserts or corrects a diagnosis which he or she previously spelled out but which thereafter was questioned by the patient. In our data, the relative proportion of extended responses is bigger after diagnoses that involve conflict.

Table 8.5 *Certainty of diagnosis and the patient's response*

	Patient's response		
Controversiality of diagnosis	None or minimal	Extended	Total
Uncertain	16	12	28
Certain	32	11	43
Total	48	23	71

Pearson chi 2 (1) = 2.3109 $p = .128$

Table 8.6 *Diagnostic turn design and the patient's response*

	Patient's response		
Diagnostic turn design	None or minimal	Extended	Total
Explication of evidence	12	16	28
Evidence indexing	9	3	12
Plain assertion	27	4	31
Total	48	23	71

Pearson chi 2 (2) = 13.5079 $p = .001$

However, this association is not statistically significant. Even weaker is the association between uncertainty in diagnosis and the patient's extended response seen in Table 8.5.

There was, however, a much stronger, statistically significant association ($p = .001$) between the type of the patient's response on one hand, and the design of the doctor's diagnostic utterance on the other. It was the way that the diagnostic utterance displayed evidence of the diagnostic conclusion that was associated with the type of response. Most of the extended responses occurred after diagnostic turns where the doctor verbally explicated the evidence for the diagnostic conclusion. The two other diagnostic turn designs (turns indexing inexplicit references to evidence and plain assertions with no reference to evidence) attracted far fewer extended responses. In particular, plain assertions were very infrequently followed by extended responses (see Table 8.6).

The explication of evidence makes it much more likely that the patient will produce an extended response to diagnosis than the two other diagnostic turn designs. Thus, it appears that by explicating the evidence for the diagnostic conclusion, the doctor proposes a particular relation between the patient and himself or herself – one where the patient's reflections of the diagnosis are relevant and welcome.

It was shown in an earlier part of this chapter that uncertainty and conflict are in turn associated with the diagnostic turn design; the explication of evidence in diagnosis is more likely when the diagnosis involves uncertainty or conflict. In other words, explication of evidence is a practice that the doctors often resort to when the diagnosis is uncertain or involves conflict.[11] Thus, it appears that the diagnostic interaction can take two different trajectories that are separated from early on. In one type of case, the doctor produces the diagnosis in "plain assertion" format, and the patient remains passive while receiving it. In the other type of case, the delivery of diagnosis is made complicated by the inferential distance between the examination and the diagnosis, or by challenges to medical authority (uncertainty or discrepancy of views). In these circumstances, the doctors often resort to implicit references to, or explication of, the evidential basis of the diagnosis; and in particular if the doctor has explicated the evidence, the patient is then in his or her turn likely to respond to the diagnosis by producing his or her own talk. The doctor's choice of design of the diagnostic utterance is in a pivotal position here: retrospectively, the diagnostic utterance constructs the preceding activity (usually the medical interview and the examination) as routine or as potentially having involved some problematic aspects in it and, prospectively, it shapes the field or relevancies for the patient's recipient action.[12]

Quantitative analysis of interaction remains, however, necessarily quite far from the actual dynamics of the momentarily unfolding actions of the people who are interacting (Schegloff 1993). In the

[11] An elaboration of the four variables involved shows that, if "uncertainty" and "conflict" are controlled, the association between the form of reference to evidence and the patient's response remains strong when the diagnosis involves neither uncertainty nor conflict, whereas it is much weaker (but does not disappear altogether) when one of these or both are involved.

[12] I want to point out that this involves an active choice by the doctor: he or she *can* construct a case routine (by merely asserting the diagnosis) even if the patient has displayed problems in it; or, alternatively, he or she can treat a case as problematic (by, for example, explicating the evidence) even if there has not been any overt and explicit indications of problems in it; see extracts (8) and (15).

final part of the chapter, we will return to qualitative case-by-case analysis. We will focus on cases where the patients present themselves as knowledgeable agents. Two types of case will be considered: those where the patient explicitly agrees with the doctor's diagnosis, and others where the patient resists it.

Patient displaying agreement

In some cases, the patients say that they agree with the diagnosis that the doctor has proffered. Extract (14) below is an example of this kind of situation. During the physical examination, the patient proffered two candidate explanations for her presenting problem (pain in the hip): cancer and infection (data not shown). In his diagnostic utterance (taking place after the exam and some paperwork and involving an indexed reference to the inferential process), the doctor does not comment upon the patient's candidate explanations. However, his conclusion corresponds to one of the patient's earlier explanations:

(14) (Dgn 24 11B3)

Dr.: Now there appears to be an (1,0) infection at the contact point
of the joint below it in the sac of mucus there [in the hip.]
P: -> [Yes right. .hh]
P: -> that's what I (think/thought) myself too that <it probably
-> must be an infection>. [.hhhh
Dr.: [And, because you have had
P: trouble this [long we will make sure and take an X-[ray.]
P: [hhhhh [Yes:.]

In lines 3–5, partially overlapping with the completion of the doctor's diagnostic statement, the patient responds with an acknowledgment and then expands her turn by saying, "Yes right. .hh that's what I (think/thought)[13] myself too that <it probably must be an infection>." By reporting her agreement, the patient treats herself as an agent capable of diagnostic reasoning. But at the same time, however, both participants also treat the domain of medical reasoning as something that ultimately belongs to the doctor. This is observable in a number of features.

[13] In the video recording, the tense of the verb "think" is ambiguous. If the patient is heard to speak in past tense, her utterance is also hearable as one that retrieves her earlier candidate explanation (Raevaara 2000).

First, the patient designs her agreement as arising from a distinct personal *perspective*. Through the turn beginning "that's what I (think/thought) myself too" she frames her agreement as a report of her own thoughts, not of "objective" realities (cf. Heath 1992; Maynard 1991c). Second, the patient formulates the diagnosis using probabilistic and non-specific terms ("it probably must be an infection"), thus portraying her conception of the illness as much more general than that of the doctor, who had given a detailed specification concerning the site of the infection (in lines 1–2). And third, it is also noticeable that by moving on to the next phase of the consultation (announcement of future action) immediately after the patient's turn, the doctor does not topicalize or otherwise take note of the patient's report of her thoughts. Through the continuation marker "And" at the beginning of his turn in line 6, the doctor frames his talk about the further examinations as a continuation of the diagnostic statement (lines 1–2) – thus "sequentially deleting" the patient's comment. Through this non-attention, the doctor constructs his own diagnostic reasoning and that of the patient as two separate processes (Raevaara 2000).

In sum, therefore, in extract (14) the patient presented herself as a knowledgeable agent in diagnostic reasoning by expressing an explicit agreement with the doctor's diagnosis. This agency had both self-imposed and externally imposed limits: the patient presented her diagnostic thinking as markedly subjective and approximate, and the doctor treated the patient's statement as not a relevant target for further talk. Hence, along with allowing for the patient's agency, the participants collaboratively treated the details of the process of medical reasoning as something belonging exclusively to the doctor's domain.

Patients resisting the doctors' diagnosis

Consider again extract (15) below, which was shown earlier as extract (8). Before the delivery of the diagnostic statement, the doctor has undertaken a long physical examination of the patient, who has complained about a sudden pain in her back. In lines 1–8, the doctor reports some of her observations while palpating the patient's back. She then withdraws from the patient (line 10) and, while returning to her seat, she tells the patient her diagnostic conclusion.

In her diagnostic utterance, the doctor first explicates the evidence for the diagnosis (lines 11–13), thereafter delivering the diagnosis proper (lines 13–14). Immediately after the diagnosis, she then moves on to speculate about the possible cause of the ailment (lines 14–16, 18). As it was pointed out above, this case does not involve any overt disagreement between the patient and the doctor before the delivery of the diagnosis; but by explicating the evidence for the non-serious diagnostic conclusion, the doctor seems to be attending to the fact that the patient has described the problem as particularly worrisome and puzzling.

(15) (Expansion of [8])

Dr.:	(But but) I really can feel these with my fingers
	here it is you see [( ) this way, a very tight=
P:	[Yes,
Dr.:	=muscle fiber,
	(1.0)
P:	Yes a little th[ere<
Dr.:	[IT GOes here from the top but
	it probably gives it (.) a bit further down then,
	(1.0)
	[((Dr. withdraws her hands from P's back))
Dr.:	As [tapping on the vertebrae didn't cause any ↑pain
	and there aren't (yet) any actual reflection symptoms
	in your legs it suggests a muscle h (.hhhh)
	complication so hhh it's [only whether hhh (0.4) you
	[((Dr. lands on her chair.))
	have been exposed to a draft or has it otherwise=
P:	=Right,
Dr.:	.Hh got irrita[ted,
P:	[It couldn't be from somewhere inside then
	as ↑ it is a burning feeling there so it couldn't be
	in the kidneys or somewhere (that p[ain,)
Dr.:	[Have you
	had any tr- (0.2) trouble with urinating.=
	=a pa- need to urinate more frequently or
	any pains when you urinate,

The patient's first response to the doctor's diagnostic statement occurs in line 17. Through her "Right," the patient receives the prior turn (concerning the possible origins of the ailment) as informative and as something that makes sense and/or can be agreed with (cf. Heritage and Sefi 1992; Sorjonen 1997). The next time the patient speaks is in line 19, slightly overlapping with the completion of the doctor's reflections about the origin of the complication. The patient's comments at lines 19–21 take up and question the doctor's diagnostic conclusion. Her utterance is constructed as a multi-unit turn.

First, in line 19, she offers (in the form of a question) a characterization of the location of the trouble that is marked as contrastive to what the doctor has said. Toward the end of her turn she specifies this location, again in the form of a Yes/No question. In between these two proposals, she proffers evidence: "as it is a burning feeling." Thus, this patient not only provides a symptom description that is presented as discrepant with the doctor's diagnosis (which she does in line 20), but she also formulates her own diagnostic proposal concerning what these symptoms possibly could be a sign of (lines 19 and 21).

However, while talking about the diagnosis (and thus displaying her knowledgeability concerning it), the patient also orients to the doctor's ultimate authority in the medical domain. Through the use of a question format in her diagnostic suggestions (lines 19–21), and through the question design that is built to accommodate a rejection of her suggestion (cf. Stivers 2000), the patient displays a commitment that the doctor's view is correct and it is the doctor who will ultimately diagnose the trouble. The way in which she formulates her diagnostic proposals concerning the location of the ailment is nontechnical and approximate ("from somewhere inside then" and "in the kidneys or somewhere"). Moreover, the evidence that the patient produces in line 20 is of "experiential" nature: by saying *as* "it is a burning feeling" the patient describes a bodily sensation to which she only has access (cf. Peräkylä and Silverman 1991). This subjective evidence is in contrast with the objective evidence produced by the doctor in lines 11–13 (cf. Maynard 1991c:479).

In spite of their cautious and subjective character, the patient's diagnostic reflections are taken up by the doctor, who withholds the move to discussion about treatment which otherwise would have been projectable here (Byrne and Long 1976; Heath 1992; Robinson 2003). Instead, in lines 22–25, she resumes a verbal examination. The new examination (focusing on possible troubles with urinating) can be seen as motivated by the patient's suggestion that the trouble might reside in the kidneys. The doctor's questions follow immediately after the patient's query and, hence, they are offered as preliminary to answering the patient's question. In resuming the examination, the doctor acknowledges the patient's response as a legitimate basis for reconsidering the diagnosis.

Extract (16) below is another example of the patient's explicit resistance to the diagnosis. In this case, the patient has come for a health check. The extract is from the beginning of the consultation. The doctor is examining papers that may have come from a nurse who has seen the patient before the doctor.

(16) (Dgn 29–21A2)

Dr.: So there's a hearing defect at some point hhhh
(0.3) ((Dr. goes through the papers))
Dr.: ((Focusing her gaze on a paper:)) or well that
doesn't actually look quite like a hearing defect that,
(0.5) ((Dr. gazes at the paper))
P: Mm::[::
Dr.: [cu:rve as there's such an even decline in the
<other ear.>
(0.8) ((Dr. gazes at the paper.))
P: Well in a way probably a defect but it is
one tha : : : :t erm (0.4) has (.) came up already
a long time ago an:d (2.0) I don't know then whether it
is : : from work of is i:t (.) from an illness
but (I don't),
(0.2)
B[ecause >you know I have< worked on a paper machine.
Dr.: [Nyeah,
Dr.: Ye:[:s,
P: [In a paper factory,
(0.5)
Dr.: Ex[actly,]
P: [So in] that sense: (0.2) it may also be from
that.
(0.3)
Dr.: .mhh
(0.5)
P: Or not from that.
Dr.: Or not from that.
(0.3)
Dr.: When was it that this was first taken
notice of do you have any: recolle[ction: of r- that,]
P: [hh mmmm hhhhhh] Might

have been s: : :a:y ten year[s ago. hhhh]h
Dr.: ['rs ago]
Dr.: Yeah,=
P: =Something was then: : (.) when the first curves
were taken then it was found that there is something
((continues))

At line 1, the doctor identifies a probable diagnosis (a hearing defect) that is likely found in the records. Subsequently, while looking at the fresh hearing test result, she corrects herself (lines 3–4) and describes the evidence that she sees in the curve (lines 7–8). Via the correction, the diagnosis becomes problematic (for the author of the records, "hearing defect" has been a plausible diagnosis, but the doctor disagrees), and the description of evidence is alive to this problem. In his response to the diagnosis, the patient at first disagrees with the doctor's corrected diagnosis by insisting on the initial one: "Well in a way probably a defect" (line 10). He then proceeds to an elaborated account concerning the history and the background of the defect (lines 10–27). After the patient's account, the doctor takes up his contrastive diagnostic proposal in her follow-up question that seeks more information about the history of the trouble and the medical attention it has previously received (beginning from lines 30–31; continuation not shown).

It is obvious that by insisting on a diagnosis that has been rejected by the doctor, the patient assumes a role in which he is capable of diagnostic thinking. However, the way in which he does his disagreement also betrays a constant orientation to the doctor's ultimate authority in this sphere. Three features of the lengthy diagnostic segment are particularly significant. First, it is noticeable that the patient's disagreement is done "in the auspices of" the doctor's initial diagnostic statement. It was the doctor who first said that there is a hearing defect, and thus the patient insists on a diagnosis that *the doctor* has first suggested, not a diagnosis that he himself would have independently arrived at.[14] Second, in his account following the formulation of the disagreement, the patient draws attention

[14] It is quite possible, if not likely, that the reference to a "hearing defect" is in the papers that the doctor has read, as a result of the patient having told the nurse about it before the consultation. Even if that is the case, the doctor nevertheless herself spells out this diagnosis, and in the current interaction the patient insists on a diagnosis that has once been spelled out by the doctor.

not only to his own understandings, but also to the expertise of other medical professionals. In lines 11–12, he tells the doctor that the alleged defect came up long time ago. By using a Finnish word ("*ilmeni*") here, the patient alludes that the defect was identified *by somebody else than himself*, thus alluding to medical professionals that have been involved.[15] And third, when the patient moves on to speculate about the origin of the alleged defect, he suggests that it is caused by him having worked on a paper machine (lines 16–23). The doctor withholds uptake (see especially lines 24–26) – and in the face of that the patient explicitly backs down from his theory (line 27), thereby receiving marked acknowledgment from the doctor, who in line 28 repeats the patient's utterance whereby he backed down. By withholding uptake, the doctor couches the patient to offer backdown, with the result that the doctor does not need to "officially" assert that the patient is wrong.

Thus, in (16), in assuming the role of an knowledgeable agent in the domain of diagnostic reasoning, the patient simultaneously acknowledged the doctor's (and the medical profession's) authority in this area. The agency that he assumed was accountably produced by himself as agency operating in a world that is ultimately defined and guarded by the profession.

Responses to diagnosis: a summary

In the latter half of this chapter, I have explored the patients' extended responses to the doctors' diagnostic statements. I started with quantitative analysis which showed that the Finnish primary health care patients respond with more than acknowledgment tokens after about one third of doctors' diagnostic statements. Comparable exact numbers of patient responses have not been provided in earlier research, but the thrust of Heath's (1992) influential

[15] The doctor hears the patient's talk this way, which is indicated by her choosing the passive form in her follow-up question in lines 30–31. She doesn't ask when the patient has taken notice of the problem but, rather, when the problem "was first taken notice of," thus implicating other persons' possible involvement. And finally, in an expansion to his answer, by referring to the time "when the first curves were taken" (lines 36–37), the patient unequivocally indicates the involvement of medical professionals (and medical technology) in the identification of the "defect."

discussion suggests that the British patients in 1980s may have been more passive than the Finnish patients in the 1990s.

In the quantitative part of this study, we also found that the extended responses are most likely to occur after diagnostic statements in which the doctors explicate the evidence for the diagnostic conclusion. This observation has direct practical implications. It suggests that if (in a particular consultation) the doctor considers the patient's participation in discussion about diagnosis welcome, one thing that a doctor can do to foster such participation is to indicate to the patient some of the evidential grounds of the diagnosis.

The fact that the patients are passive after diagnosis in two-thirds of cases may be an indication of their submission in the face of medical authority, as Heath (1992) suggested. On the other hand, two other things may also be involved here. One is the patients' possible orientation to a generic "new delivery sequence" (Maynard 1997), where an extended response is not required from the recipient, and the other is the patients' possible orientation to the "progressivity" of the consultation (Robinson 2003). By remaining passive the patients can simply show their recipiency, and/or they can indicate their expectation that discussion on treatment or other future action will ensue. But my primary interests here were the one third of the cases where the patients responded actively and thereby halted the progression of the consultation towards "post-diagnosis" phases. I noted (again, essentially in line with Heath's earlier observations) that the patients design these responses in a cautious manner, consistently displaying an orientation to the difference between their own and the doctors' ways of reasoning. The primary way for the patients to express their reservations toward the diagnosis is to offer additional observations discrepant with the diagnosis. These additional observations come from outside the realm of the physical examination or the examination of documents; they are not observations of the things that the doctor has been examining, but they are about something that the patient has direct access to (bodily sensations or reports from everyday life). If the doctors present their observations as evidence to support the diagnosis, the patients in most cases systematically refrain from any discussion concerning these observations, let alone question the inferential procedures from the observations to the diagnostic conclusion.

The extracts of extended responses that we have examined suggest that primary care patients can, and in a number of cases do, assume a degree of agency and knowledgeability in relation to their diagnoses. They have available ways for displaying agreement and disagreement with the diagnosis. But their agency and knowledgeability are intertwined and also overshadowed by the patients' and the doctors' orientation to the doctor's authority in the domain of medical reasoning. This dual orientation is perhaps most strikingly encapsulated in those cases where the patient responds to a diagnostic utterance where the doctor has explicated the evidence for his or her conclusion (and that is where most of the active responses occur). The explication of evidence "opens up" patients to talk after the diagnosis. But in their talk that follows the diagnosis, the patients systematically avoid addressing the very evidence that the doctors explicated.

Conclusion

In the beginning of this chapter, I pointed out the dilemma between the expectations concerning the doctor's authority and the patient's knowledgeability in medical consultations. The dilemma first came up through literature on medical consultations: some texts emphasize the authoritarian aspects of the relation, while others describe it as a dialogue between two differently but equally resourceful agents. The dilemma, found in texts, motivated the empirical study of diagnostic sequences which was reported in this chapter.

Throughout the chapter, I have explored different facets of this dilemma in the context of the delivery and the reception of the doctors' diagnostic utterances. Again and again we have seen how the "symmetric" or "dialogical" qualities of interaction – the ways in which the doctors systematically orient to their accountability for the evidential basis of the diagnosis and the ways in which the patients adopt an active, knowledgeable position in responding to the diagnostic statements – are intertwined and also overshadowed with the participants' orientation to the doctor's ultimate authority in the domain of medical reasoning (cf. Heritage 2005).

The upshot of these observations for medical practice is twofold. *First*, I want to suggest – in line with Atkinson (1982) and Silverman (1987) – that those versions of "patient centeredness" which assume that the patient's knowledge and experience can or should provide a frame of reference for the consultation, as an alternative to, or as an equal partner of, the doctor's expert knowledge, are out of touch with the interactional reality of medical consultation. The doctor's authority seems to be a constitutive feature of medical interaction. As far as I can see, deleting the doctor's authority would entail that the interaction would not any more be medical at all; and I see no reason to advocate that. But *secondly*, I also want to point out that the doctor's authority does not exclude the building of genuine doctor–patient partnership (cf. Roter and Hall 1992; Maynard 1991c). At least in the diagnostic sequences that I have considered in this chapter, the participants regularly find ways of accommodating the doctor's authority with his accountability and the patient's knowledgeability. In the diagnostic sequences, the doctors and the patients seem to be oriented to the maintenance of the mutual intelligibility of the evidential basis of the diagnosis. Even when the patients produce extended responses, they may be more concerned with intelligibility and evidence rather than challenging the doctors' authority, because these actions are produced and received, by both participants, in ways that systematically sustain the doctor's authority. Paradoxically, therefore, I would like to suggest that the doctor's authority is so deeply rooted in the details of medical interaction that it allows for the possibility of the doctors explaining their ways of reasoning to the patient, and the patients expressing their own ideas, possibly even more than they do today, without the doctor's authority being called into question.

9

On diagnostic rationality: bad news, good news, and the symptom residue

Douglas W. Maynard and Richard M. Frankel

"Consideration of the patient's condition," or the fourth phase of the medical interview is, according to Byrne and Long (1976), the point at which the physician – having performed introductory matters, ascertained the reason for the patient's visit, and conducted a history and exam – delivers diagnostic information. In the "three function model" of the medical interview (Cohen-Cole 1991; Lazare et al. 1995), conveying diagnostic information fits within the third function of carrying out patient education and treatment plans. To date, research on this phase and function of the interview has been minimal, and has emphasized "bad" news and the communication problems surrounding it. And this literature, as Ptacek and Eberhardt (1996) concluded in a comprehensive review, is overwhelmingly anecdotal, based on clinical experience, written from the physician's point of view, and rarely theoretically justified or accompanied by empirical investigation.[1] Moreover, the preoccupation with bad news has meant that other kinds of diagnoses, such as those that are good news or uncertain, have received virtually no study. For the medical profession, this neglect in research also means there is not much of a base on which to build curricula or standards of practice.

Recently, Frankel (1994), Heath (1992), Maynard (1991c, 2003), and Peräkylä (1998, 2002, this volume), approaching the delivery and receipt of diagnostic news as an interactional event, have employed video recordings of actual interviews as a basis for analysis. However, neither Heath's (1992) nor Peräkylä's (1998) investigations distinguish between bad or good news deliveries as such, while

[1] Girgis and Sanson-Fisher (1995) reviewed 750 papers on the topic of bad news and found only three that used controlled methods to test the effectiveness of various approaches to delivering bad news.

Frankel (1994) and Maynard (1991c) exclusively consider bad news. Our analysis in this chapter concentrates on episodes in which the delivery is produced and/or received as having a *valence* either way – as "good" *or* "bad." Further, because of their prominence in our data, we also analyze cases involving uncertainty.[2] One purpose is to demonstrate that the valence of testing of diagnostic news – whether medical information is marked as good, bad, or uncertain – matters significantly for both delivery and receipt of diagnostic news.

Beyond investigating patterns of diagnostic delivery and receipt, we are interested in applications of interaction-based research. Heath (1992:264) has argued that efforts to transform communication and other behavioral features of medical consultation need to be sensitive to interactional organizations through which participants accomplish matters such as the diagnostic presentation. Those interactional organizations are not readily transparent, in part because of the lack of empirical and theoretical grounding for the understanding of clinical discourse in general, not just diagnostic informing events (Frankel 1995b; West and Frankel 1991). With regard to these events, the little existing research suggests that doctors are generally poor at communicating diagnostic information, even when they have had video feedback training during medical school (Maguire et al. 1986). But, argues Frankel (1995b), "As education and scholarship in this area continue to develop, important questions about how best to communicate not only bad news but 'good news' and 'no news' will be addressed." Developing such a knowledge base is another aim of our chapter.

While many American and all Canadian medical schools now offer training in communication skills, only a few offer sessions specifically about the conveyance of diagnostic information.[3] If there is no formal instruction about presentational strategies as part of medical training, the skills whereby participants deliver and receive good, bad, and other kinds of news are part of a tacit or commonsense knowledge base (Garfinkel 1967; Polanyi 1958; Schutz 1962), acquired without pedagogy or practice and through everyday

[2] For an extended analysis of a single case of uncertainty, see Maynard and Frankel (2003).

[3] Fallowfield and Lipkin (1995:317) observe that there is increased teaching of communication skills in medical schools, but that "the proportion of the curriculum concerned with this important area is still woefully smaller than that given to other clinical skills."

communicative experiences. For example, by emerging and ongoing participation in society, and becoming competent at conversation, participants may learn a generic News Delivery Sequence or NDS (Maynard 1997, 2003) comprising four turns of talk – announcement, announcement response, elaboration, and assessment. We will explore how doctors and patients enact and configure this sequence in the context of medical diagnostic news.

Our analysis includes a discussion of the strong interactional asymmetries in the delivery and receipt of good as opposed to bad news. Good news, as might be expected, involves an easier path than does bad news, implicating both parties in relief and joint solidarity. Deliverers present good news in an *exposed* fashion – prefacing the news with a positive assessment, placing the news in the first turn of the NDS, avoiding disfluencies, and so on. By contrast, bad news often approaches a breakdown in solidarity and a breach in rational discourse between physician and patient. Bad news is *shrouded* – deliverers preface the news with neutral terms (or even positive evaluations) rather than negative assessments, often delay the delivery until the third turn of the News Delivery Sequence, produce the news after hesitations and other disfluencies in a turn of talk, or otherwise position it last in the turn. Moreover, compared with their immediate, evaluative reactions to good news, recipients are restrained in how they treat bad news. They may delay their responses, and often do not use a semantic term when assessing the news, but do produce expletives like "Oh, shit," or "Oh, God." The pattern of asymmetry in the interpersonal handling of news works toward the sense of a "benign" social world (Maynard 2003). Nevertheless, good news can have its own edge, for a *symptom residue* often accompanies good news in the clinic – persistent medical complaints may go unexplained when a serious diagnostic possibility is excluded. This raises the specter of indeterminacy and uncertainty in clinical medicine and thereby a different but no less significant approach to the irrational than bad news presents.

Diagnostic news deliveries in primary care

In clinical environments, the "primary" consequential figure in a diagnostic news delivery is the patient. And, although family members may be attending as well, patients are the main recipient.

In fact, this is one general way of differentiating information transfer in institutional settings from that in ordinary conversation. In conversation, participants regularly share news about others or about themselves. Most episodes, that is, are "third-party" deliveries (Maynard 2003) about relatives, friends, neighbors, acquaintances, and sometimes public persons whom the participants know in common. Or conversational episodes are "first-party" tidings in which the deliverer is the primary figure, reporting something about ego or self, as when party A tells party B, "Guess what – I haven't had a drink for eight days now" (Terasaki 1976:7). Only rarely in conversation are there episodes in which one party tells a recipient "second-party" news, or tidings about the recipient him- or herself as the primary figure. In that sense, the conversational experiences of participants are limited. However, in various organizations, professionals customarily have "second-party" news to deliver. It is our welfare workers, police, clergy, real estate agents, attorneys, and of course physicians and nurses who are regularly involved in bearing news to a recipient who is the primary figure. This feature of medical routine – the frequency with which practitioners are in the position of conveying news to the primary figure – may be at the root of arguments for medical schools needing to devote more time to training about the communication process and especially bad news (Lipkin, Putnam, and Lazare 1995). We shall argue that conveying good news and uncertain diagnostic information needs attention as well.

As a matter of everyday routine, physicians, in interaction with patients, deploy the News Delivery Sequence, but configure its four turns differently from the conversational sequence. Physicians regularly announce testing and diagnostic information by *citing or explicating the evidence* or making reference to the tests that warrant their diagnostic announcements (Maynard 1991a, 2004; Peräkylä 1998). This citing of the evidence often occurs in a first turn announcement or may appear in an elaboration turn. In either case, it represents a contrast with conversational deliveries of news. In ordinary conversation, deliverers and recipients display an orientation to the speaker's "firsthand knowledge" or at least closer-hand knowledge than the recipient. Consequently, news deliveries do not necessarily exhibit *how* speakers know about what they announce although they may exhibit *that* speakers are knowledgeable and recipients are not. For instance, when giving news about themselves, deliverers draw on and have respected their entitlement to know their own experiences (Sacks 1992b:243–8). When bearing news about third parties, deliverers announce it by assertions or declarations that display "firsthand knowledge" also deriving from their own biographies (if only having heard the news previously from someone else). Recipients, in response and without asking for any kind of displays of "practical epistemology" (Whalen and Zimmerman 1990) from deliverers, produce various kinds of newsmarks, news receipts, and assessments that show an orientation to having a "changed state" (Heritage 1984b) or having received the news and understood its valence as bad or good (Maynard 1997). In short, conversational participants exhibit an orientation to deliverers' knowing *that* something is news and possibly good or bad. In the clinic, physicians exhibit not only that they are knowledgeable but *how* they are knowledgeable.[4]

Asymmetries between good and bad news: minor conditions

The delivery and receipt of good diagnostic news, then, can closely follow a generic News Delivery Sequence, which is configured in ways to show how physicians know the basis of their diagnostic news. Additionally, while there may be generic ways for the delivery and receipt of diagnostic news, as we have seen in conversation, there are orderly asymmetries between bad and good news in the clinical setting. These asymmetries shed light on what each type of event means in relation to the *rationality* of discourse in medicine. Asymmetries between bad and good diagnostic news appear across the clinical spectrum from reports on minor procedures and conditions to more major ones.[5]

[4] Peräkylä (1998, this volume) has shown that physicians strike a balance between relatively authoritative assertions and those evidence-based formulations that work to make diagnostic news intersubjectively available and valid. That is, physicians' deliveries of news provide for the accountability of their vocalized diagnostic reports in a way that is not characteristic of conversation when someone delivers bad or good news.

[5] Asymmetries between bad and good news, as we are about to describe them, have been documented in a number of clinics. See Stivers (1998) regarding veterinary medicine, Heritage and Stivers (1999) on pediatrics and internal medicine, and Leppänen (1998) on nurses giving blood pressure and blood sugar results to adult patients. For a general consideration of these asymmetries, see Maynard (2003: Chapter 6).

As a start, we examine instances of reporting blood pressure results. In the excerpt below, which has "good" results, the patient has been sitting on the examining table while the doctor takes his blood pressure. The doctor removes the blood pressure cuff and hangs it on the wall just before the utterance in line 1 below. At line 4, the patient's reference to the "Fre:shman at Cornell" refers to the physician's son, whom they have discussed previously.

(1) CGN: 39 (3.3; p. 7:10)

Dr. G:		Have a seat. ((Doctor sits down at desk in corner of
		room; patient then sits down next to the desk, facing
		the doctor.))
Mr. T:		Fre:sh↓man at Cornell huh?
Dr. G:		Ye:ah.
Mr. T:		That's great.
		(2.0)
Mr. T:		Doesn't that time go fast (.) MAN[hh
Dr. G:		[Sure does .hhh
	1→	ONE THIRTY SIX OVER EIGHTY FOUR with yer sittin, so=
Mr. T:	2→	=Mkay=
Dr. G:	3→	=those are in good shape. [Let's get a white cell
Mr. T:	4→	[((nods head))
Dr. G:		taday,
Mr. T:		Okay.

After the side sequence about how fast the time goes, Dr. F announces the blood pressure result at arrow 1 by citing the evidence. Then, following the patient's "Mkay" response (arrow 2), Dr. G elaborates the news at arrow 3 by providing a positive assessment. Mr. T receives this assessment by nodding (arrow 4). Because the physician is the one who first assesses the news (arrow 3), he can be heard in that turn to be *interpreting* the blood pressure reading for the patient, and the patient's nodding aligns to the positive assessment rather than independently assessing the news (as often happens in the fourth turn). Notice that there is nothing hesitant in Dr. G's manner for giving either the result or the assessment, and both are produced quickly in the sense that the news represents an abrupt change from the previous topic of the physician's daughter, and is followed by a topic change, a proposal for a different ("white cell") test (line 12), which occurs in simultaneity with the patient's nodding.

This good news episode can be compared with one also involving blood pressure and in which the news is at least ostensibly bad. Neither physician nor patient assesses the news as bad, instead producing other interactional indications that the news is disfavored. The interview from which excerpt (2) is taken began with the physician and patient reviewing the patient's medications (she had come to obtain a renewal of her blood pressure medicine), and the doctor next proposed an agenda-like organization for the rest of the interview. In so doing he raised a concern about her blood pressure test. Notice how, in lines 1–3 below, Dr. L introduces the "borderline" blood pressure result. He names the feature to be reported on ("blood pressure," line 1), gives a source for the to-be-reported result, next hesitates with an "uh:" and brief pause, then offers a hedge ("was perhaps") and minimizer ("little") before stating the "borderline" result.

(2) Dr. L/Ms. B (2.1:125)

Dr. L: .hh Alright, well: let's see. An' your blood pressure
according to thuh clinic assistants:=uh: (0.2) was
perhaps (uh:) little borderline. So may- I- I think I
might like to: jus' double check that.
Ms. B: M[kay,
Dr. L: [An' then why don't I look at thuh sma:ll of your
back.

Shortly after this, Dr. L put the blood pressure cuff on Ms. B (see lines 3–6 below) and conducted the pressure check for which he had indicated his intention. In announcing the result (below, arrow 1), Dr. L cites the evidence (lines 10–11) in a very delayed fashion (a turn-initial "Well," a naming of the condition to be reported on, "your blood pressure", and a reference to the "reading", lines 7–8). Although preceding his report of the result Dr. L offers an assessment, it is mitigated ("a little higher . . ." , line 8). Furthermore, he embeds this assessment within a subsequent, moderating position-statement ("than I'd like tuh see it.").

(3) Dr. L/Ms. B (2.1:173)

Dr. L: And how old are you now?
Ms. B: Fifty (three,)
(26.0)/((Dr. L is standing and inflating and

deflating the blood pressure cuff as Ms. B sits on
the examining table. He is removing the cuff from her
arm as the following is spoken:))
Dr. L: 1→ Well, your ↑blood pressure hh by that reading would
be a little higher than I'd like tuh see it. (Itsa-)
((helping remove the cuff)) have you put your arm
through- (.) right there °okay like that°. I got
about one forty over ninety ei:ght.
(0.2)
Ms. B: 2→ Mm.
Dr. L: 3→ Which is (.) ya know a little bit higher than what
thuh clinic assistants g[ot.
Ms. B: 4→ [Mm hm.
(2.5)
Dr. L: °ah:°.hh Do you ever have thee opportunity tuh
moni[tor it at all?
Ms. B: [I do:: an' I have uh car:d . . .

Then, when Dr. L reports the result (lines 10–11), he forms it as an approximation ("about", line 11). After Ms. B's token response (arrow 2), he elaborates (arrow 3) by observing that the reading is higher than the other one, which had been suggested as "borderline" in excerpt (2) (line 3). Consequently, the news delivery is one in which the upshot that the patient's blood pressure is too high is never stated outright, and the delivery is, in various ways, cautious and circumspect. Ms. B receives the elaboration with another token (arrow 4). She neither shows a strong "change of state" in her understanding nor assesses this news. Her response, in accord with conversational news deliveries wherein a recipient is the primary figure, is restrained.[6] As in the organization of conversational tidings, diagnostic bad news is shrouded, while diagnostic good news is exposed.

[6] Indeed, Ms. B's response represents a regularity in the way patients receive relatively bad diagnostic news: they produce *stoic* responses (Maynard 2003: Chapter 5). An implication here is that withheld responses in the context of bad diagnostic news may not necessarily indicate a patient's orientation to physician authority, as per Heath's (1992:262) argument. Rather, they may display the normatively constrained fashion by which recipients handle bad news in which they are the primary figure. Stoicism in the face of one's own bad news represents a balance between showing too much *distance*, on one hand, and, on the other, too much *involvement*, which can verge on self-pity.

Asymmetries between good and bad news: major conditions

Compared to the ubiquity with which primary care physicians deliver news about relatively minor conditions, bad and good news concerning major conditions are less frequent. However, such news can take on life and death significance, result in dramatic and emotion-filled experiences for both the patient and the physician, and have profound legal, ethical, and social consequences. For such reasons alone, informing episodes involving potentially serious conditions warrant scrutiny. Beyond this, diagnostic news regarding major illness permits us to explore further the asymmetric modes of delivery and receipt for the interactional work that they perform. Along lines that Heritage (1984a:269) has suggested about how preference structure in conversation exhibits affiliation and solidarity, diagnostic news events show the importance placed on rational interchange in the doctor–patient relationship. Bad news threatens such interchange in a way that good news does not. Accordingly, preferencing forms in good news (exposing the news and visibility of its valence) and dispreferencing forms in bad news (shrouding the news and valence) work to enhance solidarity by preserving not only intersubjectivity or mutual understanding, but also a kind of public *rationality*.

We first examine an episode of good news concerning a patient's cardiovascular system, and follow this, for comparative purposes, with an example of bad news wherein a patient is told that he has cancer. In addition to verbalized aspects of this event, we explore the bodily comportment and nonvocalized behaviors of doctors and patients, which demonstrate alignment in the good news encounter and nonalignment in the bad news event, and are part of the asymmetries in delivery and receipt of the news.

Cardiovascular good news

In the good news interview, as doctor and patient work their way through a diagnostic News Delivery Sequence, they demonstrate alignment and convergence in their vocal and nonvocal interactive practices on the goodness of the news. Dr. "Donna Thomas," an internist in the primary care center of a Midwest university hospital, has been treating a patient, 50-year-old Ms. "Gayle Roberts," for various symptoms, including severe chest pain. Because of this pain, the patient was referred to a cardiology clinic for specialized testing, which is now complete. Dr. Thomas has seen the results and, after entering and seating herself in the clinic room where Ms. R has been waiting, and while paging through the patient's record, asks a standardized how-are-you question (line 1 below) that marks this as a return visit (Robinson, this volume). In answering such queries, Frankel (1995b) has observed, patients display two orientations. One is to answer in a "sociable" mode as an extension of or substitute "greeting sequence" (Sacks 1975). The other is to answer the question in a "clinical" mode, according to the specific medical complaint the patient may be bringing.[7] Here, the patient, Ms. R, initially responds sociably that she is "pretty good" (line 2) and then, in a more clinical vein, reports tentatively ("I think") that her test results have come out "okay" (lines 2–3). Without hesitation, Dr. T confirms this (line 4) and then leaves to obtain the "paper." She is gone for over two minutes (line 7):

(4) **Dr. T/Ms. R**

Dr. T:		↑How are ya doin?
Ms. R:		↑I'm doin pretty good. I ha:d- da te:↑sts::, an I
		think they all came out o↑kay.
Dr. T:		They did. Lemme go get- I had that um (0.8) uh tch
		paper on that, be right ba[ck.
Ms. R:		[°Mm°
		((physician leaves room and returns after 2:12))
Dr. T:		Did they talk to you:: at the time of
		th[e:: (.) te:st?]
Ms. R:		[No: they didn't]
Dr. T:		>Okay.<
Dr. T:	pa→	.hhh Um (.) it did come out very well.
Ms. R:	ga→	G[ood
Dr. T:	1→	[Thee: uh::m (0.4) >you know they do< two:: (.)
	|	parts of it, a::nd one part is:. hhh (.) that they,
	|	have the electrocardiogram, ((brings hands toward
	↓	chest))

[7] See also Robinson's (this volume) analysis of different ways – for example, the "open-ended" or "closed-ended" questions – in which doctors ask about patients' health problems.

Ms. R: Mm [hm]
Dr. T: | [on.] .hhh an::dt that uh they look uh:: for
| evidence of too little (0.4) blood and oxygen going
| to the heart muscle. .hhh ((leans toward Ms. R)) an
↓ that was fi:ne,=
Ms. R: =[°Mm hmm°] ((nodding))
Dr. T: | =[the elec]trocardiogram part of it, they said that
| .hhh ((reading report on desk, left hand on page))
| you: (.) um exercised very well:, with an excellent
| functional ((returns gaze to patient)) ay:robic
↓ capacity.
Ms. R: 2→ O[kay] ((smiles; nods during Dr.'s next turn:))
Dr. T: 3→ [So that] ((continuing gaze at patient)) that means
| that fo:r:.h >you know they always say for
| somebody at this particular< a:ge and a female
| per:son .hh they have kind of an a:verage or a low or
↓ a hi::gh amount of ac[tivity] (.) that they
Ms. R: [°Mm hmm°]
Dr. T: | were able to do and you were able to do a lo:t of
↓ activity.
Ms. R: 4→ That's grea:t [cause] I want to really start=
Dr. T: [Yeah]
Ms. R: ↓ =exercising a:nd reduc:e wei:ght. I [gain]ed fifteen
Dr. T: [Yeah]
Ms. R: ↓ poun:ds an .hhh the red li(h)(h)ght [is on.]
Dr. T: [((nodding)] So
.hh ((returning gaze to report)) that was good they
said a excellent functional ayrobic capa:ci[ty. hh
Ms. R: [So I
could- coul:d uh si:gn up fer aerobic classes.
(0.2) ((Dr. T looking at report))
Dr. T: Mm hmm ((nodding))

When Dr. T returns to the room, she asks if "they" had talked to the patient "at the time" the test had been performed (lines 8–9), to which Ms. A replies negatively (line 10). After acknowledging this (line 11), Dr. T produces a kind of preface to her announcement of the news (pa→, line 12), which reconfirms (using emphasis on the verb) the favorability of the results. Goodwin (1996), following Sacks (1974) on story prefaces, has referred to utterances such as this as "prospective indexicals." That is, "it did come out very well" provides a kind of headline to the upcoming news, and an indication of how to respond to it. Ms. R treats this utterance with a positive assessment that suggests a "go-ahead" (ga→, line 13) and occasions the announcement of results (arrow 1 at line 14 and continuing).

In the first part of the News Delivery, Dr. T cites and explicates the test results, and also summarizes the outcome of a thallium procedure. She prefaces her delivery by suggesting that there are "two:: parts" and referring to the "electrocardiogram" being "on" (lines 14–16, and 19). Then, referring to the thallium, Dr. T adds that "they look uh:: for . . . blood and oxygen going to the heart muscle." (lines 19–21), and produces a general assessment (line 22) that it "was fi:ne,". At this point, Ms. R produces a continuer and starts nodding (line 23). In overlap with the continuer, and looking at the file on her desk, Dr. T cites the evidence from the electrocardiogram by reading specific determinations (lines 24–28). On the words "excellent functional ay:robic capacity." she also shifts her gaze from the record to the patient. The patient responds here with "smile voice" and an "Okay" acknowledgment (arrow 2).

Now Dr. T (arrow 3, line 30 and continuing) elaborates the electrocardiogram news, proposing what the test result "means" (lines 30–34) and reporting that the patient was "able to do a lo:t of activity." (lines 36–37). Immediately (arrow 4, line 38 and continuing), the patient assesses this news positively and then provides an account for her assessment (lines 38, 40, and 42), which has to do with her "want" to exercise because of a weight gain. Dr. T, gazing at the patient, tracks this account (lines 39 and 41) and nods (line 43) at its completion. Following this, she also produces a positive assessment as part of a summarizing repeat of the findings (lines 43–45), which appears to be a device for holding the floor while further reading the report on her desk. Ms. R, however, next exhibits that her previous expression of wanting to exercise because of having gained weight may have been a tacit request for *permission* to exercise, because at lines 46–47 she explicitly asks whether she could sign up for aerobic classes. Dr. T gives her nodding assent while continuing to look at the report (lines 48–49).

Subsequently (not on the transcript above), there are brief references to back pain (which we discuss later) and then breathing difficulties the patient experienced during the electrocardiogram test.

There is also a second segment to this good news delivery, wherein Dr. T elaborates on the thallium procedure, which showed that oxygen was getting to all sections of the heart. Dr. T ended the news delivery by saying that "together" the two tests (electrocardiogram and thallium) suggested that there was no "part of the heart which looks like it's in danger," and Ms. responded with "Um that's good." For considerations of space, we are not further analyzing this second segment. The first segment – excerpt (4) – displays several characteristics that also feature in the second and permits comparison with an interview concerning a patient's diagnosis of cancer. The interview between Dr. T and Ms. R is summarized in Figure 9.1, which we discuss later, for purposes of comparison with the cancer interview.

Cancer bad news

Bad diagnostic news, we have suggested, may not be referenced or formulated as such in the course of its delivery, and that taboo-like effort itself is indicative of a disfavored status the news occupies. But doctor and patient have other ways of exhibiting how they disfavor such news, as is very apparent in our next excerpt. "Clint Jones" is a 37-year-old African-American male patient in a primary care clinic affiliated with a medical school in an Eastern state (Frankel 1994). On a Friday, he reported to the clinic with complaints about stomach pain, weight loss, and an inability to tolerate solid foods. Dr. "Edward Hoffman," a white third-year resident in the primary care internal medicine training program referred him to a gastroenterologist, Dr. Smith, for evaluation. Dr. Smith's endoscopy, for which Dr. Hoffman was also present, revealed a suspicious-looking mass in the esophagus, and a biopsy was performed. The growth proved to be malignant, and on the Monday after the procedure Dr. H arranged to see Mr. J back in the clinic. The interview started with Dr. H coming into the office where Mr. J had been seated, apologizing for Mr. J's having to wait, and explaining that he had had a discussion with the previous patient that "took longer" than he thought it would. As in the interview concerning Ms. R's cardiology results, the physician then produces a how-are-you-doing query (line 1), exhibiting an orientation to this as a follow-up visit:

(5) **Dr. H/Mr. J**

Dr. H: tch ·hhhhhhh (0.6) so howareya ↑doing.
(1.1)
Mr. J: I'm doin' good, I'm losin' weight?
(0.5)
Mr. J: °Whatever.°
(0.9)
Mr. J: What was the problem. Wha' was [(decided on).]=
Dr. H: [Sh- sh'you]=
Dr. H: =lost- yuh- you lost weight. .hhh ((turns gaze away
from patient to desk and chart on right))
(0.5)
Dr. H: ↑Uh::m.
(2.5) ((Dr. repositions note on his chart))
Dr. H: pa→ There ↑is a pro:blem. ((returns gaze to patient and
nods))
. ga→ (1.6)
Dr. H: Uh: :m: hh (1.3) tch!
(1.4)
Dr. H: (a)→ Do you re↑member what we talked abou:t at the
end o' the procedure, [you had on Fri:day::.
Mr. J: [°no:° ((shaking head))
(0.5)
Dr. H: Okay well let's- (0.1) let's go over that too:.
.hhhhh uh:m (1.6) hhh (1.2) .hhhh (0.8) .hh ya know
we put the ↑sco:pe (.) ((gestures with hand moving
down torso)) ↓down into your stomach (0.1) to look
around and see what- (0.2) what it was that we could
s:ee:. .hhhhh ↑a:nd uh: hhhhhh tch Doctor Smith an' I
were there and we looked (.) into your stomach. .hhhh
(b)→ Do you remember we said we saw something g:ro:wing
in your stomach?=
Mr. J: =Mm hm
(0.6)
Dr. H: (c)→ D'you remember that?
(0.6)
Mr. J: °Ye:ah I gue:ss.°= ((Mr. J shifts in chair, hunches
over, and looks downward.))
Dr. H: 1→ =°Oh kay.° Well that's what we did see:. We- we
| looked into your sto:ma:ch and we sa::w::
| (0.6) right at the spo:t where you feel like
| (0.2) the food is getting stu:ck,
↓ (0.1) ((Dr. puts right hand on stomach.))
Mr. J: Mm
(1.0)

45	Dr. H:	→	.hhh uh::, there is something growing in your
46			stomach.
47			(4.0) ((Mr. J sits rigidly, looking downward.))
48	Mr. J:	2→	You can't te:ll what it is?=
49	Dr. H:	3→	=I can tell you what it is °Cli:nt.°
50		↓	(0.1)
51	Mr. J:		Mm hm.
52			(0.1)
53	Dr. H:	↓	Uh: (0.2) it's a cancer.
54			(0.4) ((Mr. J brings head up and to his right))
55	Mr. J:	4→	°Jhheesuhhs:° ((whispered)) ((Mr. J swings right
56		|	elbow up and rests it on edge of edge of counter,
57		|	puts right hand over eyes, and left hand at crotch.))
58		|	(1.2)
59	Mr. J:	|	Oh:: °my gohhd°
60		|	(1.2)
61	Mr. J:	|	TCH!
62		|	(0.5)
63	Mr. J:	|	.hhh
64		|	(1.8)
65	Mr. J:	|	°Oh::no::hh°. ((Mr. J bends forward, resting both
66		↓	elbows on his knees and hanging his head low.)

When Dr. H produces the "return-visit" query (Robinson this volume) about how the patient is doing (line 1), he and Mr. J, who leans his left elbow on the desk, are facing one another. The patient first responds sociably that he is "doin' good" and then, in a more clinical vein, announces his continued weight loss (line 3). Following a softly spoken "Whatever" tag (line 5), Mr. J then occasions a news delivery by asking Dr. H about "the problem" (line 7).

Dr. H acknowledges the "lost weight" (lines 8–9) and then, after looking at the diagnostic report on his desk (lines 9–11), a turn-holding "Uh::m." (line 12), and a large silence during which he moves a small "post-it" memo (line 13), he responds to his patient's query by nodding and confirming that "there is a pro:blem." in a manner that also prefaces the announcement of findings and diagnosis to come (pa→, line 14). As a prospective indexical, this utterance and term project specification and "filling in" (Goodwin 1996:384), but, in contrast to Dr. T's preface "it did come out very well." in excerpt (4) (line 12), this preface does not contain an evaluation as such and is relatively restrained. There is, in other words, no lexical pre-indication of how "bad" the problem might be. Notice also the delays and hesitations (lines 11–13) while he moves the "post-it" note – preceding the confirmation at line 14. This confirmation meets with no response from Mr. J, who directs his gaze to the chart Dr. H was just perusing. Rather, this behavior can be said to display "recipiency" (Heath 1982a) and operates as a nonvocal "go ahead" (ga→, line 16) for the delivery of diagnostic news.

Dr. H then, hesitatingly, produces a perspective display invitation (arrow (a), line 19). This in fact, turns out to be the first of three such invitations (arrows (a), (b), and (c)). As described by Maynard (1991d) such devices initiate a presequence to the delivery of news that displays the recipient's view of a condition in advance of the news delivery. Subsequent to the display, clinicians work both to *confirm* the recipient's perspective as valid and to use it in *affirming* their own diagnostic announcement. Here, Dr. H formulates the invitation at line 19 by asking Mr. J if he remembers what they had "talked abou:t" at the end of the procedure the previous Friday, thereby asking not just for any view from Mr. J but one that reflects a previous discussion. Mr. J denies remembering (line 21), and this occasions Dr. H's suggestion for going "over that too:." (line 23); he then describes the procedure through a brief narrative (lines 23–28) and also invokes another medical observer, Dr. Smith, besides himself, as jointly witnessing the evidence (lines 28–29). Embedded in this narrative are a number of breathy hesitations and silences, which prolong a halting quality to Dr. H's presentation. Then at arrow (b) (line 30), Dr. H produces the second of his perspective display invitations, this one proposing a specification of what Mr. J should "remember". Mr. J, at line 32, responds with a minimal utterance. Subsequently, in a third invitation at arrow (c) (line 34), and showing an orientation to the minimalism of his recipient's previous utterance, Dr. H asks for a stronger display of recollection. Although Mr. J produces such a display, it is delayed (line 35), spoken quietly, and the affirmative "Ye:ah" is muted with "I gue:ss." (line 36).

When Mr. J acknowledges remembering, he also bends his torso forward in his chair and faces the floor (lines 36–37), retaining this position as Dr. H moves to deliver the news. Overall, this effort at gleaning a display of recollection proposes to "co-implicate" Mr. J's perspective (Maynard 1992), along with Dr. Smith's and his own, in Dr. H's subsequent announcement of a growth in Mr. J's stomach (arrow 1, lines 38 and continuing). Dr. H – partly through the emphasis on the deictic term "that's" and the verb "did" – produces an agreeing proposal that they saw something growing (lines 38–39) and then locates the growth in relation to what is suggested as the patient's own account of a symptom (lines 40–41). In regular fashion, he thereby suggests confirmation of Mr. J's purported "seeing" and experience of symptoms, and (after Mr. J's token at line 43) uses that perspective to affirm the diagnostic formulation at lines 45–46 that "there is something growing in your stomach." Mr. J is still bent forward during this turn of talk and, after it, is silent (line 47) until vocalizing a response (arrow 2, line 48) to the announcement, a query that prefers (Sacks 1987) confirmation that Dr. H "can't te:ll what it is?" Still, Mr. J's negative or denying response implicates the diagnostic upshot or announcement. Dr. H (arrow 3, line 49 and continuing), by suggesting that he "can tell" what it is, contravenes the proposal of his patient. After Mr. J's delayed continuer (lines 50–51), Dr. H hesitatingly declares "it's a cancer." (line 53). Mr. J immediately shifts his body posture from his leaning-forward position to a brief lean back, with his left hand over his eyes (lines 55–58). Vocally, he produces whispered expletives (line 55, 59), a tongue click (line 61), and, after an inbreath (line 63), a very soft denying utterance (line 65). Mr. J also bodily returns to a torso-forward position, more extreme than the one he had just left. This segment of the interview in excerpt (5) is summarized along with the heart interview, excerpt (4), in Figure 9.1.

Both physician and patient remain silent for over seven seconds. Mr. J is still bent forward, while Dr. H sits upright with his eyes on his patient's head and back. Mr. J breaks the silence with a question at line 1 below:

(6) Dr. H/Mr. J

Mr. J: >What does that mean.<
(0.4)
Dr. H: TCH ·hhhh (0.4) We:ll? (5.0) It mea::ns you're going
to needta see a lo:t o' do:ctors °Clint°.
(2.0)
Dr. H: °Uhhm° (1.0) You're gonna need a lo:t of medical
help.
(0.4)
Mr. J: Phh (0.6) °>Does it mean I'm gonna die::.<°
(1.5)
Dr. H: hhh
(3.7)

13 Mr. J: (Oo:↑:::::)hhh.hh ((whimper))
14 (2.6) ((Mr. J shifts feet back and starts to stand.
15 Dr. H reaches hands out touching Mr. J's left elbow.
16 Mr. J stands and swings body so that he is facing the
17 counter with his back to Dr. H))
18 Dr. H: Stay with me Clint.
19 (1.1)
20 Mr. J: How long I got.
21 (0.2)
22 Dr. H: Come on stay with me now.
23 ((Dr. H gestures toward empty chair with hand.))
24 (1.2)
25 Mr. J: How long do I got.
26 (2.4)
27 Dr. H: I don't know:.
28 (1.6)
29 Dr. H: I don't ↑know yet, there are a lo:t of questions yet
30 we haven't answered.

Dr. H answers Mr. J (lines 3–4 and 6–7) that he going to need "a lo:t" of further medical attention. Subsequently, and remaining in his forward bend, Mr. J queries (with downward intonation), "does it mean I'm gonna die::." (line 9). As Dr. H hesitates in answering (lines 10–12), Mr. J emits a kind of whimpering sound (line 13) and starts to leave his chair (lines 14–17). As he does this, Dr. H reaches out with both hands as if to grab Mr. J's elbow, but withdraws his hands quickly when Mr. J stands up fully and steps to the counter at his right (lines 14–17). Then, Dr. H asks him to "Stay with me" (line 18), but Mr. J remains standing while asking "How long" he has (line 20). Next, Dr. H intensifies his request for Mr. J to "stay" with him, both verbally (line 22) and by gesturing to the chair (line 23), and Mr. J stays standing as he re-asks his question (line 25), which Dr. H answers by his claim to a lack of knowledge (lines 27 and 29–30).

Eventually, after Mr. J returns to his seat, the physician discusses treatment options, emphasizes an immediate need for surgery, and suggests that Mr. J needs to see another doctor. It is clearly an agonizing interview for both patient and physician, in which they discuss a variety of topics, including "how long" the patient has, how to manage pain, how to handle feelings of despair, and other matters. Relevant to the shrouding of bad news, it is only at a juncture near the close of the interview, after proposing the need to "get things lined up and move quickly," that Dr. H evaluates the tidings. He says, "it's horrible news," and adds, "I'm sorry I had to give ya such upsetting news," reporting that he had "thought a lot about it this weekend, about how I would do it, and it didn't come out at all the way I thought."

Comparing good and bad news in primary care

Structurally, the interviews concerning cardiovascular good news and cancer bad news are parallel (see Figure 9.1). Both interviews proceed from the physician's (A) "how are you doing" inquiries. The patients produce socially appropriate responses first, following them with clinical responses, and then with (B) utterances that initiate discussion of the diagnostic news. The heart patient, Ms. R, tentatively *offers* an assessment that her tests "all came out okay," which works to elicit a fuller report from the physician, while the cancer patient, Mr. J, with his question about what the "problem" is, *asks for* further information regarding his tests. Then, confirming what the patient has already suggested – that the testing came out very well (heart patient), or that there is a problem (cancer patient), each physician begins a preface to an upcoming announcement. In turn, each patient produces a go-ahead signal that occasions a delivery of diagnostic news.

From this point, the interviews diverge, however, in that Dr. T indeed proceeds with a (C) News Delivery Sequence – by almost immediately (1) announcing the thallium and electrocardiogram results – whereas Dr. H inserts a Perspective Display Sequence before (C). Only after obtaining his patient's exhibit of remembering what they jointly observed does he firmly (1) announce finding a growth in Mr. J's stomach. Then, in each interview, after these announcements, the patients produce (2) responses – Ms. R produces a smiling "Okay" and Mr. J asks a question – that elicit (3) elaboration. In her elaboration, Dr. T explains what the electrocardiogram results "mean"; Dr. H elaborates by asserting that his patient's "growth" is a "cancer." Subsequently, the patients produce (4) assessment-type receipts, or broad displays of understanding of the kind of news they have received. Ms. R verbalizes a "that's grea:t" assessment, while Mr. J produces response cries of various sorts.

However, while these generic how-are-you, prefaces to announcement, and News Delivery forms are similarly deployed in each interview, there are vocal and nonvocal patterns that exhibit strong asymmetries between good and bad news. Dr. T delivers her good news in more or less immediate response to the patient's "go-ahead" signal and, in proceeding with few hesitations or pauses in her talk, is rather smooth in summarizing the thallium procedure and then citing the electrocardiogram evidence. She gives both the "that was fi:ne" thallium upshot and "excellent functional aerobic capacity" upshot during the announcement, and subsequently, in what we call a *rational* elaboration of the news, she proposes to explain what these upshots mean medically. The patient, Ms. R, also produces continuers and news receipts in an unhesitating manner. Indeed, they are often spoken at the same time as Dr. T is talking, and Ms. R produces her fourth turn assessment, "that's grea:t," immediately after the elaboration of the electrocardiogram results and provides an account for this assessment. She virtually *embraces* Dr. T's announcement and rational elaboration. Nonvocally, these two parties maintain mutual gaze for long periods and their bodies frequently are aligned to one another, each participant sitting upright on her chair (the doctor moves forward and back) and squarely facing the other.

Things are much different with the cancer patient. Dr. H delivers the cancer bad news in a hesitating, delaying, halting fashion that is consonant with the manner in which conversational participants produce "dispreferred" utterances in response to various kinds of initiations.[8] Moreover, Dr. H produces the citation of evidence concerning "something g:ro:wing" in the patient's stomach through invoking, in a very deliberate manner, a Perspective Display Sequence, thereby aligning the patient's experience to this announcement (and vice versa) before producing the announcement. And the focal part of the news – the upshot that Mr. J has cancer – appears in turn three or elaboration of the News Delivery Sequence. This delays the attempt at rational explication of the news – explaining what it means medically – until after Mr. J's assessment turn.

Mr. J's responses to the diagnostic news, as well, involve delays, silence, and minimal utterances. In a word, they appear *resistive* to

[8] Recall that the physician in each interview delivers the diagnostic news in answer to solicitations from the patient; i.e., as a responsive activity. As Schegloff (1988:446) succinctly observes, the sequential and temporal feature of preferred and dispreferred responses is that "preferred comes early, dispreferred is commonly delayed."

	Sequencing	BAD NEWS Dr. C with Cancer Patient	GOOD NEWS Dr. H with Heart Patient
A. Introductory	Inquiry	So howareya doing?	How are ya doing?
	Response	I'm doin' good, I'm losin' weight	Pretty good, tests all came out okay
B. Preface to announcement	Prefacing headline	There is a problem	It did come out very well
	Go-ahead	((silence))	Good
(Insert) Perspective-Display Pre-Sequence	Perspective-Display Inquiry	Do you remember ...we saw something growing in your stomach? ... Do you remember that?	
	Reply/perspective display	Yeah I guess.	
C. Diagnostic News Delivery Sequence	1. Announcement	Okay. Well that's what we did see... there is something growing in your stomach.	blood and oxygen...was fine ... excellent functional aerobic capacity.
	2. Announcement response	You can't tell what it is?	Okay.
	3. Elaboration	I can tell you what it is, Clint. It's a cancer.	So that means ...you were able to do a lot of activity.
	4. Receipt/assessment	Jhheesuhhs. Oh my god...Oh no.	That's great cause I want to really start exercizing and reduce weight.

Figure 9.1 News delivery sequences

the trajectory of the news. He at first *denies* remembering, and then only reluctantly recalls the endoscopy and the discussion about it when a growth in his stomach was first witnessed. Subsequent to Dr. H's announcement that there is indeed this growth, Mr. J occasions the elaborating pronouncement about cancer with a *negatively formed* proposal that the doctor "can't tell what it is." Finally, after the "cancer" upshot, Mr. J appears agitated as he emits a series of expletives and a *disavowing* "Oh::no::hh." In terms of body posture, throughout the interview the gaze of doctor and patient rarely meet, and they only face one another briefly. After the initial "howareya doing" sequence, the patient is mostly bending forward in his chair, looking at the floor, while the doctor glances back and forth between the report on his desk and the patient's head. After the cancer pronouncement, the patient is leaning back, bending over again, standing up, and walking about, while the doctor sits in his chair, making slight moves toward his desk or toward the patient and asking his patient to "stay with him."

Once again, these asymmetries point toward good news as something to be exposed – forthrightly, even boldly delivered and received. Bad news is shrouded – the participants in the interview are extremely discreet in its treatment. Two facets of this contrast between good and bad news deserve further attention. One is related to how, in citing his evidence for Mr. J's stomach growth, Dr. H works to co-implicate *both* his patient-recipient and his colleague, Dr. Smith, in asserting the observability of the growth in Mr. J's stomach. Consequently, there is an effort to establish the diagnosis intersubjectively by publicly invoking a convergence or "reciprocity of perspectives" (Schutz 1962) within the medical interview itself. Dr. T's presentation, in contrast, only refers to an anonymous "they" as she describes what was looked for and what was found with Ms. R's electrocardiogram and thallium procedures. Neither she nor the patient is portrayed as having evidence related to the diagnostic upshots. Accordingly, the intersubjective status of these upshots – their truth for the physician and patient in the present situation – appears to derive from an authoritative perspective that is anchored outside of this situation but that can be permissively asserted within it.

Another facet of the contrast between bad and good news involves a semantically *positive* delivery and receipt of good news and a semantically *neutral* handling of the diagnostic bad news. That is, the announcement about Ms. R's heart is preceded with mildly positive assessments from both doctor and patient, including Ms. R's "Good" by which she solicits delivery of the news. Dr. T interjects "fi:ne" when announcing the thallium results, and "excellent" as she reads the electrocardiogram results. Ms. R marks her receipt of this report with "that's grea:t" and goes on to offer an account for her assessment. Slightly later, after Dr. T further elaborates on the thallium results (transcript not shown), Ms. R claims to be "happy" about the diagnostic news, because she had been nervous, there was a family history of stroke, and she "now" knows that she can ride the bike. Thus, positive assessments and this claim of happiness proliferate in the good news delivery and receipt about the patient's heart. In the cancer episode, however, doctor and patient appear to refrain from producing overt negative assessments and evaluations – neither formulates an assessment of the "badness" of the news, that is, in the context of its delivery – and at no point does Mr. J state or define how he is affected by the news. Rather, the "bad" valence is mostly exhibited in other practices, such as the withholding of reference to that valence, and the dispreferencing modes whereby the parties present and receive the news, and the co-implicating manner of citing the evidence. It is only near the end of the interview that Dr. H acknowledges verbally how "terrible" the news is.

We find caution, circumspection, or shrouding with regard to bad diagnostic news, then, and boldness, assertiveness, or exposure with good diagnostic news. Why the difference? What is the interactional work of these asymmetric modes of delivery? It seems apparent that, from the physician's point of view, good news is something that needs relatively little buildup, preparation, or "forecasting" (Maynard 1996). Largely, physicians seem to depend on and often receive patients' unmediated affiliation to the news and to its valence. This means that patients can and do follow what the news "means" in a discursively rational way, accepting the physician's explanations and offering accounts of their own that build topically on those explanations. Furthermore, these rational elaborations often involve reciprocal displays of positive affect on the part of the participants. In short, good news is regarded as enhancing the social bond between physician and patient.

Contrariwise, physicians seem oriented to the possibility of disaffiliation from the news when it is bad. Shrouding bad news represents restraint on the part of physicians and can encourage restraint on the part of their recipients, who may be at risk of otherwise "flooding out" upon the pronouncement or confirmation of diagnosis.[9] If Goffman (1978) is correct, response cries like those occurring as receipts of bad news are indications of this propensity for emotional loss of control. Response cries, that is, are something like "self-talk" as a kind of "externalized inward state." As relatively brief emotional expressions of pain, they do not overwhelm their producer. Nevertheless, they are enough to threaten mutual intelligibility, and physicians are therefore concerned to "contain" the scene to which they respond and in which they may be emitted (Goffman 1978:795; Sudnow 1967:141).[10] We observed that, in dealing with Mr. J's response to the cancer diagnosis, including his response cries, his question about what it means and if it means he is "gonna die::," and his pacing around the room, Dr. H, in proceeding to discuss meaning, prognosis, treatment, and other matters, remains seated. He urges his patient, "Stay with me, Clint," thereby calling his patient back to the discourse of rational medicine. In short, the asymmetries between good and bad news in clinical environments, in which participants behaviorally and interactionally exhibit the favoring of good news and the disfavoring of bad news, are structures that enhance the possibility of order over disorder, intersubjectivity over a descent into the subjectivity of emotion, and explanatory rationality over emotional displays as a kind of irrationality.

Good news, indeterminacy, and uncertainty: the problem of symptom residue

Unbounded response cries and displays of emotion represent only one potential kind of irrationality in the delivery of diagnostic news.

[9] For examples of such flooding out, see the example in Maynard (2003:79–85) of a mother who cries and sobs when hearing the diagnosis of "mental retardation" for her son, and the example of a woman who shows what Quill and Townsend (1991) call "rage" and "terror" when she finds out that she has been diagnosed with AIDS.

[10] For a study of how strong displays can impede the work of professionals in an organizational setting, see Whalen and Zimmerman (1998). They analyze the use of "hysteria" as a label that 911 call-takers apply to those callers whose behavior overwhelms the interactional demands of gathering information necessary for the dispatch of help.

Another potential irrationality is evoked when physicians *don't know* or are *uncertain* about the answers to medical questions.[11] In the cancer interview, Dr. H had difficulty with Mr. J's questions about what his diagnosis meant. These are questions of prognosis, which notoriously raise problems of indeterminacy and uncertainty when someone is diagnosed with a given disease. But even when diagnostic news is ostensibly good, there is often a *residue of symptoms* for which there is no account, and this also can send physician and patient to the edge of rationality.[12] Consider the continuation of excerpt (4), involving the cardiology patient. After Dr. T affirms that Ms. R can sign up for aerobic classes, she introduces a complaint about her back (lines 50–51 below). Dr. T acknowledges and receives this as information and, continuing to read from the file, quotes others who observed that, during the electrocardiogram, the patient was fatigued and had chest pain (arrows below at lines 53–56):

(7) Dr. T/Ms. R: continues excerpt (7)

Dr. T: . . . excellent functional aerobic capa:ci[ty .hh
Ms. R: [So I
could- coul:d uh si:gn up fer aerobic classes.
(0.2) ((Dr. T looking at report))
Dr. T: Mm hmm ((nodding))
Ms. R: The o(h)(h)nly thing is a:fterwards the ba::ck was
really bo[t h e r i n g m e] but.hh hh
Dr. T: [Oh is that ri:ght.] ((gazing at Ms. R))
Dr. T: → ((returns gaze to file on desk)) .hh Now: they
→ said that um you sto:pped because you were,
→ fatigue:d and that you al:so did have an aching kind
→ of che[st pai]n is that cor[rect]
Ms. R: [Mm hmm] [Mm hmm]

This symptom residue occupies a great deal of attention during the interview after the delivery of this good news diagnosis of excellent aerobic capacity and about the thallium test. In this way, in the immediate environment of a good news delivery, the problem of

[11] Researchers and scholars have devoted considerable attention to the problem of uncertainty in medicine. Traditionally, the emphasis has been on the anxiety that uncertainty produces in physicians (Buckman 1984), and how they have attempted to conceal their lack of knowledge from patients (Fox 1957; Katz 1984). Such problems are not our focus per se, although they also point to forms of irrationality associated with medical uncertainty.

[12] See Abbott's (1988:42–4) discussion of how, within any professional classification symptom, there can be "areas of unclassified, residual problems."

indeterminacy can rear its head, which Frankel (1995b:252) has described as stemming from physicians' approach to illness as one that attempts to *rule out* various possible conditions. When, in Ms. R's case, heart disease is ruled out, the question remains as to the source of her pain:

(8) Dr. T/Ms. R (normalized transcript)

Dr. T: The um the fact that you did have chest pain that came on is a little bit disturbing to me . . . all these things are good that it doesn't show that there's any major thing that's wrong with it. Um I think it may be that you know sometimes people get chest pain from other things, from their muscles for example.

At such a point, the physician may have to construct ad hoc explanations ("muscles") for the symptom or difficulty that a patient experiences. And Dr. T recommends that if Ms. R feels fatigued or has some "extra" chest pains, or if the pain otherwise does not go away, she should call back.

In this example, the patient first complains about her back, and then it is the *physician* who brings up the problem of fatigue and chest pain. More regularly, it is the *patient* who, after receiving diagnostic information that a physician has presented as good news, refrains from any positive assessment and brings up remaining symptomatic or other health concerns that the good news diagnosis leaves unexplained. In one interview, a physician presented results from a number of diagnostic tests to the patient (Maynard and Frankel 2003). At lines 1–2 below, "Dr. Kallberg" reports on his patient's pap test, and "Ms. Victor" receives this as good news (line 3). Together lines 1–3 constitute a prototypical *two-part* rather than four-part News Delivery Sequence (as per arrows 1 and 2):

(9) Dr. K/Ms. V: 1.5:235

Dr. K: 1→ Yer pa::p (.) is negative?
(0.4)
Ms. V: 2→ Oh good.
Dr. K: 1a→ Yer: leg ex ray is negative?
(1.0)
Ms. V: ?→ So di- So are you gonna tell me what's wrong with my
leg [then?]
Dr. K: [I alrea]dy told you what's wrong.
Ms. V: Oh just tendinitis?

Then, the production format for Dr. K's announcement about the leg X-ray at arrow 1a closely parallels the previous announcement containing the pap report (line 1). But Ms. V responds very differently. Instead of a relatively close-positioned positive assessment, there is a substantial silence (line 5) following the announcement, and then a query about what's wrong with the leg (lines 6–7). The doctor's answer is one that occasions the patient's guess about tendinitis (line 9) and then some joking about whether the patient has tendinitis or bursitis (data not shown). Our point is that the problem of a symptom residue may disrupt a good news delivery sequence.

When this disruption happens, it may be no laughing matter, especially when the symptoms are potentially serious, as in excerpt (10) below. Dr. L, reading from the report on his desk, announces the mammogram result at arrow 1, the patient responds with a nodding continuer at arrow 2, and then Dr. L elaborates the report with a kind *best case* formulation[13] at arrow 3, which proposes how good the news is. In the sequential position (?→, line 11) where the patient's assessment could occur, Ms. S initiates a question.

(10) Dr. L w/Ms. S (2.3)

Ms. S:		An' then: you were going tuh tell me tuhday about thuh
		mammiogram.
Dr. L:		Tlk.hh That's right. A:nd I think thuh report on that
		was good. ('t) did cross my desk.
		(1.0) ((Dr. looking through file))
Dr. L:	1→	((reading:)).hh Uh: uncha::nged appearance. ((shifts
		gaze to patient:)) No evidence for cancer.
Ms. S:	2→	Mm hm. ((nodding))
Dr. L:	3→	((returns gaze to report:)) So: it's- it's thuh:: .hh
		°b:est° uh: report you can find. [(You just uh-)
Ms. S:	?→	[.hh Now: wouldju
		answer a question for me. [On thuh=m-) thuh mammiogram.
Dr. L:		[I'll try.
		(.)
Dr. L:		[Mm hm,
Ms. S:		[°eh°- thee: extent of what it examines is thee::=uh
		.hhh tissue of thuh breast itself.
		(0.5)

13 See Pomerantz's (1986) discussion of "extreme case formulations" and the way they are used to "legitimize claims."

Dr. L: Corre[ct.
Ms. S: [Correct?
Dr. L: Right.
Ms. S: Does it reach beyo:nd it.
Dr. L: It doesn't really reach up in thuh arm pits. if that's
what you're: [were thinking of.
Ms. S: [Well I'm concerned (.) that there is uh
lump, an' it is growing.

It turns out that the patient has a concern about a "lump" in her armpit. The mammogram has not covered that area, which means that the doctor must further consider the possibility of a cancer. The symptom residue occurs here because a diagnostic test is not comprehensive enough. And that residue of symptoms appears to interfere with the patient producing an agreeing assessment with what the doctor proposes to be good news.

In short, when some disease is ruled out, it can be "good news" from a clinical point of view. That point of view may or may not be one that the patient shares, and at times physicians may appear insensitive "to the context of patient experience," as Frankel (1995b:252) puts it, especially when the patient does have some residue of pain or other symptoms.[14] In these circumstances, argues Heath (1992), the incongruence between doctor and patient can mean that patients will feel compelled to recount their experience of illness in order to justify having visited the doctor (Halkowski this volume; Heritage and Robinson this volume). The practitioner may reorient from delivering news and managing closure toward re-examining the patient and possibly referring the patient for further diagnostic testing. Frankel (1995b:254) similarly proposes that the physician must "extend the assessment" of the patient by

[14] In a study involving 38 patients referred by their cardiologists for echocardiography, all of whom received the news that their results were normal, 21 patients (more than half) reported residual doubt and anxiety about the condition of their hearts (McDonald et al. 1996). Of the 38 patients, 10 were referred for the test because they came to the clinic with worries about palpitations or pain or both, and all 10 had doubt and anxiety after their favorable tests. Out of the 28 who were referred to cardiologists, and by them for testing, because a primary care physician detected a systolic murmur during routine examination, 11 had residual doubt and anxiety after the test. In another study, which involved a sample of patients who were referred for neurological examinations because of headache, 40 percent were still worried three months after they received "reassuring results" from the specialist that their symptoms did not reflect serious disease (Fitzpatrick and Hopkins 1981).

ordering further tests. Therefore, while physicians may have a high level of diagnostic certainty regarding the tests already performed and what has been ruled out, they nevertheless can be faced with symptoms of indeterminate origins and consequently must deal with *un*certainty about a larger medical picture of the patient surrounding one particular episode of diagnostic news.

In our data, the problem of symptom residue appears with great regularity. Good news can and does go hand in hand with indeterminacy and certain forms of uncertainty. Let us recall Heath's (1992) argument that physicians announce their diagnoses in ways that are authoritative, and that patients, when receiving diagnostic news, are largely passive and silent such that they display an orientation to this authority. At most, when there is incongruence between doctor and patient, the patient attempts to *justify* having sought the doctor's help. Peräkylä (1998) has suggested something else: physicians regularly and carefully provide evidential reasons for their diagnostic conclusions, in ways that display the intersubjective rather than authoritative grounds for their diagnoses. Our investigation of good news and the problem of symptom residue adds a further dimension to previous work, for this problem puts physicians and patients at the edge of rationality where authority and intersubjectivity are in jeopardy. Despite the good news that some disease is not present, patients still have their pains and symptoms, and doctors cannot yet assert anything definitive to account for them. That is, while institutional medicine can rule out possible conditions and provide good news to patients, it neither can give a name to nor explain a vast amount of symptom residue, and patients' experiences may be otherwise unintelligible to the doctor.

Conclusion

The delivery and receipt of diagnostic news is literally a defining moment in the medical interview, an integral part of the "third function" where physicians are to educate patients about their conditions and possible treatments. Where, in the past, this phase of the interview has lacked for research, we add to a number of conversation-analytic investigations demonstrating the orderliness and organization of diagnostic informing events. We have shown that a generic, four-part News Delivery Sequence is adapted to the clinical setting, although articulated asymmetrically according to whether physicians have bad or good testing and diagnostic news to report. When the news is good, deliveries are dependably upbeat and rational, at least initially and before a possible symptom residue may be exposed in the talk. The participants are not at immediate risk of any rupture in mutual intelligibility and understanding. When the news is bad, however, physician and patient appear on the edge of rationality, insofar as the news may evoke a strong emotional reaction in the patient, whose display both parties often work to avert. Consequently, physicians deliver bad news in a more circumspect manner than good news, and patients may resist the news and be restrained in response. The ways in which doctor and patient exhibit the shrouding of bad news may work on behalf of preserving the interview as a rational dialogue or one that avoids the disorder and descent into subjectivity that strong displays of emotion are perceived to entail.

After all, the emotional realm is one that authoritative medicine has so far minimized in the training of students, in part because of the value placed on clinical detachment and affective neutrality (Frankel 1995a; Parsons 1951:458–9; Spiro 1992). Recently, however, there is growing recognition of the importance of empathy in the doctor–patient relationship. An implication from our analysis is that, at the point where bad news is delivered, when patients provide clear although contained displays of emotional distress, there emerges what Suchman et al. (1997) call an "empathic opportunity." Instead of asking the patient to *stay with him* (as in our cancer episode in excerpts 8 and 9), the physician can consider *going with the patient*. In other words, before turning to the rational assessment of prognosis and treatment, the physician could at least acknowledge expressions of affect and invite their exploration in a manner that facilitates understanding in the realm of emotional response.

Our analysis might end with the interactional asymmetries involved in coping with bad news as compared with sharing good news, and the need for physicians' expressions of empathy when patients show distress upon receiving bad news. At first glance, good news appears to be largely unproblematic, as both doctor and patient interactionally handle such news in a relatively smooth and upbeat manner. However, good news can approach another territory of the irrational besides the emotional one. This area is one of indeterminate and uncertain knowledge, where authoritative medicine, having ruled out one or more candidate diseases or conditions, cannot name or explain symptoms a patient experiences and presents. In that sense, good news in medicine can have a kinship to bad news.[15] Therefore, just as investigators have advocated research and training on bad news, we argue that good news and uncertainty demand similar attention.[16] In terms of medical education and curriculum design, at least three skill sets need to be developed. First, because we have barely more than a glimmer of understanding of the psychological processes that physicians must navigate in order to inform patients successfully, physicians will benefit from training in self-awareness (Novack et al. 1997). Second, it is important for physicians to determine patients' needs and desires for information and to ensure that there is agreement about what has been conveyed. Finally, besides integrating awareness of self and other, medical curricula can incorporate learning about the specific devices that effective practitioners use when they deliver diagnostic news.[17] Our aim is to contribute to a research base revealing the interactional dynamics that must be understood for diagnostic news delivery and related skill sets to be effective.

[15] And vice versa. That is, sometimes "bad" news, because it provides relief from situations of indeterminacy, is experienced as relatively "good" news. See, for example, Fallowfield (1991:39).

[16] In a *British Medical Journal* editorial, Fitzpatrick (1996) refers to the McDonald et al. (1996) and the Fitzpatrick and Hopkins (1981) studies showing that normal examination results (and hence good diagnostic news) do not always relieve patient anxiety (see note 14). Fitzpatrick (1996:312) suggests that poor communication is the "usual culprit" in the failure to reassure patients, and calls for physicians to engage in "direct discussion of patients' concerns." But medical curricula, as we have noted, do not ordinarily provide training in how to conduct such discussions. Teaching about the conveyance of good news is probably more neglected than the problem of bad news. Furthermore, Hewson et al. (1996) suggest that, because the handling of uncertainty is also rarely articulated in the medical curriculum, physicians in practice end up using a set of undeveloped, taken-for-granted and tacit skills when having to communicate about indeterminate conditions.

[17] However, see Buckman (1984), Frankel (1994), Maynard (2003: epilogue), and Quill and Townsend (1991), for example.

10

Treatment decisions: negotiations between doctors and parents in acute care encounters

Tanya Stivers

When people seek medical attention for an illness, they are generally looking both for an explanation of the illness and for a solution to their or their child's medical problem (Robinson 2003). Acute medical encounters typically include both a phase of the interaction that is concerned with the diagnosis delivery and a phase that is concerned with treatment for the medical condition (Byrne and Long 1976; Robinson 2003; Waitzkin 1991). Although both the diagnosis delivery and the treatment recommendation involve the physician imparting knowledge to the patient/parent,[1] the two actions have a rather different sequential structure and are treated differently by physicians and parents. This chapter will demonstrate that, in acute medical encounters, the final treatment decision is negotiated by physicians and parents – whether implicitly or explicitly. While parents typically do not respond to diagnosis deliveries, they do routinely accept treatment recommendations. Furthermore, in contrast to diagnoses, if parents do *not* accept a treatment recommendation, this is treated as resisting the recommendation. Resistance – passive and active – is a problematic behavior with both interactional

Portions of this chapter were presented at the Institute in the Qualitative Case Study in Communication Research, University of Washington, Seattle, Washington in 2002; at the International Communication Association Convention in San Diego, California in May 2003; and at the National Communication Association Convention in Miami, Florida in November 2003. Correspondence concerning this article should be addressed to the author at the Max Planck Institute for Psycholinguistics, PB 310, NL-6500 AH Nijmegen, The Netherlands, or electronically at Tanya.Stivers@mpi.nl.

[1] In order to keep things concise, I will generally refer to parent(s) because most of the data I am relying on are pediatric. However, points being made usually refer to both patients and parents unless otherwise specified.

and medical consequences. Finally, I will discuss alternative formats for delivering the treatment recommendation, and show that it may be possible to reduce the likelihood that parents will resist the initial treatment recommendation.

Data

This chapter draws on several corpora of video- and audiotaped medical encounters from internal medicine, orthopedics, and pediatrics collected between 1996 and 2001. However, the original analysis of the practices outlined in this chapter was based exclusively on pediatric encounters (see Stivers et al. 2003 and Stivers 2005a for a full description of these samples). Relying heavily on previous analyses (Stivers 2005a, 2005b), this chapter makes use of this broad range of data in order to document that treatment is oriented to as negotiated across primary care. The examples chosen for this chapter – whether from pediatrics or from the adult context – are representative of and qualitatively similar to the cases in the original analyses on which this chapter is based.

Background

Patient participation in health care

Many countries are recognizing that the role that patients play in their own health care is an important and consequential one. Because of this, there has been much emphasis within health care policy on encouraging physicians to involve patients/parents in treatment decisions. Within the United States, the primary government health care policy document states that patients who participate actively in decisions about their health care can positively impact national health (see US Department of Health and Human Services 2000 for a description of these data). And many health policy researchers assert that patients should, whenever possible, be offered choices in their treatment decisions (Brody 1980; Butler et al. 1998; Deber 1994; Emanuel and Emanuel 1992; Evans et al. 1987; Fallowfield et al. 1990; Kassirer 1994; Levine et al. 1992). A number of American medical associations now recommend that physicians explicitly involve patients in their decision-making. For instance, the American Cancer Society, the American Urological Association, the American Gastroenterological Association, the American College of Physicians, and the National Institutes of Health (NIH) all recommend shared decision-making for decisions surrounding cancer screening (Frosch and Kaplan 1999).

The primary rationale for these recommendations has two facets: patients have a right to, and want to, participate in the decision (Blanchard et al. 1988; Cassileth et al. 1980; Emerson 1983; Ende et al. 1989; Faden et al. 1981; Thompson et al. 1993); and patients have improved outcomes when they participate in medical decision-making, including satisfaction (Brody, Miller, Lerman Smith, and Caputo 1989; Brody, Miller, Lerman, Smith, Lazaro, and Blum 1989; Evans et al. 1987), patient health (Brody 1980; Greenfield et al. 1988; Kaplan et al. 1989; Mendonca and Brehm 1983; Schulman 1979), and patient mental well-being (Brody, Miller, Lerman, Smith, and Caputo 1989; Evans et al. 1987; Fallowfield et al. 1990; Greenfield et al. 1988). Although researchers suggest that in the acute primary care context, doctors are much less likely to involve patients in treatment decision-making (Braddock et al. 1999; Elwyn et al. 1999; Tuckett et al. 1985), this appears to be based on the assumption that a patient must be explicitly invited to participate by a physician in order to be involved in the decision process. In what follows I will show not only that parents do, typically without invitation, affect the treatment outcome through participating in a negotiation process, but also that their participation is treated by physicians as conditionally relevant.

Analysis

Responses to diagnosis deliveries and treatment recommendations

Parents and physicians alike orient to diagnoses as within the physician's domain of expertise. This is primarily evidenced by the fact that when physicians deliver diagnoses they are routinely not even minimally responded to (Heath 1992; Peräkylä 1998; Stivers 2005b). Further, physicians do not pursue parent uptake of their diagnoses. This normative environment sustains diagnosis delivery as complete and permits movement into the treatment recommendation. By contrast, both parties orient to parents (perhaps more than adult patients) as having the right to accept or reject the treatment proposal. Thus, while diagnoses are oriented to by the participants as within the physician's domain of responsibility, treatment decisions are oriented to as the responsibility of both parties.

It has previously been argued that participants are typically oriented to treatment as the final activity of the project of solving patients' new medical problems (Robinson 2003). However, a physician's presentation of a treatment recommendation is *not* generally treated by either doctors or parents/patients as sufficient for activity closure. Both physicians and parents/patients display an orientation to parent acceptance of the treatment recommendation as relevant upon completion of the treatment recommendation (Stivers 2005b). Thus, the sequential structure of treatment recommendations typically involves a recommendation followed by parent/patient acceptance, and only then a shift to other business or closure of the encounter. For example:

(1) 2002 (Dr. 6)

1	DOC:		.hhh Uh:m his – # – # lef:t:=h ea:r=h, is infected,
2		->	(0.2)
3	DOC:		.h is bulging, has uh little pus in thuh
4		->	ba:ck, =h
5	DOC:	->	Uh:m, an' it's re:d,
6	DOC:		.hh So he needs some antibiotics to treat tha:t,
7	DAD:	=>	Alright.
8	DOC:		Mka:y, so we'll go ahead and treat- him: <he has
9			no a- uh:m, allergies to any penicillin or anything.

Having just completed her examination of the child, the doctor here explains the child's diagnosis (lines 1–5). Although the doctor comes to possible turn completion most notably at the end of line 1 but also at the end of line 4 and at the end of line 5, the parent does not respond. By contrast, after the physician offers her treatment recommendation in line 6 the father accepts this with "Alright." immediately upon possible completion of that turn constructional unit (TCU). Also notice that, once the parent has accepted, the physician, at line 8, moves from the generic discussion of "antibiotics" to determining which type of medication can be prescribed.

Another example is shown in Extract (2). Here, the mother receipts the doctor's diagnosis of an ear infection with "Mm:." (line 3). This token offers only minimal acknowledgment of the diagnosis (Gardner 1997).

(2) 1183 (Dr. 1)

1	DOC:		Well I think what's happened is is that she
2			ha:s this: uh- (.) .h ear infection in her left ear?,
3	MOM:		[Mm:.
4	DOC:	->	[And we'll put her on some medicine and she'll [be fine.
5	MOM:		[Okay.

However, the parent's response to the treatment recommendation, is "Okay." (line 5). This token – particularly with final intonation – accepts the doctor's recommendation, thereby treating it as a proposal which makes acceptance relevant, and not as an informing. The parent's two different receipt tokens offered in close proximity provide evidence that parents orient to diagnoses and treatment recommendations as actions that make relevant different sorts of responses.

Withholding acceptance as passive resistance

That parents routinely accept physicians' treatment recommendations but not diagnoses is one form of evidence that treatment is a domain of joint responsibility and that parents participate in treatment decisions in a way that they do not participate in diagnosis. Further evidence lies in physicians' pursuits of acceptance when none is forthcoming. For instance, see Extract (3) from an internal medicine practice. The diagnosis is delivered across lines 1–7. The patient receipts the information with continuers at lines 3, 6, and 9. In line 10 the physician moves into her treatment recommendation, which is also receipted with continuers in lines 12, 14, and 16. Note that the physician shifted from diagnosis delivery to treatment recommendation in the face of having received only continuers from the patient. Once in the treatment recommendation phase, however, the physician pursues the patient's acceptance.

(3) SG 1211

```
 1 DOC:       I don't ^think- to be honest I think you
 2            probably had this infection_ .hh=
 3 PAT:       =M[m hm,
 4 DOC:         [an:d=uh it's- whatever you had it's: vi ral
 5            infection:, your bo[dy is trying to get rid of
 6 PAT:                          [Mm hm,
 7            it,
 8 DOC:       .h[h
 9 PAT:         [Mm h[m.
10 DOC:              [An' you just need uh little bit of push_
11            (0.4)
12 PAT:       [Mm hm,
13 DOC:       [to help you to get over this cough:.
14 PAT:       Mm hm,
15 DOC:       I don't think you need antibiotics?,
16 PAT:       Mm hm,
17 DOC: ->    I (didn't)/(don't) see any si:gns .h indicati:ng
18      ->    (.) ya know- (.) uh: for thuh [antibiotics.
19 PAT:                                     [#huh huh# ((cough))
20 PAT:       hm [kay,
21 DOC:          [.hh Uhm you probably need some strong cough
22            medicatio:n=so[me
23 PAT:                     [Mm hm,
24 DOC:       expectorant, stronger expectorants, [.hh ai- to=
25 PAT:                                           [Mm hm,
26 DOC:       =clear your airways from thuh phle:gm,
27 DOC: ->    .ml[h and uh: (m) also at ni:ght I would use uh=
28 PAT:          [Mm hm,
29 DOC: ->    =cough suppressant which I usually: (.) am hesitant
30      ->    to u:se_
31 DOC: ->    .hh [but only at ni:ght_ (.) so you can go t:o s:-=
32 PAT:           [Mm hm,
33 DOC: ->    =[uh to slee:p an:' not wake up with (th') cough.
34 PAT:       =[Mm hm,
35 PAT:       Mm hm?,
36 DOC: ->    Okay?
37 PAT:       Mkay.
```

First, at lines 17–18 the physician offers a rationale for her assertion that the woman does not need antibiotics. She accounts for the recommendation, which is one way of pursuing acceptance (Stivers 2005b). In response, the patient offers "hm kay," but with continuing intonation, this offers acknowledgment but does not fully accept the treatment. Second, the physician offers an alternative medication ("strong cough medicatio:n", lines 21–22, 24, and 26), but this is receipted only with continuers. Thus, the patient here treats the physician as not yet done with her recommendation. The physician then goes on to recommend a third medication beginning at line 27 ("also at ni:ght"). Note that this recommendation is offered only after no uptake following line 26. Although it is not uncommon for physicians to offer multiple recommendations, it is notable that additional recommendations frequently appear at interactional junctures such as this, where there has not been an acceptance of the treatment proposal. This is further pursued with the reinvocation of "only at ni:ght." in line 31, which works to recomplete the sequence and thus pursues sequence closure (Schegloff, in press). Finally, at the end of the treatment in line 35, the patient still offers only a continuer in response. At this point the physician overtly solicits acceptance with an upward-intoned "Okay?" in line 36.

Extract (4), from a pediatric encounter, is an example which shows that silence or continuers communicate a withholding of acceptance in a sequential environment where acceptance is normatively required. At this point, the physician has completed an in-office throat culture and is waiting for these culture results. She begins her treatment recommendation with suggestions that are irrespective of these culture results. Throughout this explanation the parent says very little. At each single arrowed line there is an opportunity for the parent to respond to the physician's recommendation – acceptance is a relevant action. However, in each case the parent does not offer acknowledgment, let alone acceptance.

(4) 2020 (Dr. 6)

1 DOC: #Mkay:::.# so::,=h (0.5)
2 DOC: Tlk=.h Let's see: what=thuh results of this i:s,=h
3 while we're waiting for tha:::t,
4 DOC: .h So no matter what the result i:s, h she does
5 ha:ve uh:m hh redness in 'er throa:t, an' looks
6 like she has pharyngitis, <whether it's from bacterial
7 -> or from virus,

8	DOC:	->	.hh So:: uhm I want her to do mouthwashes?,
9	DOC:	->	.h Gargling at ho:me?,
10	DOC:	->	Really deep gargling. (.) All the way back.
11		=>	#Aghghghgh.# All thuh way back of thuh throat, okay:?,
12	DOC:	->	.hh Do it as many as- time as you can.
13			(.)
14	DOC:	->	Three:_ four times uh day. Especially after eating.
15		=>	Mkay,
16	DOC:	->	.h That clears it out an' that makes it feel better.
17			Mkay,=you can do it with salt water:, you can do it
18		->	with Sco:pe,
19	DOC:	->	.hh whatever mouthwash: flavor that she likes.
20	DOC:	->	.hh So lets do tha:t,
21	DOC:	=>	.hh Give 'er uh soft die:t?, Mkay:, Don't
22			give her anything heavy, nothing oily:,
23		->	French fries, (.) fried chicken_ hamburgers,
24	DOC:	=>	.hh Nothing spicy.=h for uh couple days. Okay:,
25	DOC:		.h Cuz it's gonna hurt every time she swallows those
26		->	kind uh stuff.
27	DOC:	->	.hh Let's give 'er lots of liquids at ho:me,
28			(0.6)
29	DOC:	->	.hh Give 'er: water, jui:ce, whatever she wants to drink.=h
30	DOC:	->	Ice cream is okay:, That will make her feel better:,
31	DOC:	->	.h Popsicles,
32			(.)
33	DOC:	->	That makes you feel better,
34	DOC:	=>	.h Mkay:?,
35	DOC:	->	.h Maybe some mashed potatoe::s, you know
36		->	(so)/(it's uh) soft diet. as uh general.
37			(.)
38	DOC:	=>	Yogur:t, things like that. Nkay:,
39	DOC:	->	.hh Uh:m_ and you're just gonna have to rest.
40			(.)
41	DOC:		You know?,
42			(.)
43	DOC:		She's gonna have to rest.
44	MOM:		Yeah.=
45	DOC:		=No more running arou:nd an' – (.) ya know staying
46		->	up la:te, an' things like that.
47	DOC:		.h You're just gonna have=t' take lots of na:ps,
48		->	an' re:st, throughout thuh weekend.
49	DOC:	=>	.h Mkay:, ((Doc moves to look at rapid strep culture)

This physician seeks acceptance of her recommendations for mouthwashes (line 8), a soft diet (line 21), liquids (line 27), and rest (line 39). We can see this in several ways. First, similar to Extract (3), she provides accounts for her recommendations (e.g., lines 16, 25, 30, and 33). She also restates her treatment recommendations (e.g., lines 10–11, 35–36, 43, and 47–48). Third, she adds additional treatments (lines 21, 27, and 39). Fourth, she can be seen to pursue acceptance with rising intonation at the end of TCUs such as in lines 8, 9, and 21 (Sacks and Schegloff 1979; Schegloff 1996d). That these locations were designedly in pursuit of acknowledgment can be seen, for example, in the doctor's repeat of lines 8 and 9 in line 10 and the respecification with "All the way back." (also in line 10). There is still further pursuit in line 11, first with the demonstration of gargling, and second with the redoing, yet again, of "All thuh way back of thuh throat," and then with a more direct request for acceptance with "okay:?,".

Similarly, through the physician's use of three-part lists the physician also hearably invites the parent's uptake because these lists project completion and have been shown to be strongly designed for recipient uptake (Heritage and Greatbatch 1986; Jefferson 1990). For example, at the end of line 19 the doctor reaches the third item of her projected three-part list and thereby implicates confirmation. A similar list is in line 29, but, as before, the parent does not offer any uptake.

As in Extract (3), the physician actively pursues the parent's acceptance through other means. For example, in the double arrowed lines, the doctor can be seen to pursue acceptance with various forms of "okay." The physician also changes her addressee from the mother to the child (see lines 33 and 39). This change in addressee also appears to be designed to elicit acceptance even if that is from the child.[2] And, in line 41, the physician pursues a response with "You know?,". However, it is not until line 44, after multiple pursuits and a change in addressee back to the mother, that she minimally agrees with the doctor's treatment recommendation of rest.

In this section I have shown that physicians work diligently to elicit parent acceptance before closing the activity of recommending treatment. We saw that their pursuits of acceptance

[2] If the physician had elicited agreement from the child – which is explicitly sought – this might have helped get a somewhat coerced acceptance by the mother. It is in this sense that I see this as a practice for pursuing *parent* acceptance.

include extending the activity with accounts, returning to prior activities such as diagnostic findings in support of the treatment recommendation, offering additional recommendations, pursuing acceptance with rising intonation, or, more explicitly, with variations on "Okay?". Thus, a failure to accept is heard as withholding acceptance; and physicians regard it as passive resistance (Heritage and Sefi 1992) to their proposed treatment. Thus, passive resistance is one interactional resource through which parents/patients initiate a negotiation of the treatment decision. This argument relies on a normative structure of treatment recommendations to suggest that even "doing nothing" in a particular sequential environment can be a consequential form of participation and can affect treatment decisions.

Active resistance

Whereas passive resistance works purely in a second/responsive sequential position, active resistance makes relevant a next action by the physician, so it is both a responsive and an initiating action. This makes it a stronger type of resistance. Despite these differences, either form of resistance puts the physician in a position of working to "convince" a parent to accept the proposed treatment recommendation, or offering the parent possible or actual concessions because of the normative orientation that parents/patients must accept treatment recommendations before physicians proceed to the next activity in the visit. Through either type of resistance, parents hearably take a position against the treatment they are being offered. In the pediatric data in particular, parent resistance is typically against an over-the-counter or non-prescription treatment plan. In the following instance, the entry into a negotiation is brought to the surface of the interaction. Here, after the physician states his position against antibiotics in line 4, the father resists by offering a narrative of his own illness experience (lines 6, 10, 12, 14, 17–18, 20, 23, 25, and 27).

(5) 32–28–03

1 DOC: I th:ink from what you've told me (0.2) that this is
2 pro:bably .h uh kind of (0.2) virus infec[tion,
3 DAD: [Uh huh,

4 DOC: (0.4) th:at I don't think antibiotics will ki:ll,
5 (0.2)
6 DAD: -> Well-
7 DOC: [Thee other-
8 DAD: [( )
9 DOC: >Go=ahead_<
10 DAD: -> Yeah. .hh ( ) I had it- I had thuh symp[toms
11 DOC: [I understand.
12 DAD: -> Three weeks ago.
13 DOC: [Right.
14 DAD: -> [.hh An:d I've been taking thuh over the counter cough
15 -> [( )
16 DOC: [(Good_)
17 DAD: -> Uh s- ( ) coughing syrup, Nothing take away. hh
18 -> Especially my sor- my [th- my throat was real=
19 DOC: [Mm hm
20 DAD: -> =sore [for (awhile- et- that) w:eek.
21 DOC: [Uh huh
22 DOC: °Right,°
23 DAD: -> an:d (.) I start taking thuh antibiotic (0.5)
24 INF: eh he ((cry))
25 DAD: -> Yesterday.
26 DOC: Right,
27 DAD: -> And it (.) seemed to take care of the problem.
28 DOC: [(Well) that's why we're doin' a throat [culture.
29 DAD: [( ) [Yeah.
30 DOC: [is TUH SEE if they need antibiotics.
31 DAD: [( ) Yeah yeah.
32 (0.2)
33 DOC: Cause <I don't th::ink they do.
34 DAD: O[kay,
35 DOC: => [Now if you (.) absolutely insist_ I will give you
36 => antibiotics_ but [I don't think that's the right=
37 INF: [#eh::#
38 => medicine for 'em,
39 DAD: No I'm not saying- I'm not saying it- (0.2) don't
40 get me wrong but- I'm sta- trying tuh tell you the
41 [history of ( )
42 DOC: [I understand, I- I heard [you when you told me,
43 DAD: [Yeah.
44 DOC: I under[stand,
45 DAD [Uh huh,
(INF = infant)

In lines 23, 25, and 27, the father builds a case that antibiotics solved his own illness. This narrative is positioned at a place where acceptance of the treatment recommendation is due, and thus is hearably resistant. Through the narrative, the father implies that antibiotics would be helpful for his two sons, who are ill with "the same thing" (as he mentioned earlier in the encounter). The physician's response shows his understanding of this implication as he explains that antibiotics are a possible treatment, and that this is why he performed a throat culture. Moreover, in lines 35–36 and 38, the doctor offers to prescribe antibiotics against his medical judgment if the parent insists. Note that the physician here overtly acknowledges the impact of parent pressure: if the parent continues to press, he will provide the antibiotics despite the fact that they would, in his opinion, be ineffective and thus inappropriate.

This case thus offers two types of evidence for the importance parent/patient participation plays in these encounters. (1) The parent displays in his active resistance that his stance towards the treatment matters. He takes a position which, though implicit, displays himself to be in favor of antibiotics and opposed to over-the-counter treatment. (2) The doctor's explicit acknowledgment that he will prescribe if pressured, offers evidence that for physicians, parent participation matters and can alter a treatment decision even when that participation takes this form rather than a response to an inquiry about preferences.

Another example is taken from an orthopedic clinic where a physician is seeing a woman for shoulder pain. Here, the physician recommends two types of treatment, beginning in line 1. The first involves physical therapy (lines 1–5). Although there is no verbal uptake at line 6, note that the physician had projected at least two treatment recommendations through his numbering of them. Using "number one" implies that there will be a next. Thus, acceptance is not due yet, though the patient nods in provisional (or "thus far") acceptance (line 6). The second type of recommendation is "tuh let me give ya uh little injection right here." (lines 7–8). In response to this recommendation, the patient bodily recoils (line 10), and vocally offers a very affective high-pitched "Mm::." (line 11), which is treated immediately by the physician as resistance.

(6) SG 901

1 DOC: SO WHAT I'D LIKE- what I would recommend
2 that we do is number one is that you get

3 some formal physical therapy tuh work on
4 some exercises.an' I have uh little
5 [sheet that we'll go over,
6 PAT: [((nodding))
7 DOC: .hh And number two I'd like you tuh let me give
8 ya uh little injection [right here.
9 DOC: [((pointing at shoulder model))
10 PAT: [((wraps arms around body; leans back))
11 PAT: -> (↑↑Mm::.) ((high pitch))
12 DOC: If you don't wanta do it we don't [(hafta do.)
13 PAT: [No: no no.
14 (I- i- if you hafta you hafta I- I)
15 just #ugh#.
16 (0.5)
17 DOC: If you wanna wai:t (.) I mean we can do it
18 next ti:me,
19 (.)
20 DOC: But it- I- I think most of thuh time what
21 happens is is I put three medicines in
22 there oka:y,

Immediately following this active resistance, the physician backs down from his recommendation for an injection. He shifts from offering it as what he'd "like" to do, to making it contingent on her own wishes (line 12). Slightly later, after the patient exhibits resigned acceptance (lines 13–15), he offers to at least delay the injection until another visit (lines 17–18). Although ultimately the patient does agree to the injection in line with lines 13–15, both of the physician's modifications to what he originally proposed underscore that the treatment outcome is a product of negotiation.

That physicians respond to parent resistance with concessions (whether that be delaying a particular recommendation or eliminating it altogether, both of which were seen in the extract above, or offering treatment that had not been previously offered at all) is potentially problematic not only from an interactional perspective but also from a medical perspective. For instance, in some cases, physicians alter their treatment recommendations from one type of medication to another, and this can be particularly concerning when that change involves a medication such as addictive pain relievers, medications with known side effects, or antibiotics, (Extract 5) because of the current national and international issue with bacterial resistance to antibiotics (Baquero et al. 2002; McCaig and Hughes

1995; Neu 1992; Reichler et al. 1992; Schwartz 1999; Whitney et al. 2000; Wise et al. 1998) which has been escalated in no small part by inappropriate prescribing of antibiotics for viral infections (Cristino 1999; Deeks et al. 1999; Gomez et al. 1995; Nava et al. 1994; Watanabe et al. 2000).

Although complete reversals in treatment recommendations are rare, that they happen at all provides strong evidence for the power of parent resistance and the critical role that parent/patient acceptance of the treatment recommendation plays in the treatment decision. The negotiation activity, in order to generate parent acceptance, can be quite protracted, and concessions on the part of physicians are dramatic. An instance is shown in Extracts (7a)–(7f). Here, in lines 1–2 of (7a), the physician recommends against antibiotics, but there is no parent acceptance. The physician expands her treatment recommendation against antibiotics in line 3 with an increment concerning the duration of antibiotic treatment that would be required (Schegloff 2001). The parent does not accept here, either. The physician then offers an alternative type of treatment: eye treatment (line 4). This is not accepted, and a third treatment is offered in line 5 (a decongestant). This recommendation is followed by an account (lines 7–8).

(7a) 2019 (Dr. 6)

1 DOC: .hh So: uh:m a- at this time I don't wanta commit 'er to:
2 antibiotics.
3 DOC: Like two weeks, or three weeks, or whatever:?
4 DOC: .h I thi:nk I'll go ahead and treat her for the eye:s?,
5 an' I wanta give her some decongestant.
6 (.)
7 DOC: .hh So that would, suck out all that, um,
8 secretions?=

During the next 45 lines of talk (data not shown) the parent continues to withhold acceptance and thus passively resists the non-antibiotic treatment being proposed. She inquires about decongestants and what forms they come in (i.e., liquid or pill) but does not accept them. Then, at line 54, she inquires about the treatment for her daughter's eyes. The next component is shown in Extract (7b):

(7b) ((45 lines following 7a))

54 MOM: [And then for conjunctivitis is there [(another one?,) or_]
55 DOC: [She needs uh:m_]
56 She needs eye drops.
57 (0.4)
58 DOC: Antibiotic eye drops.
59 (.)
60 DOC: Mkay:,=h=An' she's gonna hafta put- you're gonna hafta put-
61 (.) few drops i:n_ several times uh da:y.
62 DOC: .hh An' that will clear her redness:, an' that (will) get
63 rid of all that goopy: stuff. that she's having.
64 (1.0)
65 DOC: Mkay:?
66 (0.2)
67 DOC: .h ^But otherwise her ears look really goo:d,
68 MOM: Yeah [(her) ears alwa[ys look good.
69 DOC: [.hh [Her: chest sounds goo:d,
70 DOC: Uh:m, .hh- Ya know i- She doesn't look like uh:m (.)
71 Why don't we go ahead and try thuh decongestant first.
72 (.)
73 DOC: Mkay:,
74 DOC: An' if you don't think there's any: improvement with
75 thuh decongestan:t, .h an' you think she still has s:-
76 you know (-) getting all the secretions ba:ck, .h [you know=
77 MOM: [Mm hm.
78 DOC: =an' if she has:=signs of fever:, .h you know at that ti:me
79 we'll go ahea:d, but at this ti:me, you know she's (uh)
80 she's afebrile no[:w,

Here again, the parent passively resists the treatment suggested for conjunctivitis (following lines 56, 58, 61, and 63). Similar to other instances, the physician works to secure her acceptance. Note in particular the account for the eye drops recommendation in lines 62–63 and the questioning "Mkay:?" (line 65) which is positioned following a full second of silence and still does not receive acceptance. Here the physician retreats to her examination findings, restating them (lines 67 and 69). The mother resists this as a rationale for the treatment by stating that "(her) ears always look good." (line 68). The physician does not take up this resistance from the mother, but instead reasserts her treatment recommendation in line 71. The parent again passively resists even after further explicit pursuit (line 73). The physician then moves into a point at which she would consider offering antibiotics – a future concession. This future concession would be possible if the child, as the doctor says, has secretions or a fever. However, these are precisely the symptoms which brought the parent in to the physician in the first instance. The parent actively resists this since, as a condition for prescribing, the parent conveys her understanding that the condition has already been met. See Extract (7c):

(7c)

81 DOC: . . . afebrile no[:w,
82 MOM: [(Well) she's had uh low-grade temp f- on
83 [an' off (for) thuh past couple day:s_ (.) Uh:m_ (0.5)
84 DOC: [Mm hm:,
85 MOM: She never- She- (0.5)
86 DOC: Mm hm[:,

The mother actively resists the denial of antibiotics (most recently invoked through the mention of "at that ti:me we'll go ahea:d, but at this ti:me," lines 78–79). She actively resists citing that the condition of fever, which the physician indicates might, if present, be enough to warrant a prescription, has been present at home (lines 82–83). She then recounts previous experiences where medical encounters have failed to detect a temperature when one did exist (beginning in line 85 and extending six lines beyond – data not shown).

The mother then returns to her active resistance on the count not only of a fever being present (line 93) but also on the grounds that her daughter is otherwise behaving abnormally (lines 95 and 97).

(7d) ((six lines following [7c]))

93 MOM: But anyway she's had low-grade temp [(an' uhm),
94 DOC: [Mm hm.
95 MOM: (1.1) just really hasn't been hersel:f. It's- it's- It's:=
96 DOC: =M[m hm.
97 MOM: [(ya know)/(even) more than: uhm (1.5) thee eye thi:ng.
98 DOC: Uh huh:,
99 MOM: <I mean I usually don't- I- I usually wait to bring her in
100 at least until [( ).
101 DOC: [You wait unti- Yeah:,.
102 DOC: .hhh Uh:[m-
103 MOM: [Cuz it's such a big deal to come here [( )
104 DOC: [Yea:h,=h

```
            I mean: if you wa:nt ya know- I mean she looks.=
MOM:        =Can I at least have thuh prescription an' I'll decide
            whether or not to fill it, i[n a couple day:s,
DOC:                                  [.tlk
DOC:        For the antibiotics[:?
MOM:                           [Ye[ah.
DOC:                              [Uh::m_ I really don't like to do tha:t,
            because: I mean .hh She doesn't look: like she has sinusitis:.
            Ya know?,
            (.)
DOC:        Uhm, if you really wanta be su:re we can go ahead and
DOC:        take: x rays to make su:re if it's really opacify:,
        - >
DOC:        .hh cause unnecessary treatment for sinusitis: she can
        - > get resistant to uh lot of those antibiotics?,
        - > uh lot of those bugs. I mean.
DOC:    - > .hh An:d it's- it's not really good for her:.
        - > (1.0)
DOC:        So:: we try to minimi:ze ya know- treatment until
        - > it's really necessary.
        - > (.)
```

The implicit claim being made by the parent in lines 95 and 97 appears to be that the girl is "sicker" than the doctor's treatment recommendation would suggest. In lines 99–100 and 103, the mother claims to normally "wait" before visiting the doctor, thus displaying "troubles resistance" (Jefferson 1988), that she is not a mother who rushes her child to the doctor (see also Halkowski this volume; Heritage and Robinson this volume). Again, the implication is that the child's condition is more serious than the doctor's treatment recommendation would suggest. In response, the physician begins a turn that appears more concessionary. She first agrees with the parent with "Yea:h," (line 104) and then with "I mean: if you wa:nt ya know-". Note that, as a turn beginning, this is very similar to "If you absolutely insist" discussed in Extract (5). Both beginnings frame the forthcoming response as a responsive concession and thus co-implicate the parent in the revised treatment recommendation. So far, the parent has not yet explicitly stated anything that she wants or expects, but she has passively resisted the physician's treatment recommendation by withholding acceptance, and actively resisted the treatment recommendation by implying that her child is sicker than the doctor is prepared to recognize.

However, the concessionary frame is abandoned in favor of a less concessionary "I mean she looks.", which, given the no-problem physical examination that preceded this discussion, is likely to be heard as headed for an evaluation consistent with this, and inconsistent with prescribing antibiotics. It is at this point that the mother's strongest form of treatment resistance comes – an overt request for antibiotics in lines 106–107. This not only calls into question the treatment recommended so far but specifically challenges the physician's assertion earlier in Extract (7a) that she does not want to commit the girl to antibiotics at this point.

The mother's request "Can I at least have thuh prescription" treats the prescription as a minimal form of action. This is accomplished with "at least" and by coupling this initial proposal with a second unit of her turn "an' I'll decide whether or not to fill it, in a couple day:s," claiming some measure of autonomy and discretion (i.e., that she would not immediately fill the prescription and give her child antibiotics and could further determine whether and when to fill the prescription). The doctor denies her request in line 111, but does offer a concession: they could perform an X-ray that would potentially clarify whether or not the child should *appropriately* be treated for sinusitis (lines 115–116). In addition, the physician cites the inappropriateness of treating this condition with antibiotics and the general need to avoid inappropriate prescribing as an account for her recommendation against antibiotics. Note that here the account, part of a typical dispreferred turn insofar as it works to deny a request (Pomerantz 1984a), also works to pursue parent acceptance since, once again, acceptance is relevant.

The mother accepts neither the physician's rejection of antibiotics nor the concession. At each arrowed line the mother withholds acceptance of the physician's recommendation. The mother continues active resistance across the next stretch of interaction (see below). Here, after the doctor again returns to outline a situation in which she would concede and prescribe antibiotics – if the girl "looks really -ba:d," (line 126) – the mother asserts that her daughter never looks bad (lines 128–129). She goes on to claim that her daughter is not herself, thus implying (again) that her daughter is sicker than the physician is recognizing. This begins in line 128 with "I mean she can be really sick and she never looks-" and continues across the 20 lines of data not shown.

(7e)

123 DOC: So:: we try to minimi:ze ya know- treatment until
124 -> it's really necessary.
125 -> (.)
126 DOC: You know of course if she's s- you know looks really -ba:d,
127 [then I'll go ahead.
128 MOM: [(see she ne-) she never looks: ba:d. I mean
129 [she can be really sick and she never looks-
130 DOC: [Mm hm:,
131 DOC: Mm hm[:,
132 MOM: [You know: I've taken her in here with:

((20 lines: examples of girl not acting sick but having infections))

153 MOM: And plus it's her (t=her:) uhm (0.6) tlk (0.4)
154 Uh:hm_(0.5) °What'm I tryin' t' say:_° Emotionally.
155 MOM: (I [mean she's been) .hh (0.8) t- you know more 'n more=
156 DOC: [Mm hm:,
157 MOM: =tire:[d,
158 DOC: [Mm [hm:,
159 MOM: [And more 'n mo:re (.) upset easily_ [an' stuff:
160 DOC: [Mm hm,
161 MOM: over thuh past couple weeks, [an' it's- it's just been
162 DOC: [Mm hm:,
163 MOM: =building an' building an' bui[lding.
164 DOC: [Mm hm.

The mother appears to escalate her claims about how sick her daughter is by invoking the emotional and psychological realm (lines 153–155, 157, 159, 161, and 163), especially through her repetition and intensification of "building" (line 163).

Finally, the physician works to close the activity after what is now over 160 lines of negotiation over treatment. Note that if the mother had agreed readily to the treatment following the recommendation shown in Extract (7a), this activity might well have been closed virtually immediately. Now, the physician offers yet another concession – a willingness to talk to the girl's regular physician (lines 167 and 170).

(7f)

163 MOM: =building an' building an' bui[lding.
164 DOC: [Mm hm.
165 DOC: .tlkhh Who: usually sees her.

166 MOM: Doctor Hilton.
167 DOC: .hh Uh:m lemme call him an' see what he uhm says.=
168 MOM: =Oh is h[e around (today?)
169 DOC: [Okay?
170 I don't know if he's arou:nd but I'll=lemmme try to call
171 him. .hh because: uh:m_
172 MOM: He's not [( ).
173 DOC: [Tlk I really don't want to treat 'er.
174 (0.5)
175 DOC: Uhm but then I've only seen her first time.
176 DOC: This is my first time seeing her so I really don't
177 know how she (.) you know i:s,
178 DOC: .hh So let me call 'im an' see: what he sugge:st,
179 DOC: h An' the:n we'll go from there.
180 (.)
181 DOC: [Does that sound okay?
182 MOM: [°Okay.°
183 MOM: Sure, if you [can (reach) him £it sounds great.£

Even here, after proposing to call the child's regular doctor, the mother is resistant (line 174) when the physician re-raises her treatment recommendation in line 173. However, when she proposes, as an alternative, that she will "see: what he sugge:st," in line 178 and make a decision at that point (line 179), the mother acquiesces to the proposal only when the doctor pursues acceptance in line 181 with "Does that sound okay?" Even then the acceptance is conditional (in line 183 with "Sure, if you can (reach) him £it sounds great.£"

Ultimately, the physician cannot reach the girl's regular doctor, and she prescribes antibiotics for the girl despite having diagnosed only conjunctivitis, having explicitly rejected a sinusitis diagnosis, and having repeatedly expressed a desire not to treat the girl with antibiotics.

This section has focused on a second type of resistance – active resistance – to a physician's treatment recommendation. We have seen that active resistance is stronger than passive resistance because it initiates new sequences and thus makes a response from the physician conditionally relevant. This puts the physician in a place where he or she must deal with closing the treatment recommendation sequence as well as with securing acceptance from the parent before the visit can progress to the next activity and/or visit closure. Because of this, resistance can be understood as a communication practice through which parents can, intentionally or unintentionally, place pressure on physicians to alter their treatment recommendation. This is a critical form of patient/parent participation that may not ordinarily be recognized as playing a role in shaping treatment outcomes.

So far, this chapter has shown that treatment recommendations involve a negotiation between physicians and patients/parents. When treatment proposals are accepted, the relevance of that acceptance is not readily observable. It is thus primarily through deviant cases where acceptance is not forthcoming, and resistance – whether passive or active – is present, that the sequential structure and thus the relevance of parent participation becomes observable. The cases shown here provide evidence that treatment recommendations are not the result of an algorithm based on clinical findings alone but rather are subject to the influence and pressure of parent behavior and must be worked out in the medical encounter through the interaction.

This analysis has been based primarily on evidence from pediatric encounters, but a brief examination of internal medicine and orthopedic interactions – as illustrated in Extracts (3) and (6), respectively – suggest that negotiations and the practices involved are characteristic of treatment recommendations across acute primary care encounters. One of the issues this raises has been adumbrated already. What are the dangers of negotiations between physicians and patients? Previous research in pediatrics shows that when parents actively resist a physician's treatment recommendation, physicians are more likely to report that they perceived the parent to expect antibiotic treatment (Stivers et al. 2003). Because prior research has shown physicians to be more likely to prescribe antibiotics inappropriately when they perceive a parent to expect antibiotics (Mangione-Smith et al. 1999), there are both medical and social reasons for wanting to avoid or minimize parent resistance. The next part of this chapter examines alternative formats for delivering the treatment recommendation that appear directly related to whether or not parents actively resist the treatment recommendation.

The format of treatment recommendation

If we return to examples already shown in this chapter, we can see that physicians tend to offer their treatment recommendations in one of two main ways: either as a recommendation *for* or *against* a particular treatment. The most common delivery format for treatment recommendations is for the physician to recommend *for* what is to be done for the patient's problem. We observed this format in Extracts (1), (2), and (6). See Extract (8), previously shown as Extract: (1)

(8) 2002 (Dr. 6)

1 DOC: -> .hh So he needs some antibiotics to treat tha:t,
2 DAD: Alright.
3 DOC: Mka:y, so we'll go ahead and treat- him: <he has
4 no a- uh:m, allergies to any penicillin or anything.

In line 1, the physician delivers her treatment recommendation, formatted as a recommendation for how the boy should be treated (line 1).

In contrast to the recommendations *for* treatment, physicians also relate treatment recommendations negatively – by recommending *against* treatment. Recommendations that are formatted in this manner recommend against either a class of treatment or a particular treatment, as in Extracts (3), (4), (5), and (7). Here is Extract (9) as an example, which is Extract (5) repeated:

(9) 32–28–03

1 DOC: I th:ink from what you've told me (0.2) that this is
2 pro:bably .h uh kind of (0.2) virus infec[tion,
3 DAD: [Uh huh,
4 DOC: -> (0.4) th:at I don't think antibiotics will ki:ll,
5 (0.2)
6 DAD: Well-

Here, the physician identifies a treatment but then negates it with "tha:t I don't think antibiotics will ki:ll," (line 4). Although the named treatment is potentially relevant, treatment is being oriented to as relevant, the parent is not offered a solution but rather is told which solution is not an option.

As mentioned early in this chapter, previous research has argued that parents and physicians alike orient to the relevance of treatment following a diagnosis delivery. When treatment is not immediately forthcoming, patients pursue a treatment recommendation (Robinson 2003). Although this pattern is present across the different primary care data I have examined, more prominent is that some treatment recommendations are proposed by physicians but are responded to by parents as though they are insufficient. In what follows I will expand on what parents treat as minimally sufficient as compared to insufficient.

Insufficient treatment recommendations. Parents respond to treatment recommendations as insufficient when the recommendation – whether implied or stated – "1) fails to provide an affirmative action step, 2) is non-specific, or 3) minimizes the significance of the problem" (Stivers 2005a). For instance, see Extract (10). Having just reported non-problematic physical examination findings for a girl who presented with upper respiratory cold symptoms, the physician states "she's gonna get better on her ow:n," (line 1). With this statement, the physician orients to the relevance of "treatment-related actions" (Robinson 2003:45); however, he does not provide a treatment recommendation that is oriented to as sufficient by the caregiver.

(10) 16–07–07

DOC: 'Uhm: she's gonna get better on her ow:n,
(.)
DOC: I don't see any ear or throat infection,
GPA: -> So just (.) f:lu:ids and °you know°.=
DOC: =Fluids an' re:st an' kinda thuh (0.4) common
sense kinda things,
GPA: Sh:e's okay to go to school tomorrow_

Evidence is provided in the grandfather's response: he inquires about treatments that *could* be provided (line 4). This action displays his orientation to the physician's intimation of no treatment as an insufficient treatment recommendation and, moreover, makes relevant an affirmative and specific treatment recommendation from the physician. The physician does then provide this in line 5. However, he maintains a rather vague orientation towards the sort of mundane treatments that could be used in such a case. These types of treatment recommendations are routinely problematic, and here, although it is adequate for sequence closure, it nonetheless yields continued confusion regarding the health status of the child as evidenced by the grandfather's question in line 7.

This example suggests that parents are oriented to a minimally sufficient treatment recommendation as necessarily including a specific next action step. I argue that it is precisely for this reason that treatment recommendations that recommend *against* particular treatment are more likely to be resisted. If a treatment is ruled out, then by definition no specific next action step is provided, which leaves parents in a position of pursuing a sufficient treatment recommendation. For example, see Extract (11). After the physician recommends against antibiotics (line 5), the mother inquires about a medication that she can provide (line 9).

(11) 32–27–08

1	DOC:	.hh So: I think it's just (.) one uh thuh (.)
2		thi:ngs: kids get one thing after another sometimes,
3	MOM:	M[kay.
4	DOC:	[Nothing serious here,
5	DOC:	.mh Nothing that I can see that an antibiotic would help,
6	MOM:	Okay;
7		(.)
8	DOC:	[Uh:m
9	MOM: ->	[So uh:m (.) should I continue with thuh Tyleno:l? er_
10	DOC:	Tylenol if he's uncomfortable.
11		(.)
12	DOC:	[With fever 'n (0.2) headache,
13	MOM:	[('kay)
14	DOC:	or anything [like that.
15	MOM:	[(Okay.)

Also see Extract (12):

(12) 17–08–02

1	DOC: ->	Uh::m o- nl- unfortunately we probably can't give her
2	->	stuff .hh like Sudafed.
3		(.)
4	DOC:	Because that'd crank her blood pressure up_
5		an' we don't need tha:t.
6	MOM:	Right.
7		(1.0)

8 MOM: -> Okay: so give her Tylenol?,=
9 DOC: =Yeah.
10 (0.2)
11 DOC: for discomfort.

In this case, after the physician recommends against an over-the-counter cold medication (lines 1–2), the mother inquires about another form of non-prescription treatment that she could offer her daughter (line 8), and the doctor agrees to this (lines 9–11).

Parent responses to alternative treatment recommendation formats

Parents' responses to treatment recommendations vary depending on whether the recommendation is formatted as *for* or *against* treatment. Whereas parents are more likely to accept positive announcements of treatment recommendations, resistance is more likely to be engendered by a recommendation against a particular treatment. For instance, note that two of the more extreme active resistance examples shown earlier both involved an initial recommendation against antibiotics – Extracts (5) and (7a)–(7f). In particular, return to Extract (5). Here, although the physician may have intended to go on to offer affirmative action steps, once a ruled-out treatment recommendation was on the table in line 4 the parent's acceptance was due in line 5. Instead, passive (line 5) and then active resistance (beginning in line 6 and extending through to line 27) must be managed before an affirmative action step can be proposed. I argue that the root of this issue is the lack of an affirmative and specific treatment recommendation. This becomes even more visible as the root issue in cases where no treatment is offered, as in Extract (13). Here, the physician implies a recommendation against any medication through her diagnosis of a cold and her statement that the mother does not "have to be so concerned about it" (data not shown). The mother's response is a type of active resistance: she states her concern that the illness may get worse over the long weekend ahead (lines 1–2 and 4).

(13) 15–06–04

1 MOM: -> I just was worried with thuh Thank- thuh long
2 -> weekend ahead of us I wasn't su[re if he was=

3 DOC: [Yeah:_
4 MOM: -> =gonna get worse [or no:t.
5 DOC: [Yeah:.
6 DOC: .hh No I:- I:- (.) I'm [thinking he p'obably=
7 MOM: [Okay.
8 DOC: =gonna get better.
9 DOC: .h but he pro'ly s- gonna still have uh cou:gh,
10 MOM: O[kay:.
11 DOC: [Or uh runny no:se. but I don't think he should-
12 be having uh fever anymo:re.
13 DOC: .hh unless: he start developi:ng <other: kinda
14 infections> like uh pneumo:nia or uh sinus infection
15 .hh things like that.=
16 MOM: =If: his fever continues thuh next few day:s?,
17 DOC: Mm hm:, I would bring him back Monday.
18 (0.8)
19 MOM: But that's like three four days ahead [of me I mean=
20 BOY: [Mommy
21 MOM: =do I stick it ou:t?, or [do I call an' will somebody=
22 BOY: [Mommy:
23 MOM: =prescribe [an' antibiotics [or something?,]
24 DOC: [Oh ye^ah. [.hh If you ca:ll,]
25 DOC: they might not
26 BOY: (Mommy [ )
27 MOM: [Give him any[thing
28 DOC: [You may- They may not give you
29 (many) a- anything.
30 DOC: .h any antibiotics.
31 DOC: It(s) just depend on how high the fever is.
32 MOM: Okay.

The parent's resistance to a no-treatment recommendation in lines 1–2 and 4 makes relevant a statement from the physician about what to do in such a situation. Instead the physician's recommendation is only to return Monday if things worsen. This visit takes place on the Wednesday before the Thanksgiving holiday. Since the office will be closed for the holiday and the Friday following, this recommendation delays the possibility of treatment for five days. In this sense, similar to other no-treatment recommendations (such as recommendations against treatment) this suggestion fails to provide the parent with an affirmative next action step since the plan is too far removed from the current circumstances. This is evidenced by the mother's next round of resistance: "But that's like three four days ahead of me" (line 19). In particular, the "but" preface of this turn treats what follows as in conflict with the physician's plan to bring him back Monday if the illness persists. She resists further with an inquiry about whether someone will provide her with an affirmative treatment of antibiotics if her child worsens (lines 21 and 23) – a question that overtly lobbies for antibiotics (Stivers 2002a).

The pattern of resistance to recommendations against particular treatment is not uncommon. In Extract (14), following the physician's recommendation against treatment in lines 1–2, the mother requests confirmation of what she takes to be the upshot of the physician's recommendation: a recommendation against antibiotics – "so no antibiotics." (line 3). Like Extract (13), this form of resistance is particularly strong because it explicitly questions the physician's no treatment proposal (see Stivers [2002a] for a full discussion).

(14) 15–12–01

1	DOC:	(Now there's) no- particular treatment that's
2		neces[sary.
3	MOM: ->	[(intres-) so no antibiotics.
4	DOC:	(uhm-) No no.
5		(.)
6	DOC:	Nuh nuh nuh no. That would make (diarrhea) worse.
7	MOM:	U(h)h h(h)uh.

The physician not only confirms the negative implication (line 4), but after a micropause (line 5) he treats her lobbying for antibiotics as unnecessarily persisting in a course of action with the repeat of "no" (first in line 4 and then more strongly in line 6) (Stivers 2004). Similar to the physician in Extract (7) who denied the mother's request, here too the physician offers an account for his rejection of the parent.

Relying on interactional evidence, we have seen that treatment recommendations that are delivered negatively are more likely to engender resistance. We can now examine this and associated patterns in the pediatric data quantitatively.

Distributional evidence. Table 10.1 shows the bi-variate relationship between treatment recommendation format and parent resistance restricted to cases where antibiotics were neither prescribed nor given as an in-office injection. In particular, cases were coded as

Table 10.1 *Treatment format by parent resistance*

	No resistance	Parent resistance	Total
No recommendation "against"	95.1% (n = 349)	4.9% (n = 18)	367
Recommendation "against"	82.8% (n = 24)	17.2% (n = 5)	29
Totals	373	23	396
p = .02			

having a recommendation against a treatment if the initial treatment recommendation included this format, and resistance was coded as present only if the parent actively resisted the initial treatment recommendation. As can be seen in Table 10.1, parents were significantly more likely to resist the treatment recommendation if it was presented using "recommendation against" format than if it was presented without such a format (17 percent versus less than 5 percent p = .02 single-tailed Fisher's exact test). This evidence further suggests that resistance is typically minimized following recommendations for particular treatment.

Securing parent acceptance. Physicians generally treat prescription medication as desired by patients. One type of evidence for this is that such medication is generally presented using a "recommendation for" format when it is recommended (e.g., pain relievers or antibiotics). An interactional dilemma is posed when physicians do not plan to offer prescription medication – or if they are not providing the most desired of medications. It is this environment which provides a solid context to examine how delivering a less than optimal (from a parent perspective) treatment can be made most palatable. It appears that an initial recommendation for treatment (whether or not a subsequent recommendation against a particular treatment is delivered) offers the best chance of securing parent acceptance because it offers the parent a concrete way to solve or at least address the medical problem. This is in accord with the evidence so far presented.

Extract (15) shows an example of a physician presenting a non-antibiotic treatment using an affirmative format. Following a diagnosis of a cold (line 1) and the explication of the evidence for that diagnosis (lines 2–7), the physician goes on to affirmatively recommend treatment: cough medicine (lines 8–10 and 13–14), and this is non-antibiotic.

(15) 15–06–14

1	DOC:		Looks like he has a co:ld,=h
2	DOC:		It's just uh virus, not uh bacteria;=his lungs sound
3			really good,=it's just .h all irritation up here;=
4			=(and)/(that) he's coughing thuh- .h throat looks
5			uh little red_ but there's no puss or anything;
6	DOC:		.hh ear is just uh little (.) slightly pi:nk and .h
7			it's uh combination for with thuh stuffy no:se_
8		->	.hh so=w:e have=to .h clear thuh nose.
9	DOC:	->	Ya know like ((exhaling noise))/(0.2)
10		->	reduce thuh congestions that will help him uh lot.
11	DOC:		[.hh
12	DAD:		[>Mm hm;<=
13	DOC:	->	=An' I'm gonna give you some cough medicine that has
14		->	some decongestant in it.
15	BOY:		((whispering))/ ((DAD nods))
16	DAD:	=>	Mkay.

The physician suggests a type of cough medicine (lines 13–14). This is accepted both visibly (line 15) and vocally (line 16). In these situations, the cough medicine may or may not turn out to be prescription, but what appears to be important in whether or not resistance is likely to be engendered is that a specific recommendation for action has been made. Although the cough medicine is not named, the physician states that she is going to "give you some" (line 13) and specifies that it has "some decongestant in it" (line 14). Both of these aspects of the turn indicate that she has in mind a particular medication and in this way she is being specific in her recommendation.

In cases like this, the physician delivers the treatment recommendation in a way which satisfies the conditions outlined earlier for a sufficient treatment recommendation – they are affirmative, specific, non-minimized treatment recommendations. Because recommendations *for* treatment by definition satisfy the criteria of being affirmative, this may explain why they are less likely to be resisted generally. When recommendations *for* treatment are resisted, they typically fail on one of the latter two dimensions. That is, they typically either involve a vague/non-specific treatment recommendation or the physician minimizes either or both the child's diagnosis and the treatment recommendation. In Extract (16), the physician has recommended against antibiotics and, with no parent uptake, has affirmatively suggested using "whatever your favorite cough medicine is," (lines 4–5). He has further downgraded the recommendation with the TCU-initial "Simply" (line 4), which depicts the treatment as elementary.

(16) 17–08–12

1 DOC: -> As you know they're viral infections, so there's
2 -> no point in any a- any ant- antibiotics.
3 (0.5)
4 DOC: -> Simply control thuh cou:gh with .hh whatever
5 -> your favorite cough medicine is,
6 (1.8)
7 DOC: #hmg hmg#=h[h
8 DAD: => [That's what I figured. (0.5) it
9 => was her mo:m who called.
10 DAD: => I said you got (tuh be k(h)idd(h)ing) he's probably-
11 => .hh heard about: couple hundred cases already=
12 => =there's not much he's gonna be able to do: so_
13 DOC: .hh (only make her uh little) more comfortable of course.
14 DAD: Yea:h,
15 DOC: You take your=uhm (0.8) #uh:m# (0.8) Tylenol for thuh
16 discomfort_ .hh Now #hmh#=hhhh (1.0) (° °)
17 (1.0)
18 DOC: There's- (0.5) Triaminicol has uh new thing ou:t_
19 (1.0) there's uh Triaminicol soft chews they're
20 called, (11.5)
21 DOC: Uh:m they taste goo:d, 'n they c'n chew them up.
22 DOC: It's got uh cough suppressant, thuh nose dryer upper_
23 DAD: Yeah, (o[kay.)
24 DOC: [which'(ll) make 'er feel better;

The parent responds by first claiming his own expertise (line 8) and then placing blame on the child's mother for the medical visit (lines 8–12). By retroactively casting the child's mother's concerns as unnecessary, he displays his own understanding that the legitimacy of this visit has been threatened. The physician takes up this dimension of the father's utterance stating that he can offer expertise for making her "more comfortable" (line 13), and goes on to affirmatively suggest specific treatment of Tylenol and Triaminicol.

Treatment recommendation formats: implications for health care practitioners

The previous section shows that practitioners who format their treatment recommendations as *against* treatment are more likely to encounter resistance. Thus, one communication option would be for physicians to recommend treatment positively, never recommending against treatments. If negatively formatted treatment recommendations are more likely to engender parent resistance, an argument might be made that there is no reason for physicians to use them at all. However, at least in the case of antibiotics, prior research suggests that physicians are more likely to recommend against antibiotics following particular parent behaviors (e.g., after offering a bacterial candidate diagnosis) that indicate they are seeking antibiotics (Stivers 2002b). In such contexts, recommending against antibiotics appears to be designed as an interactionally responsive, and thus potentially validating, behavior.[3]

A second purpose of recommendations against particular treatment is parent education. When ruling out the need for a potentially desirable medication like antibiotics, physicians very often provide an account for this recommendation – see Extracts (5), (7), (12), (14), and (16). In doing so, physicians at the very least convey that they considered prescribing it and decided against it – something that may reassure parents who were concerned about the necessity of the medication. In some cases, following a recommendation against particular treatment, physicians go on to explain why they are not prescribing the drug. When this is done prior to an affirmative and specific treatment proposal, the educational dimension is likely to be lost – see Extract (5). However, when it is done subsequent to an affirmative and specific recommendation, such as Extract (17), it can work not only to provide education but also to solidify acceptance of the proposal. Note that the parent is resisting the treatment that is proposed. She offers only provisional acceptance with her nod in line 12. It is in this environment that the physician recommends against antibiotics and offers an account for this.This is successful

[3] Note that I do not mean that a physician who denies a parent's candidate diagnoses is validating him or her. However, when a parent has stated a concern about a particular condition, when a physician recommends against the treatment for that condition, this at least conveys that the physician considered the treatment. It is in this sense that the physician validates the parent's concern.

at least insofar as the mother inquires about one of the treatments, thereby taking it seriously.

(17) 30–26–01

1	DOC:		(I'll) control it with (.) #uh::# motrin (or fe-) for
2			high fever?,
3		->	(0.5)
4	DOC:		Tylenol,
5		->	(0.6)
6	DOC:		Lots of fluids, (.) rest,
7		->	(0.5)
8	DOC:		an:d (.) cough an' cold medicine.
9		->	(1.0)
10	DOC:	=>	That's all.
11		->	(0.2)
12	MOM:		((nods))
13	DOC:	=>	Okay?,
14			(0.2)
15	DOC:	=>	There's no need for antibiotic; (this is like) viru(s).
16			(0.5)
17	DOC:	=>	Sometimes gets worse with thuh antibiotic.
18			(.)
19	MOM:		So thuh main thing is just thuh liquids.

Accordingly, recommendations against particular treatment are not to be discounted entirely, since they provide physicians with a resource for communicating two important matters: that their treatment recommendations for the patient's problems are responsive to their/the parent's concerns of whether a particular medication was necessary; and education about when a potentially desirable medication like antibiotics may not be appropriate. But they are best done following an affirmative and specific treatment recommendation.

Discussion

This chapter has shown that, contrary to what might be expected, the treatment recommendation phase of acute medical encounters requires parent participation. That is, following physicians' treatment recommendations, both parents and physicians have been shown to treat parents as having the right and the responsibility to accept the treatment recommendation offered by the physician regardless of whether that recommendation is explicitly formatted to invite their participation or not. When parents do not accept the physician's recommendation, physicians pursued such acceptance even to the point of offering (sometimes major) concessions and inappropriate prescriptions. In the last sections of this chapter, I argued that physicians who offer their initial treatment recommendation as *against* a particular treatment are more likely to be met with parent resistance. This was observed to be part of a larger pattern of behavior which suggests that parents orient to treatment recommendations as sufficient only if they include an affirmative and specific next action step.

As mentioned early in this chapter, the data were diverse – internal medicine, orthopedics, and pediatrics. The fullest analysis was done with a large corpus of acute pediatric encounters. However, the practices involved in negotiating treatment appear to be present in the adult context(s) as well. That said, it may be the case that children are nonetheless special insofar as they are oriented to by physicians and parents as a shared responsibility. The two "caregivers" may, however, have competing goals. The physician may see not putting the child on medication as better for the community and for the child in the long run, insofar as most of these cases involved a decision of whether or not to prescribe antibiotics. The parent may see putting the child on medication as important for making the child feel better in the here-and-now because he or she is responsible for attending to the child when he or she wakes up during the night or is in pain. Therefore, the process of negotiation, though present in both adult and pediatric contexts, may be particularly salient in pediatrics.

An implication of this chapter for practitioners is that parents are already participating in decisions about their treatment even if they are not being overtly invited to do so. Practitioners report feeling pressured by parents for certain types of treatment and sometimes to prescribe inappropriately, and normally assume this behavior to be overt (Barden et al. 1998; Palmer and Bauchner 1997; Schwartz 1999; Schwartz et al. 1997). In fact, most parental pressure (at least in the US context) appears to be covert or tacit such as the resistance types discussed here (Stivers 2002a). Both passive and active resistance affect physician behavior even to the extent of altering what physicians prescribe. Therefore, minimizing resistance is an important strategy for physicians. One mechanism for minimizing resistance (and consequently inappropriate prescribing) is to offer patients/parents a concrete next action step as an initial treatment recommendation (even if this is not medication). This provides patients/parents with a solution to their medical problem and may help to legitimate their having sought medical help in the first instance (Stivers 2005a).

This chapter contributes not only to our understanding of how patient participation can affect treatment outcomes but also to our understanding of what patient participation is. Through this chapter I hope to have made a case that in both the health care research and the practitioner communities, we should broaden our conception of patient participation. This chapter also offers a cautionary note with respect to patient participation. While current research celebrates the many benefits of patient participation, the potential costs have been less well documented. This chapter suggests that, although patient participation is certainly important (and, moreover, patients are participating currently anyway), in certain contexts their participation may involve pressure for outcomes that are detrimental either to themselves or to the larger society. Therefore, patient participation should be actively encouraged, but practitioners should also be educated about both eliciting this participation and recognizing more passive and implicit forms of participation in order to determine how best to deal with pressure for inappropriate and risky forms of treatment.

11

Prescriptions and prescribing: coordinating talk- and text-based activities

David Greatbatch

Introduction

Toward the end of the medical consultation, doctors often prescribe medicines, appliances or dressings. In addition to writing a prescription, they may provide patients with information concerning the name, form, strength, dosage, use, effectiveness, and/or side effects of the items they are prescribing. Sometimes doctors do this before or after preparing a prescription. Thus, for example, in Extract (1) the doctor has prescribed a cream to treat a rash around a child's groin. As he hands the prescription to the child's mother, he tells her how often, when, and for how long she should apply the cream (lines 2, 4, 6, and 8–9).

(1) [H3: 4/9/91:0.17.20: Hostel]

1 (1.7) *Dr. signs prescription slip and hands it to the patient*
2 Dr.: -> Right use that (.) u::hm (0.2) at least twice a da:y.
3 P: Yea[:h
4 Dr.: -> [U:hm but u:hm: (0.4) preferably at- at each nappy change.
5 P: Yeah.
6 Dr.: Okay?
7 P: Okay.=
8 Dr.: -> =Cover all of the reddened area involved. And continue it for about two

This chapter builds on research conducted with Christian Heath, Paul Luff and Peter Campion, which was funded by Rank Xerox Cambridge EuroPARC and the Economic and Social Research Council. I would like to express my gratitude to Christian Heath, Paul Luff, Peter Campion, Doug Maynard, and John Heritage for their comments on earlier versions of this chapter and for their discussions on the issues it addresses. I am also grateful to Jon Hindmarsh, Neil Jenkins, Doug Maynard, David Middleton, Alison Pilnick, Jack Whalen, and Marilyn Whalen for their comments and suggestions during a data analysis session held at Nottingham University in April 1996.

9 or three days after the rash [has gone.
10 P: [Yeah.
11 (.)
12 P: Okay.

Doctors also provide patients with information about prescribed medicines and appliances as they write prescriptions either by hand or by computer. For instance, in Extract (2) the doctor prescribes cream and tablets for the patient's penile infection (line 1). As he writes the prescription by computer, he tells the patient how often to apply the cream (line 3) and, in responding to the patient's question at line 5, where to apply it (lines 6–7).

(2) [C3: 29/8/91:1.03.40: Thrush]

(The computer monitor and keyboard are located on the lefthand side of the desk, next to the patient)

1 Dr.: I'll give you cream and tablets.
2 (5.2) *Dr. typing; P looking toward keyboard*
3 Dr.:-> Three times a da:y the crea::m. *Spoken as he types*
4 (1.9) *Dr. typing*
5 P: Just[on the outside or:: [or:
[*Dr. gazes at monitor* [
6 Dr.:-> [Well under the=
[*Dr. gestures*
7 -> [skin ([[ ). Spread it around.
[*Dr. looks at P* [[*Dr. looks at screen; P immediately looks toward keyboard* [
8 P: [Yeah.
9 (1.7) *Dr. uses keyboard*
((Continues))

During exchanges such as these, doctors try to ensure that patients will use prescribed items in the ways they intend. They also justify their prescribing decisions, convey medical certainty, offer reassurance and/or placate difficult patients. However, despite the importance of these activities, there are few systematic studies of the actual processes through which doctors communicate prescription-related information to patients. Even those studies which examine the impact of prescribing behaviour on patients' compliance with medication regimes (e.g., Haynes 1979; Brown et al. 1987) shed little light on this issue, for they compare doctors' explanations against abstract idealized versions of information delivery without considering how the doctors' explanations are shaped with respect to contingencies that arise within the consultation.

In this chapter, I examine how prescription-related information is delivered in consultations conducted in a medical practice in England. Specifically, I consider how doctors communicate information to patients while concurrently using a computer to write a prescription. By speaking and typing at the same time, doctors can reduce the length of their consultations and break up what would otherwise be lengthy silences as they prepare prescriptions. However, they run the risk that their interactions with patients could disrupt, or be disrupted by, their computer-related activities. Below, I show how both doctors and patients attempt to circumvent this problem by adapting generic practices for the coordination of talk-based and text-based activities to a particular computer-based textual medium.

The study is based on video recordings of eighty consultations conducted by four general practitioners (GPs) in an inner-city medical practice in northwest England. The recordings are part of a larger corpus of video recordings which were collected before and after the introduction of a computerized medical record system into the practice. They were made over one year after the system was introduced, by which time the doctors were familiar with its operation, constraints, and potential. In approximately fifty consultations, two cameras were used – one focused on the participants, the other on the computer screen. In the other consultations, a single camera was positioned to record both the participants' actions and the changes on the screen. Consequently, the recordings allow detailed analysis of the relationship between the doctors' use of the computer and their interaction with patients.

The computer system

The computer system used in the practice is IGP VAMP ("Value-Added Medical Products"). By the early 1990s, VAMP had been installed in approximately 2,200 practices in the UK (Nazareth et al. 1993; Jick et al. 1991). The system allows the doctor to document and retrieve medical information concerning the patient, and to issue and record prescriptions.

In order to issue a prescription, the doctor summons the patient's therapy file. The screen displays the patient's personal details, a list of past prescriptions and, along the bottom of the screen, a prompt line comprising the fields into which doctors enter details of each new prescription. The layout of the screen is shown in Figure 11.1.

The prompt line requires details such as the name (Pharmaceutical name), form (Frm), strength (Strength), dosage (Dosage), and quantity (Qty) of the item(s) being prescribed. The doctor usually begins by typing an abbreviation of the item they are prescribing into the Pharmaceutical name field.[1] They then enter details into the Form (Frm) and Strength fields, whereupon the system attempts to match the information they have entered to an item in a database containing details of drugs, appliances, and dressings. If the system fails to recognize the doctor's input, or two or more names in the database match an abbreviated entry, then the system requests clarifications or corrections of input. After an item has been selected and confirmed, the doctor enters information into the remaining fields, the first of which is the Dosage field.

As he or she progresses along the prompt line, the doctor presses the carriage return <CR> key to move to a subsequent field or the control key in conjunction with a character key to return to a previous field. In some cases, moving to a new field involves the relocation of the cursor; in others, more substantial changes on the screen occur, including the presentation of prompt lines. After the doctor exits the final field, the system issues a prescription and updates the patient's prescription history.

Below, I show how both doctors and patients synchronize their prescription-related talk with these computer-related actions. First I examine how doctors communicate information to patients that corresponds to the details they are required to enter into the computer fields. Subsequently, I consider how they deliver prescription-related information that is not required by the computer system. Finally, I explore how the patients' responses are organized with respect to the doctors' computer-related activities.

[1] Alternatively, the doctor may summon a list of the items contained in the database and choose an item from this list. This is often done, for example, when doctors are uncertain about which item to prescribe.

```
------------------------------------------------------------------------------------
JONES            JOHN THOMAS        84y    Male   Permanent: 17 RAILWAY COURT
THERAPY HISTORY Repeat till 23/04/88                75+ exam:Eligible   21/07/81
   Date          Pharmaceutical name Frm  Strength  Dosage days  Qty  op  Rp Is

1 06/09/84       ALUPENT              SYR   10.00    5-10MLPRN   300           -  DM
2 11/06/85       PARACETAMOL          TAB  500.00    2TDSPRN     100       3  1
3 14/06/85       ALRHEUMAT            CAP   50.00    2 BD        100       3  1
4 03/07/85       ALRHEUMAT            CAP   50.00    2 BD        100
5 25/04/88       PARACETAMOL          TAB  500.00    2TDSPRN     100
6 12/06/89       AMOXIL               CAP  250.OO    QDS          20           - *DM
------------------------------------------------------------------------------------


Allergic to: SEPTRIN
Date   Pharmaceutical name  Frm  Strength  Dosage  Days  Qty  op  Rp Is  P/N/+
06/09/90
------------------------------------------------------------------------------------
```

Figure 11.1 Layout of the computer screen

Communicating prescription-related information that corresponds to details entered into the computer fields

Sometimes doctors communicate to patients information which corresponds to the details they are required to type into the computer fields. In particular, they inform patients about the name, form, strength, dosage, and/or quantity of the items they are prescribing. When they do this, the doctors routinely seek to reconcile the potentially competing demands of their talk-based and computer-based activities by minimizing the disjuncture between them. In particular, they speak when the cursor is located in computer fields which require the self-same information that they communicate to patients. Thus, for example, in Extract (3), the doctor tells the patient how many repeat prescriptions he will be given (line 7) just after the cursor arrives in the Repeats field – that is, the field into which he is required to enter this information.

(3) [H2:21/5/91:Parkinson's disease]

(The patient suffers from Parkinson's disease and is new to the practice.
The computer monitor and keyboard are located in the center of the desk)
1 Dr.: Do you have the u::h[m effervescent u::hm ( ) or=
[*Dr. starts keying*
2 Dr.: =the- or the: [er
3 P: [The capsules.
4 (0.7) *Dr. using computer*
5 Dr.: (I'll just give you) capsules.
6 (4.7) *Dr. typing*
7 Dr.: -> And I'll put you down for four repeats initially so::
8 P: Mh[m
9 Dr.: [Unless we need to see you for anything else we'll
10 [see you again in [four- in four months time.
[*Dr. looks at P* [*Dr. looks at screen*
11 Dr.: Okay?
12 P: [Yeah
[*Dr. keying*
13 (4.7)
((*Dr. completes prescription; sits back in chair; printer starts*))

[Detail: Position of cursor at the beginning of line 7]

Repeats
|
v

Date Pharmaceutical name Frm Strength Dosage Days Qty op Rp Is P/N/+

In some cases doctors establish a still closer fit between their talk and keyboard actions. For example, consider Extract (2) below, in which the doctor announces that he is going to prescribe cream and tablets for the patient's penile infection (line 1).

(2) [C3: 29/8/91:1.03.40: Thrush]

(The computer monitor and keyboard are located on the lefthand side of the desk, next to the patient)

1 Dr.: I'll give you cream and tablets.
2 (5.2) *Dr. typing; P looking toward keyboard*
3 Dr.:-> Three times a da:y the crea::m. *Spoken as he types*
4 (1.9) *Dr. typing*
5 P: Just[on the outside or:: [or:
[*Dr. gazes at monitor* [
6 Dr.: [Well under the=
[*Dr. gestures*
7 [skin ([[ ). Spread it around.
[*Dr. looks at P* [[*Dr. looks at screen; P immediately looks toward keyboard*
8 P: [Yeah.
9 (1.7) *Dr. uses keyboard*
((Continues))

[Detail: Position of cursor at the beginning of line 3]

Dosage
|
v

Date Pharmaceutical name Frm Strength Dosage Days Qty op Rp Is P/N/+

[Detail: Lines 1–3]

1 Dr.: I'll give you cream and tablets.
2 (5.2) *Dr. typing; P looking toward keyboard*
3 Dr.: [Three times a da:y] [the crea::m.] [*Silence*]
[*Types in Dosage details*] [*Screen change*] [*Skips Days*]
finger movement *prompt*

Having remained silent as he enters abbreviated details of the name, form, and strength of the cream and then accepts the item which the computer selects from the drugs dictionary on the basis of this information (line 2), the doctor tells the patient how often he should apply the cream (line 3). Like the doctor in Extract (3), he minimizes the disjuncture between his talk-based and computer-based actions by speaking when the cursor is positioned in the field which requires the self-same information that he communicates to the patient, namely the Dosage field. However, he establishes a still closer fit between his talk and his keyboard actions by: uttering the numerical details concerning dosage as he types them into the Dosage field; and then identifying the item to which he is referring ("the crea::m") as the system processes the information he has entered and advances the cursor to the next field.

Two more examples of a doctor establishing a close fit between their talk and their keyboard actions are located in Extract (4). In this extract the doctor is prescribing medication to treat an eye problem. The patient is standing behind the doctor, dressing.

(4) [P2:3b]

1 (12.0) *Dr. entering information into computer*
[*Typing into Dosage field*]
2 Dr.: -> [Just one tablet a da:y (1.0)] for the: (0.4) eye[s, see if it'll=
3 P: [Mm mm
4 Dr.: =help the itch.
5 (0.4)
6 P: ((Sniffs))
7 Dr.: It may not help at all we'll [have to see.
[*Skips Days field*
8 (.)
9 Dr.: -> I'll just give you [twenty for now.
[*Starts typing into Quantity field*
10 (0.6)
11 P: So they won't clash with one another.
12 (.)
13 Dr.: [No.=
[*Dr. shakes head*
14 P: =[No.[Good.
[*P* [*looks away from Dr.*
[*Dr. types in details of next item*

[Position of the cursor at the beginning of line 2]
Dosage
|
v
Date Pharmaceutical name Frm Strength Dosage Days Qty op Rp Is P/N/+

[Position of the cursor at the beginning of line 9]
Quantity
|
v
Date Pharmaceutical name Frm Strength Dosage Days Qty op Rp Is P/N/+

The doctor provides the patient with numerical information concerning dosage (line 2) and quantity (line 9), while the cursor is positioned in the Dosage field and the Quantity field respectively. In the case of dosage (line 2), the doctor starts to speak and type at the same time. Like the doctor in Extract (2), he coordinates his talk and his typing by: providing the patient with numerical details concerning dosage ("Just one tablet a da:y") as he types them into the Dosage field; and then identifying the item to which he is referring, by mentioning the problem for which it is being prescribed – "for the: (0.4) eyes" – as he waits for the system to advance the cursor to the next field.[2] In the case of quantity (line 9), the doctor minimizes the gap between his talk-based and computer-based actions by delaying starting to type. This enables him to enter numerical information into the Quantity field at the same time as he specifies it in his utterance.

Sometimes the doctors coordinate the communication of prescription-related information to patients by reference not only to the entry of details into the computer fields but also to the patient's visual conduct. Thus, for example, in Extract (5), the doctor is prescribing a gel for a woman who has severe neck pain.

(5) [H3:4/9/91: Neck pain: 1.29.58]

(The computer monitor and keyboard are located at the center of the desk)

1 Dr.: You'd probably be better off without [a pillow for a little while.
                    [*Dr. gazes at P*
2 P: Mm: I've- [I've tried without, tried with two, tried with (.) one=
          [*Dr. returns gaze to medical record cards*
3 P: =and this: seems to be the .hhh best of the lot. The one that I
4 bought.=It's not feathers or (.) I don't know what it is (   ).
5 (0.5)
6 *Dr. puts pen down and shifts attention to computer*
7 (0.2)
8 Dr.: [One of these man-made fibers.
  [*Dr. starts to use computer*
9 P: Mm:
10 (7.0) *Dr. types information; P shifts gaze to Dr. after 6.5 seconds*

[2] Having simultaneously typed and uttered numerical information concerning dosage, the doctor remains silent for approximately one second as he finishes typing in the Dosage field. He thus appears to delay the referent of his talk, which he is not required to enter in the Dosage field, until he has finished typing in the numerical information that he has just conveyed to the patient.

11 Dr.: -> And put this- rub this in three times a da:y.
12 P: Mm mm *P nods and then averts gaze from Dr.*
13 (2.5) *As Dr. types, P looks at keys, then looks down in front of her*

[Detail: Position of cursor at the beginning of line 11]

Dosage
|
v

Date Pharmaceutical name Frm Strength Dosage Days Qty op Rp Is P/N/+

[Detail: Lines 10–13]

10 (7.0)
(a) After 6 seconds Dr. accepts drug name and prepares to enter details into Dosage field
(b) After approximately 6.1 seconds Patient begins to shift gaze to Dr., following pronouncement movement of the Dr.'s hand after he has pressed the <CR> key to accept the item displayed by the system
(c) After approximately 6.2 seconds Dr. begins to enter details into Dosage field
(d) After approximately 6.8 seconds Patient's gaze arrives, as Dr. makes second keystroke
(e) After approximately 6.9 seconds Dr. makes third keystroke
11 Dr.: -> [And put this- rub this in three times] a da:y.
12 [*Dr. makes three more keystrokes into Dosage field*]
13 P: Mm [Mm
[*Dr. makes two <CR> keystrokes to exit Dosage (op) field and to skip Days field*

As the doctor types information into the Pharmaceutical name, Form, and Strength fields, the patient looks at the keyboard and then down toward the floor in front of her. However, after just over six seconds, she starts to move her gaze toward the doctor, apparently in response to a pronounced movement of the doctor's right hand across the keyboard – see Detail: *(b)* in line 10. As the doctor types the second of six symbols into the Dosage field, her gaze arrives at his face – see Detail *(d)* in line 10. Following his next keystroke, the doctor provides her with instructions concerning Dosage (line 11). Thus the doctor appears to orientate not only to the positioning of the cursor in a particular field (Dosage), but also to the visual actions of the patient. Indeed it is possible that the doctor's utterance is occasioned by the patient's actions, which render his current orientation to the computer problematic by establishing the relevance of some form of response from him.

In summary, doctors routinely minimize the disjuncture between their talk-based and computer-based activities when providing patients with prescription-related information which corresponds to the information that they are required to enter into the computer fields. In particular, they speak when the cursor is located in computer fields which require the self-same information that they communicate to patients. Sometimes they also establish a close fit between their talk and their keystrokes. By using these practices the doctors minimize the likelihood that their talk-based and/or computer-based activities will be disrupted due to them speaking while they use the computer.[3]

Communicating prescription-related information which does not correspond to details entered into the computer fields

Sometimes doctors communicate prescription-related information which does not correspond to the details they enter into the computer fields. For example, they describe the side effects of drugs, explain how they react with other medications, and assess their effectiveness. When they do this the doctors seek to reconcile the

[3] It should be added that the doctors do not always straightforwardly convey to patients the "bare bones" of the information that they type into the computer fields, as does the doctor in Extract (2) when he informs the patient that the cream should be used three times a day. Often they convey additional information to patients by assessing, clarifying, or qualifying the details that they are concurrently entering into the computer and verbally communicating to patients. In so doing, the doctors reassure patients, signify that treatments are on trial, indicate whether particular numbers represent a little or a lot, and/or refer to the ways in which items should be used. Thus, for example, in Extract (3) above the doctor characterizes the four repeat prescriptions as an initial allocation ("initially," line 7), thereby leaving open the possibility that more may be provided at a later date, but without committing himself to this. Similarly, in Extract (4) the doctor does not merely tell the patient that she should take one tablet a day (line 2) and that she is to be given twenty tablets (line 9). Instead, he presents these numbers as small amounts ("*Just* one tablet," "I'll *just* give you twenty"), and indicates that additional tablets may be prescribed in the future ("I'll just give you twenty *for now*"). In addition, information concerning the form of drug is embedded in the instructions concerning dosage ("Just one tablet a da:y"). Thus the doctor designs his utterances concerning dosage and quantity to convey particular interpretations of the factual details that he is concurrently entering into the computer and communicating to the patient. Similar phenomena are observable in Extracts (3) and (5). In Extract (3) the doctor characterizes the four repeats as an initial allocation (line 7) before drawing out the implications of this with respect to the timing of the patient's next appointment. In Extract (5) the doctor embeds information concerning the application of the cream he is prescribing ("rub this in") in his instructions concerning dosage ("three times a da:y." line 11).

potentially competing demands of their talk-based and computer-based activities by: speaking where the cognitive and physical demands of using the computer are relatively low; and/or configuring their use of the keyboard to accommodate their talk.

An example of a doctor speaking when his or her computer-related activity is relatively undemanding is located in Extract (6). In this extract the patient hands a list of her repeat medications to the doctor and asks him to prescribe them along with the painkillers he is giving her for a recurrent back problem.

(6) [OB:10/9/91:0.00.00:Rheumatologist]

(("He" at line 6 refers to consultant rheumatologist that the patient has visited))

1	P:	mhm mhm I wanted you to give me them (.) while I was
2		here [as well please doct[or.
3	Dr.:	[Yeah. [Yeah. All right.
4	P:	The Quinine.
5		(0.5)
6	P:	He was telling me as well they don't know what causes this cramp.
7		(.)
8	Dr.:	No[:
9	P:	[I thought when I had the operation on the foot I was going to get
10		over that.
11		(0.2)
12	Dr.:	Yea:h.
13	P:	It's not-
14	Dr.:	N[o:
15	P:	[it's gone worse actually it's creeping a bit further up my leg.
16	Dr.:	Yea:h.
17		(0.7)
18	Dr.:	Now you need thu- wu- which- how many of these,=you need all of these
19		no:[w.
20	P:	[Those three top ones [please mhm=
21	Dr.:	[Ri:ght.
22	Dr.:	
23	Dr.:	=i- Use if you're using uhm (0.5) the Coproximal don't use the
24		(hydrocordin) or if you're using the (hydrocordin) don't use the
25		Coproximal.
26	P:	Oh ri[ght. Okay.
27	Dr.:	[u:hm Don't take them together.=
28	P:	No right. Okay. As long as I know.
29		(2.7)
30	Dr.:->	[They're likely to make [you feel quite groggy=
31		[*Just after <CR>* [*<CR> accepting item*
32	Dr.:	if [you (0.6) if you do.
33		[*Starts to enter details at Dosage prompt*

34 P: mhm mhm?
35 (6.7)
((*Printer starts*))

[Position of the cursor at the beginning of line 30]

System searching drug dictionary
|
v
Date Pharmaceutical name Frm Strength Dosage Days Qty op Rp Is P/N/+

As the patient hands the list of medications to the doctor, she mentions one of the items, Quinine (line 4), by name and then, as the doctor types details of the painkillers into the computer, refers to the problem it is being used to treat (lines 6, 9–10, 13, and 15–16). After the doctor finishes typing in the details of the painkillers, he looks at the list and abruptly shifts topic to ask whether she needs all of the items on the list (lines 18–19). Then, following the patient's confirmation that she does, he warns her against taking one of the items together with the painkillers (lines 23–25 and 27). As his utterance nears completion, he starts to type details of one of the repeat prescriptions into the computer.

Just over two and a half seconds after the patient's response (at line 28) to the doctor's directive, the doctor describes the untoward effects of combining the two drugs (lines 30–31 and 32). His utterance conveys prescription-related information which is not required by the computer for the production of the prescription. However, the doctor speaks at a point at which the cognitive and physical demands of using the computer are relatively low – namely, a fraction of a second after the cursor exits the Strength field. At this point, he is obliged to wait for the system to match the information he has entered to an item in its drugs database. Moreover, unless there is a problem, his next task will simply be to press the <CR> key to accept the details which the system displays on the screen, and to move the cursor to the Dosage field. Interestingly, it is only when he begins the more demanding task of typing information into the Dosage field (line 31) that he displays (by hesitating and restarting his utterance) difficulty interweaving his interaction with the patient with his use of the computer.

An example of a doctor configuring his use of the keyboard to accommodate the production of talk which is not directly related to the fourteen computer fields is observable in Extract (4), in which the doctor appends such talk to his instructions concerning dosage.

(4) [P2:3b]

```
 1              (12.0) Dr. entering information into computer
                [Typing into Dosage field  ]
 2  Dr.:  -->   [Just one tablet a da:y (1.0)] for the: (0.4) eye[s, see if it'll=
 3   P:                                                         [Mm mm
 4  Dr.:        =help the itch.
 5              (0.4)
 6   P:         ((Sniffs))
 7  Dr.:        It may not help at all we'll [have to see.
                                             [Skips Days field
 8              (.)
 9  Dr.:  -->   I'll just give you [twenty for now.]
                                   [Starts typing into Quantity field
10              (0.6)
11   P:         So they won't clash with one another.
12              (.)
13  Dr.:        [No.=
                [Dr. shakes head
14   P:         =[No.[Good.
                 [P  [looks away from Dr
                     [Dr. types in details of next item
```

[Position of the cursor at the beginning of line 2]

```
                                                       Dosage
                                                         |
                                                         v
Date Pharmaceutical name Frm Strength Dosage Days Qty op Rp Is P/N/+
```

[Position of the cursor at the beginning of line 9]

```
                                            Quantity
                                               |
                                               v
Date Pharmaceutical name Frm Strength Dosage Days Qty op Rp Is P/N/+
```

As noted earlier, the doctor provides the patient with dosage instructions, completes the entry of information into the Dosage field, and then explicitly identifies the item he is referring to by mentioning the condition for which it is being prescribed – "for the: (0.4) eyes,". Following this, he recommends that the patient monitor the effects of the drug ("see if it'll help the itch." lines 2 and 4), explicitly asserts that the drug may not alleviate the condition ("It may not help at all" line 7), and then reasserts the need to monitor it's effects ("we'll have to see."). Although the doctor continues to gaze at the computer screen as he conveys this information, he does not resume typing until his utterance at line 7 nears completion, whereupon he presses the <CR> key to move the cursor from the Days field to the Quantity field. Thus the doctor appears to configure his keyboard actions so as to provide a slot within which to furnish information which does not correspond to any of the details he enters into the computer.

It is worth adding here that doctors also use these practices when, in contrast to Extracts (2)–(5), they deliver prescription-related information which corresponds to the details that they enter into the computer, either before the cursor reaches or after the cursor leaves the corresponding computational fields. Consider Extract (7), in which the doctor is prescribing tablets to treat the patient's depression.

(7) [C3:29/8/91: Strange things]

1 Dr.: [.h h h h [h h *Dr. sits back after pressing return key. P shifts gaze to Dr.*
[
2 P: [(Terrible [eff[ect).
3 Dr.: [*P looks at Dr.* [[If I give you tablets for two weeks:
[*P looks away*
4 P: [Ye::s.
[*P looks at keys*
5 Dr.: Could you [come back in two weeks.
[*Dr. shifts gaze to P*
[*P looks at Dr.*
6 P: [Ye:[s. [(I'll do that). ( ).
7 Dr.: [Okay. [*P looks at system*
[*Dr. looks at system*
8 (0.7)
9 Dr.:-> And just take two at night.
10 P: Yea:h.
11 (1.2) *Dr. completes prescription and sits back. Printer starts up.*
12 Dr.: Uhm (0.9) When I say at night (0.2) probably about (0.5) seven or eight
13 o'clock

[Detail: Position of cursor at the beginning of line 9]

Repeats
|
v

Date Pharmaceutical name Frm Strength Dosage Days Qty op Rp Is P/N/+

[Detail: Lines 8–9]

8 (0.7) *Types number into Qty (op) field and then <CR>;*
9 Dr.: -> [And just take [two at night.
[*Skips Repeats*

The doctor asks the patient if it is appropriate for him to prescribe tablets for a fortnight (lines 3 and 5).[4] Following the patient's affirmative answers (lines 4 and 6), the doctor enters a number into the Quantity field, and then advances the cursor to the Repeats field. As the cursor comes to rest in the Repeats field, he initiates his utterance concerning dosage (line 9). Subsequently, as he provides the patient with dosage instructions, he advances the cursor to the next field by pressing the carriage return key. Here, then, the doctor communicates information concerning dosage not as he enters details into the Dosage field – as do the doctors in Extracts (2), (4), and (5) above – but rather as he bypasses the Repeats field. Notice, however, that his utterance coincides with a series of simple keyboard actions. Since it is not necessary for the doctor to enter information into the remaining fields, he has only to make a short series of <CR> keystrokes to complete the prescription. Consequently, he speaks in a context in which his computer-based activities place relatively low cognitive and physical demands upon him.

We have seen that doctors routinely coordinate the delivery of prescription-related information with their computer-based activities, and that they thereby minimize the likelihood of their talk-based and computer-based activities disrupting each other. We now turn to consider the patients' responses, paying particular attention to the ways in which the patients orient to audible and visible features of the doctors' conduct.

Patients' responses

Often patients acknowledge or accept what doctors tell them without either expressing an opinion or initiating further discussion about their treatment. Thus, for example, in Extracts (3), (5), (6), and (7), the patients produce minimal acknowledgments.

(3) [H2:21/5/91: Parkinson's disease]

(4.7)
Dr.: And I'll put you down for four repeats initially so::
P: -> Mh[m

[4] In addition to soliciting details that are relevant to the entry of information into the Quantity field, the doctor's question at lines 3 and 5 informs the patient about the number of tablets he is to be given (enough tablets to last two weeks) and of the implications of this (a consultation with the doctor in two weeks' time).

Dr.: [Unless we need to see you for anything else we'll
[see you again in [four- in four months time.
[*Dr. looks at P* [*Dr. looks at screen*
Dr.: Okay?
P: [Yeah
[*Dr. keying*
(4.7)
((*Dr. completes prescription; sits back in chair; printer starts*))

(5) [H3:4/9/91: Neck pain:1.29.58]

(7.0) *Patient starts to shift gaze to doctor after approx 6 secs*
Dr.: And put this- rub this in three times a da:y.
P: -> Mm mm *P nods and then averts gaze from Dr.*

(6) [OB:10/9/91:0.00.00: Rheumatologist]

Dr.: [They're likely to make [you feel quite groggy=
[*Just after <CR>* [*<CR> accepting item*
Dr.: if [you (0.6) if you do.
[*Starts to enter details at Dosage prompt*
P: -> mhm mhm?
(6.7)
((*Printer starts*))

(7) [C3:29/8/91: Strange things: Detail]

Dr.: And just take two at night.
P: -> Yea:h.
(1.2) *Dr. completes prescription and sits back. Printer starts up.*
Dr.: Uhm (0.9) When I say at night (0.2) probably about (0.5) seven or eight o'clock

When patients produce minimal responses they generally either look away from the doctors, as in Extracts (3), (6), and (7), or withdraw their gaze from them either during or immediately after responding to the doctors' utterances, in Extract (5). In these ways the patients exhibit an orientation to the doctors' continuing use of the computer, avoiding actions which might elicit the doctors' gaze and disrupt their computer-based activities.

Alternatively, patients may respond by asking the doctors for additional information, as in Extracts (2) and (4).

(2) [C3: 29/8/91:1.03.40: Thrush]

3 Dr.: Three times a da:y the crea::m. *Spoken as he types*
4 (1.9) *Dr. typing* [*Potential juncture; P shifts gaze to Dr; and does circular gesture with hand*

5 P: -> [Just [on the outside or:: [or:
[*Dr. gazes at monitor* [
6 Dr.: [Well under the=
[*Dr. gestures*
7 [skin ([[ ). Spread it around.
[*Dr. looks at P* [[*Dr. looks at screen; P immediately looks toward*
keyboard [
8 P: [Yeah.
9 (1.7) *Dr. uses keyboard*
((Continues))

(4) [P2:3b]

9 Dr.: I'll just give you [twenty for now.
[*Starts typing into Quantity field*
10 (0.6)
11 P: -> So they won't clash with one another.
12 (.)
13 Dr.: [No.=
[*Dr. shakes head*
14 P: =[No.[Good.
[*P* [*looks away from Dr*
[*Dr. types in details of next item*

When patients ask doctors questions about their treatment, they usually minimize the likelihood that they will disrupt the doctors' computer-based activities by delaying their questions until potential junctures in the doctor's use of the computer. Because the patients have limited access to, and understanding of, the doctors' computer-based activities, they anticipate these junctures on the basis of visible and audible aspects of the doctors' conduct – such as the relative intensity of keystrokes, the movements of the doctor's hands and fingers and shifts in the doctor's orientation and gaze (Greatbatch et al. 1993, 1995a, 1995b; Luff et al. 1994). For example, consider the patient's question in Extract (2).

(2) [C3: 29/8/91:1.03.40: Thrush: Detail]

((Line 4 shows final three keystrokes only of keyboard activity in 1.9-second silence))
3 Dr.: Three times a da:y the crea::m. *Spoken as he types*
4 (1.9) op Rp/Is P/N/+
| | |
v v v
<CR> <CR> <CR>
[*P shifts gaze to Dr.; and gestures towards his groin*

5 P: [Just [on the outside or:: [or:
[*Dr. gazes at monitor* [
6 Dr.: [Well under the=
[*Dr. gestures*

Almost two seconds after being told by the doctor that he should apply the cream "three times a da:y" (line 3), the patient asks the doctor to explain *how* it should be applied to the penis (line 5). The patient's question occurs immediately after the third in a sequence of three <CR> keystrokes. After this keystroke, which completes the prescription for the cream, the doctor stares at the screen as he waits for the system to process the information he has entered. Thus the patient appears to coordinate his question with a juncture in the doctor's keyboard actions.

Several aspects of the doctor's witnessable conduct as he makes the three <CR> keystrokes which precede the patient's utterance may combine to enable the patient to project a potential boundary in the doctor's use of the keyboard. First, the keystrokes are louder, made closer together, and, consequently, involve more pronounced and rapid hand movements than those which precede them. Second, as the doctor makes the keystrokes with his right hand, he holds his left hand still above the keyboard and thus gives no indication that he might be about to use it to press another key. Third, after pressing the <CR> key for the third time, the doctor moves his right hand abruptly away from the key. Upon the completion of the sound of the third return keystroke, the movement and comportment of the doctor's right hand suggest that he will not immediately use it to make another keystroke. Taken together these features suggest potential disengagement from the use of the keyboard and, as noted above, a lull does follow.

Similar patterns of conduct are observable in Extract (4), in which a patient again asks a doctor a question following a sequence of three <CR> keystrokes.

(4) [P2:3b]

(The doctor gazes at the screen throughout this extract. The Patient is standing behind him)

9 Dr.: I'll just give you [twenty for now. *P averts her gaze from Dr.*
[*Starts typing into Quantity field*

10 (0.6) op Rp/Is P/N/+
| | |
v v v
<CR> <CR> <CR>

11 P: So [they won't clash with one another.
[*P gazes at Dr.*

12 (.)

13 Dr.: [No.=
[*Dr. shakes head*

14 P: =[No.[Good.
[*P* [*looks away from Dr.*
[*Dr. types in details of next item*

As in Extract (2), the patient's question occurs in a context in which the doctor's actions are consistent with a lull in his use of the keyboard. The doctor makes the three <CR> keystrokes which precede the patient's question in rapid succession (line 10), thrusting his forefinger back down towards the <CR> key immediately after both the first and second of the keystrokes. Upon releasing the <CR> key for the third time, however, he holds his finger still above the <CR> key, while holding his other hand motionless over the alphanumeric keys. His actions are thus consistent with a brief lull in his use of the keyboard: the sudden stilling of his finger above the key, together with the inactivity of his other hand, marking out a potential juncture in his typing.

The patients' bodily movements as they ask questions

In each of the examples above the patient's bodily movements display their understanding that they are speaking at a potential juncture in the doctor's use of the keyboard. Thus, in Extract (2) the patient does not look at the doctor while he is entering details of the cream into the computer (line 3). Even when the doctor tells him how often he should apply the cream, the patient continues to gaze at the keyboard, thereby leaving the doctor free to focus exclusively on the computer-based task in hand.

However, as the patient asks the doctor a question, the patient gazes at the doctor and produces a circular gesture around his groin with his left hand. The patient's actions establish the relevance of, and perhaps solicit, a gaze shift by the doctor away from the computer to the patient. Consequently, the patient's actions, together with the question which accompanies them, exhibit the patient's understanding that the doctor has reached a potential juncture in his keyboard actions.

In Extract (4) the patient also shifts her gaze to the doctor as she produces her question. As the doctor types, the patient stands to one side (and slightly behind) the doctor rearranging her clothing. Immediately after the doctor tells her to take "one tablet a da:y" (line 2), she looks directly at the side of his face. However, he continues to focus on the screen and, following his utterance concerning quantity (at line 9), she averts her gaze as he makes the first of the three <CR> keystrokes which precede her question (line 10). Then, just after she initiates her question (line 11), she returns her gaze to the side of the doctor's face. Thus, as in Extract (2), the patient's bodily movements establish a "participation framework" (Goffman 1981; Goodwin 1981; Heath 1986) within which it would be appropriate for the doctor to gaze at the patient rather than at the computer and, in so doing, she displays her understanding that she is speaking at a (potential) juncture in the doctor's use of the keyboard.

The patients' bodily movements during the doctors' responses

Although patients often solicit doctors' visual attention when they ask them questions, they immediately avert their gaze if it becomes apparent that the doctors are preparing to resume typing. By doing this, they lift the relevance of the doctors gazing at them and thereby leave the doctors "free" to continue with the computer task in hand as they respond to the patient's question. Thus, for example, in Extract (4), the doctor's actions suggest that he is preparing to type in further details, for, as he responds to the patient's question, he not only continues to gaze at the screen but also repositions his fingers over the keyboard (line 13).

As the patient acknowledges his reply, she shifts her gaze away from him (line 14), with the result that when the doctor resumes typing in the midst of her talk she is no longer looking at him. Thus when it becomes apparent that the doctor is preparing to continue typing, the patient withdraws her gaze from him and thereby reduces the interactional demands she is placing upon him.

A similar pattern is observable in Extract (2), even though in this case the patient initially succeeds in attracting the doctor's visual attention.

(2) [C3: 29/8/91:1.03.40: Thrush: Detail]

((Line 4 shows final three keystrokes only of keyboard activity in 1.9-second silence))
3 Dr.: Three times a da:y the crea::m. *Spoken as he types*
4 (1.9) op Rp/Is P/N/+
| | |
v v v
<CR> <CR> <CR>
[*P shifts gaze to Dr; and gestures towards his groin*
5 P: [Just [on the outside or:: [or:
[*Dr. gazes at monitor* [
6 Dr.: [Well under the=
[*Dr. gestures*
7 [skin ([[ ). Spread it around.
[*Dr. looks at P* [[*Dr. looks at screen; P immediately looks toward keyboard*
8 P: [Yeah.
9 (1.7) *Dr. uses keyboard*
((Continues))

As noted above, as the patient produces his question concerning the application of the cream (line 5) he looks at the doctor and gestures towards his own groin.

Initially, the doctor continues to gaze at the monitor as the computer processes the information he has entered. Subsequently, however, as the patient stretches and repeats a word ("or"), actions which are also associated with the solicitation of gaze (Goodwin 1979, 1981), the doctor not only responds to the patient but also lifts his hands away from the keyboard and undertakes a circular gesture with his right hand which seems to mirror the patient's gesture (line 6). Then, holding out his hands in a horizontal position, as if to give emphasis to what he is saying, he gazes at the patient (as the doctor utters the word "skin", line 7). A fraction of a second later, just after the doctor utters the word "skin," a change takes effect on the screen. This means that the system is now ready to receive details of the tablets that the doctor is prescribing, along with the cream to treat the patient's penile infection. A moment later, having talked across the patient's response at line 8, the doctor looks back to the computer screen and prepares to resume typing. The patient immediately averts his gaze and looks at the keyboard. Consequently, upon the completion of the doctor's utterance, both parties are looking at the computer. After a brief pause, the doctor presses another key.

In summary, when patients respond to doctors' prescription-related statements by asking questions, they coordinate their questions with potential junctures in the doctors' keyboard actions. Although they sometimes seek to secure the doctors' undivided attention by gazing at them, they immediately withdraw their gaze from the doctors if it becomes apparent that the doctors are preparing to continue typing. In these ways they minimize the interactional demands that they place upon the doctors when the latter are typing, and thereby minimize the likelihood of their actions disrupting the doctors' computer-based activities.

Discussion

The delivery of prescription-related information by doctors can be critical to the management of health and illness. By communicating this information to patients, doctors seek to ensure that patients understand treatment regimens. They also try to increase the likelihood that patients will comply with such regimes by, inter alia, describing their side effects, assessing their effectiveness, and/or explaining how they react with other medications.

In this chapter I have examined how information concerning prescribed medicines is delivered by doctors and received by patients in medical consultations conducted in a medical practice in England. In so doing, I have concentrated on cases in which doctors communicate information to patients as they write prescriptions via a computer. As noted earlier, by doing this the doctors can reduce the length of their consultations and break up what might otherwise be lengthy silences as they use the computer. However, they also run the risk that their talk-based and computer-based activities will undermine each other.

I have shown that the doctors routinely coordinate their verbal delivery of prescription-related information with their progress through the computer fields. Thus, for example, they speak either while the cursor is located in computer fields concerning the selfsame information that they communicate to patients or when the cognitive and physical demands of using the computer are relatively low. Alternatively, they configure their use of the computer so as to establish "gaps" within which they can furnish information that does not correspond to the details they enter into the computer fields. These practices enable the doctors to reconcile the potentially competing demands of interacting with patients and writing prescriptions. That is to say, they allow the doctors to communicate information to patients as they write prescriptions without seriously disrupting either their talk-based or computer-based activities.

As for the patients, they seek to minimize the likelihood of their responses disrupting the doctors' text-based activities. When they merely acknowledge what the doctor tells them, they avoid visual actions which might attract the doctor's gaze and thus interrupt the computer-based task in hand. When they respond by asking questions, they coordinate both their talk and their gaze with potential junctures in the doctor's use of the keyboard. Moreover, if the doctors continue typing, they leave the doctors free to do so by withdrawing their gaze from them.

Video recordings of consultations conducted before the introduction of the computer system show that doctors and patients used similar practices when prescriptions were written by hand. Thus, for example, the doctors communicated prescription-related information to patients as they wrote the self-same information on prescription forms. They also configured their writing to create "space" for prescription-related talk which did not correspond to the details they were required to write on the prescription forms. In the case of the patients, they coordinated their actions with potential junctures in the doctors' text-based activities, which they identified on the basis of audible and visible aspects of the doctors' conduct, such as the doctors' movement of their pens from one part of the prescription form to another. This suggests that doctors and patients adapt generic practices for the coordination of talk-based and text-based activities to the constraints and opportunities which derive from the tools that are being used to inscribe the texts (keyboard/monitor or pen/paper) and the organizational features of the textual medium in use (e.g., the layout of documents, the form in which information is recorded, and the order in which it is written or typed).

It is important to note that the coordination of interpersonal communication and computer use can operate to maximize, as well as to minimize, the disjuncture between talk-based and computer-based activities. Sometimes this occurs due to patients "misprojecting" junctures in the doctors' computer-based activities. More commonly, however, it results from the doctors' privileging their text-based activities in one or more of the following ways:

1. Either remaining silent or restricting their contributions to minimal, largely undifferentiated responses as they type, write, or read – even though a patient's utterances may have invited a range of possible reactions such as assessments, advice, laughter, or expressions of sympathy or surprise.
2. Delaying, or pausing in the midst of, their utterances until they have written or typed a segment of information or checked something in their paper-based or screen-based documents.
3. Confining their visual attention to either the prescription form or the monitor and keyboard.
4. Abruptly shifting away from immediately preceding topics (which may concern the prescription per se or other issues such as the state of the patient's health, other medical matters, or psychosocial issues) in order to elicit information concerning their text-based activities.
5. Abruptly withdrawing their gaze from patients in order to inscribe or read paper-based or screen-based text.

Of course, these phenomena do not necessarily mean that doctors are *unable* to interleave their text-based activities with their interaction with the patient. While text-based tasks may sometimes place constraints on doctors which undermine their ability to simultaneously participate in discussions with their patients, the doctors may use their involvement in text-based activities as a warrant for curtailing discussion of the topics of prior talk.[5]

With this said, however, it is noteworthy that displays of preoccupation with text-based activities are more common in consultations in which prescriptions are produced via computer than in consultations in which they are written by hand. In general, then, the computer appears to undermine the doctor's ability to produce prescriptions in ways in which they can simultaneously display sensitivity to the ongoing demands of the interaction with the patient. There are at least three reasons for this. First, paper-based prescription forms are inanimate and provide no response to the doctors' use of the media. Consequently, doctors do not have to monitor paper documents to discern whether information has been "accepted." In the case of the computer system, however, the doctors often need

[5] It should also be noted that such conduct may on occasion encourage, as opposed to inhibit, talk by patients, since it can provide space for them to discuss issues at length.

to closely monitor the operation of the computer to ensure that the appropriate responses have been elicited, as well as to enable them to coordinate their own actions with the movement of the cursor along the prompt line and other changes on the screen. Doctors are also required to attend output messages, such as requests for clarification, corrections to inputs, and warning "beeps."

Second, paper documents collocate reading and writing. Doctors are able to read where the pen touches the paper. With the computer system, however, the keyboard and monitor separate spatially and visually the domain in which text is inscribed and manipulated from the domain in which it is read. The physical separation of reading and writing demanded by screen and keyboard, and the ongoing shifts in visual orientation it necessitates, appear to undermine the doctors' ability to delicately coordinate reading and writing with the ongoing and contingent demands of the interaction.

Third, paper documents are ecologically mobile. The small A6 prescription pad used in general practice can be easily moved around the desk and the consulting room. This means that the prescription pad can be placed between doctor and patient on the desk so that only a minor shift in orientation is required for the doctor to shift gaze from one to the other. With the computer, however, shifts in gaze and bodily orientation are more marked, especially if the screen is placed away from the patient at the center or far end of the desk. Together with the other "constraints" of system use noted above, this can in some situations reduce the doctor's ability to simultaneously participate in discussions with the patient whilst writing prescriptions.

As for the patients, they generally display a greater sensitivity to the possibility of interrupting or disrupting an activity in progress when the computer is being used. Thus the coordination of patients' talk with potential junctures in the documentation and retrieval of information is more common when the computer is being used than it is when the doctors are using paper. This may be due to the observably interactive character of the doctors' use of the computer and to the ways in which the system observably places, or is constituted as placing, demands on the doctor that do not apply when prescriptions are being directly produced by hand. Thus, the extent to which patients attempt to synchronize their conduct with the visible and audible aspects of system operation and use appears to depend largely on the way in which the doctor uses the system. For the most part, patients coordinate their actions with the use and operation of the system in situations in which the doctors exhibit a preoccupation with the computational task at hand. The more doctors "background" the use of the computer as they interact with patients, the less likely patients will treat system-based conduct as immediately consequential to production and delivery of their talk.

In conclusion, primary care information systems are designed to enable individual doctors to document and retrieve medical information alone. However, as we have seen, their use in medical consultations is ineluctably interrelated with the interaction between doctor and patient. Doctors and patients coordinate their communicative actions with their text-based activities. Consequently, the competencies involved in the accomplishment of text-based tasks are in many cases inseparable from those which underpin the doctor–patient interaction. Further research is needed to determine the extent to which the use of different primary care information systems, with different physical and organizational properties, facilitate or impede the accomplishment and coordination of talk-based and task-based activities.

12

Lifestyle discussions in medical interviews

Marja-Leena Sorjonen, Liisa Raevaara, Markku Haakana, Tuukka Tammi, and Anssi Peräkylä

Introduction

Earlier research

It is widely acknowledged that issues of lifestyle – such as diet, drinking, smoking, and exercise – have a significant impact on the health of individuals, and that promoting healthier patient lifestyle choices is an important task for primary care doctors. In spite of its importance, this part of the consultation has been focused upon in only a few empirical observational studies. The main studies so far have been made in the United States and in the Nordic (Scandinavian) countries.

These studies report that in American and Nordic consultations alike, lifestyle is talked about in 30–50 percent of encounters in primary care (Waitzkin and Britt 1993; Russel and Roter 1993; Johansson et al. 1995; Engeström et al. 1989) and in internal medicine (Larsson et al. 1987). But the existing literature seems to suggest that practices of talking about lifestyle may be rather different in different countries.

One important difference concerns the *activity types* through which lifestyle gets discussed. Nordic studies report that talk about lifestyle involves primarily *elicitation of information* concerning the patient's habits; Nordic doctors do *not* often give patients information about the health-related consequences of their lifestyle (Larsson

This research was made possible by a grant from the Finnish Foundation for Alcohol Studies in a project co-directed by Anssi Peräkylä and Marja-Leena Sorjonen. We are grateful to John Heritage and Douglas Maynard for their most insightful comments on earlier drafts of this chapter.

et al. 1987; Johansson et al. 1994). In America, by contrast, Russel and Roter (1993) report that, in 60 percent of cases, talk about lifestyle takes the form of *counseling* which involves the doctor's attempts to influence the patient's behavior. In the transcripts presented in the qualitative papers on American practice by Waitzkin and Britt (1993) and Freeman (1987), doctors do not confine themselves to asking questions about patients' lifestyle, but also give quite explicit advice aimed at changing the patient's lifestyle.

Regarding the *location* of the lifestyle talk in consultation, a Nordic study (Larsson et al. 1987) reports that lifestyle was almost exclusively addressed during the *history-taking phase* of the consultation.[1] The American studies give a somewhat different picture. Russel and Roter (1993) reported in their large quantitative study (439 interactions between primary care doctors and chronically ill patients) that lifestyle was often also discussed during the physical examination and in the conclusion of the visit.

The Nordic studies point out the shallowness of the discussions: descriptions of lifestyle given by patients and accepted by doctors are vague and imprecise (Larsson et al. 1987; Engeström et al. 1989). The picture given in the American studies varies more. As already mentioned, Russel and Roter (1993) claim that American doctors often get involved in lifestyle counseling. However, Freeman (1987) pointed out that longer sequences of talk about lifestyle usually took place when lifestyle was directly connected with the patient's medical problem. By contrast, when there was no such connection (i.e., when the doctor attempted to initiate the discussion in terms of "general" health promotion), the patients were resistant and discussions died out quickly.

In sum, the research published so far seems to suggest that the American doctors are more inclined to engage in more extensive discussions on lifestyle, and to give advice – possibly also with "moral" tones (cf. Waitzkin and Britt 1993). Nordic doctors, by contrast, may focus on information-gathering and be more reluctant to give information and advice. However, these studies have operated at a

[1] Johansson et al. (1995) report that in Swedish primary care consultations, physical exercise is also often discussed during the concluding phase of the visit. However, they define lifestyle in very broad terms and it remains unclear whether these discussions concern the patient's habitual exercising or specific physical exercise recommended as the treatment for particular medical problems (such as stretching of muscles after an operation).

relatively gross level of precision. The American studies do not give explanations as to *how* and *why* in some consultations the participants return to lifestyle topics when concluding the consultation and in others they do not; nor as to *how* and *why* in some consultations, participants engage in extensive lifestyle counseling and in others they just briefly mention the issue. In a similar fashion, the earlier reports on Nordic practices make a most important contribution by pointing out that lifestyle is usually described in a relatively shallow manner and that doctors tend to withhold information and advice; but the studies do not show *how* and *why* they end up doing this.

Lifestyle discussions in our data have features that are grossly similar to those already identified in earlier studies on Nordic consultations: doctors predominantly ask questions without engaging in advice-giving or information delivery about the medical significance of the patient's lifestyle. This is, however, only the starting point of our analysis: what we primarily want to offer is an empirical analysis that shows how the Finnish doctors and their patients collaboratively build up their interaction so that (in most cases) advice or information concerning lifestyle never becomes a relevant interactional option; or (in some cases) so that advice concerning the lifestyle is a logical outcome of the talk. It turns out that certain features of interaction – the location of the doctor's question concerning the patient's lifestyle, and both ways in which the patient describes her or his lifestyle and ways in which the doctor receives the description – establish participants' problem or no-problem orientation and thereby create relevancies for advice to occur.

We will start by outlining different environments within the consultation in which doctors ask the patient about her or his lifestyle. Thereafter, we will discuss how the patient's lifestyle gets treated as non-problematic or as problematic. Finally, we will talk about advice-giving and the way in which a problem orientation established during the questioning phase creates relevancies for advice to occur.

Data

Our database consists of some 90 videotaped and transcribed primary care consultations in four primary care health centres in Central Finland. This database involves 14 doctors; there is a different patient in each visit. Out of this corpus, we have collected all segments where the patients' eating, drinking, smoking, or exercising habits are discussed. In this chapter, we will focus exclusively on segments that were initiated by the doctor's question and where the given aspect of lifestyle is addressed for the first time, i.e., it has not been addressed in earlier consultations. The number of cases we have is 38 and they come from 25 different consultations.

The discussions on lifestyle that we will focus on take place almost exclusively in *acute* or *follow-up* visits. These are visits where the patient's medical problem is presented for the first time, or where the patient meets the doctor for a follow-up after having undergone tests or treatment related to an acute problem. Only one of our data segments (number 14) involves a *routine visit* involving monitoring of a medical problem that has been identified some time ago.

Visits in which the patient's lifestyle gets discussed for the first time are crucial in terms of the way in which the patient's lifestyle gets treated later, for it is there that a stance toward the medical relevance of the patient's lifestyle is first formulated. By asking about the patient's lifestyle, the doctor indicates that lifestyle may have an impact on the patient's health and therefore it may be medically problematic. The point of the question is to find out whether there is a problem or not.

Environments and forms of lifestyle questions

When the doctor asks about the patient's lifestyle for the first time, the question ordinarily aims at finding out whether a given aspect of lifestyle is problematic or not in terms of the patient's ailment (cf. Raevaara 1996b). The questions can be located in two different places relative to utterances, where the medical problem is being brought up or formulated: either subsequent to such utterances, or further away from them. The analysis will show that the former type of questions are understood to suggest a closer linkage between the patient's lifestyle and her or his current ailment.

Questions that are asked subsequent to a formulation of a medical problem

In 12 cases of our collection of 38 topic-initial lifestyle questions, the doctor asks the question subsequent to or in close proximity to a verbal formulation of a medical problem. The problem formulation may have been done by the patient himself or herself as a description of problematic symptoms, often concerning an issue presented as subsidiary rather than the main reason for the visit. Or it may have been done by the doctor, as a formulation of problematic test results or findings in the physical exam. We will show an instance of a latter case as example (1) below. In the transcripts, the first line of each numbered line provides an idiomatic translation, the second line offers the Finnish original, and the third line presents a word-by-word gloss of the Finnish.

(1) [1A6:3–4]

1	D:		*.hh Cholesterol eight point ↑one in other words it has*
			.hh Kolestrooli kaheksan pilkku ↑yks elikkä se on
			cholesterol eight comma one in.other.words it is
2			*a bi- (0.2) again gone ↑up a bit,*
			p- (0.2) taas pikkusen ↑noussu,
			a.little.bit again a.little.bit gone up
3			*(0.2)*
4	D:		*>And triclyserids four point ↑ze:ro blood sugars*
			>Ja triklyseridit neljä pilkku ↑nol:la veren sokerit
			and triclyserids four comma zero blood sugars
5			*four point ↑seve:n,*
			neljä pilkku ↑sei:tsemän,
6			*(5.0)*
7	D:		°*Ye::s.*°
			°Joo::.°
8			*(1.1)*
9	D:		*Hemoglobin hundred and thirty-five which is ↑good,*
			Hemoglobiini satakolmeviis mikä on ↑hyvä,
			hemoglobin 135 which is good
10			*(0.8)*
11	D:	=>	*↑How much,h (.) sugar do you use.*
			↑Kuinka paljon,h (.) käytätte sokeria.
			how much use.you sugar
12	P:		*Well< (.) no:t much really.*
			No< (.) en: oikeestaan paljoo.
			well not really much
13			*(0.2)*
14	P:		*Like with coffee not at all and<*
			N'ku kahvin kanssakaa en ollenkaa ja<
			like coffee with not at.all and
15			*(0.8)*

16	P:		*What there is then in the food but usually I don't*
			Mitä sitte noissa nyt ruuissa on mut en mä yleensä
			what then those now foods is but not I usually
17			*(0.2) (like) (0.2) use sugar.*
			(0.2) (siis et) (0.2) käytä sokeria.
			so that use sugar
18	D:	=>	°*Yeah:.*° *What about fats.*
			°Joo:.° Entäs rasvoja.

In lines 1–5, the doctor reads aloud test results from the computer screen. She (line 2) points out the rise in the cholesterol level since the last test (the numerical values of cholesterol and triclyserids are high). The announcement of the test results is followed by questions concerning the patient's eating habits in lines 11 and 18. By placing the questions after an indication of a problem, the doctor indexes an understanding that lifestyle is a probable factor behind the problem. Thus the location of the question suggests a specific linkage between lifestyle and the medical problem: too much use of sugar or fats may have caused the rise in cholesterol.

Questions that are asked further away from the formulation of the medical problem

In some other cases, however, the doctor's question is located further away from the formulation of a medical problem. Such placement of the question indexes a less specific linkage between the lifestyle and the patient's medical problem: lifestyle is presented not as a primary factor, but as a factor among many others that may be associated with the ailment. These questions form the largest subgroup in our collection: 26 instances out of 38 topic-initial lifestyle questions.

Questions are located further away from the problem formulation most often in cases where the patient presents the relevant problem at the beginning of the consultation as the reason for his or her visit. Example (2) below is a case in point. The patient has presented a recurrent abdominal pain as the reason for his visit. The doctor has started the history-taking with a series of questions about the pain, followed by questions that focus on possible other symptoms (such as diarrhea) and medication. He then asks about travel (line 1). In line 6, he moves to ask about lifestyle:

(2) [5A2:5–6]

1 D: => *You haven't been ab↑road,*
↑Ulkomailla ette oo ollu,
abroad not.you be been
2 P: *No.*
En.
3 *(1.0)*
4 D: *<I see,>*
<Ahah,>
5 *(0.5)*
6 D: => *Do you smoke,*
Tupakoitteko,
smoke.you
7 *(1.0)*
8 P: *Oh do I smo>ke<,*
Jaa tupa>koinko<,
smoke.I
9 D: *Yes,*
Ni,
10 P: *No,*
Eh,
11 *(0.3)*
12 D: *Not at all,*
Ette ollenkaa,
not.you at.all
13 P: °*No,*°
°Eh,°
14 *(0.2)*
15 D: [*I see,*]
[Jaha,]
16 P: [*I've been already*] *(.) thirteen years*
[M' oon ollu jo] (.) kolometoista vuotta
[I have been already thirteen years
17 *without. .mhhh A bit more, >no< fou:rteen.*
ilman. .mhhh Vähä enempi, > eiku< nel:jätoista.
without a.bit more no.but fourteen
18 D: => *What is your diet like.*
Minkäslainen se teiän ruokavalio on.
what.kind the your diet is

Here the questions about lifestyle (lines 6 and 18) initiate new topical areas and they do not display any connection to their prior talk. However, because these questions occur prior to diagnosis, they can be understood as in search of possible factors behind the medical problem. Furthermore, since lifestyle questions tend to be raised after other kinds of diagnostic questions, they treat lifestyle as a factor of less than primary importance for the patient's ailment.

Treating lifestyle as non-problematic

In the vast majority of cases in our database, the patient responds to the doctor's question with an answer that treats the lifestyle as non-problematic; this is especially so when the question is asked away from the formulation of a medical problem. Furthermore, despite the fact that after such answers talk about lifestyle in most cases gets extended, a treatment of lifestyle as non-problematic is sustained in the subsequent talk – in the doctors' requests for specification and in the patients' responses to them.

Types of no-problem answer

There are several different kinds of answers through which the patients claim that there is no problem in their lifestyle. The type of the answer is associated with the type of question asked by the doctor and the kind of behavior being talked about.

Flat-out rejections. When the question is formulated as a Yes/No question, which is the case especially with smoking and when a female patient is asked about drinking,[2] a straightforward "no" is hearable as a no-problem answer, as in the following example:

(3) [10A3:18]

1	D:	*.h Do you smoke.*	*O[r*	*] have you*	*ever*	*smoked.*
		.h Tupakoitko.	T[ai	] ootko	koskaan	tupakoinu.
		smoke.you	or	] have.you	ever	smoked

[2] When asking about drinking, the doctors vary the question form according to the gender of the patient. When asking a female patient about drinking for the first time, the question is designed as a Yes/No question ("Do you drink"), whereas in the case of a male patient, it is built up as a *wh-* question ("How much do you drink"). Thus with the male patients the assumption and starting point is that the patient drinks alcohol and the doctor's task is to find out the details of the behavior, whereas with the female patients the doctor starts with an inquiry that seeks to find out whether the behavior exists at all.

2 P: => [*No.*]
[En.]
3 P: => *No.*
En.
4 *(0.7)*
5 D: *Yea::.*
Joo::.
6 *(1.3)*
7 D: *Do you use alcohol at all.*
Käytätkö alkohoolia yhtää.
use.you alcohol at.all

By contrast, after *wh-* questions the features of no-problem answers vary. What is common to answers, however, is that they are unspecific: they do not provide any details (e.g., frequency or amount) of the behavior.

Claims of normality. Some *wh-* questions invite a description of the patient's behavior without specifying any parameters for it. In the following, the patient gives a no-problem answer to such a question concerning drinking:

(4) [5A1:9–10]

1 D: *.mhh And what about the use of alcohol,*
.mhh Ja mitenkäs sulla alkoholin käyttö on,
and how you alcohol use is
2 P: => *Quite nor:mal y'know so,*
Semmosta ihan nor:maalia °että°,
such just normal so
3 D: *Which means,*
Eli,

In his answer in line 2, the patient describes his habit of drinking alcohol with the adjective "normal." Through it he treats his behavior as ordinary and thereby implies its nothing-to-be-reported and non-problematic character.

Minimizing and maximizing answers. The doctor can also inquire about the amount and/or frequency of a given behavior. This is especially the case when asking about exercise and specific food substances. In responses to these questions, the patients characterize the behavior by using unspecified descriptors (e.g., "much," "little," "sometimes"), as in the following examples:

(5) [1A6:3–4]

1 D: ↑*How much,h (.) sugar do you use.*
↑Kuinka paljon,h (.) käytätte sokeria.
how much use.you sugar
2 P: => *Well< (.) no:t much really.*
No< (.) en: oikeestaan paljoo.
well not.I really much
3 *(0.2)*
4 P: *Like with coffee not at all and<*
N'ku kahvin kanssakaa en ollenkaa ja<
like coffee with.also not.I at.all and

(6) [8A3:5–6]

1 D: *.mhh How much exercise do you, h*
.mhh Mitenkäs paljo te liikuntaa, h
how much you exercise
2 P: *.mth [hhh*
3 D: *[perform,*
[suoritatte,
4 P:=> *Well definitely some every day, h*
No kyl[lä minä joka] päivä jonkun verran, h
well definitely I every day some amount
5 D: [*(do,)*]
[(teette),]
6 *(0.2)*
7 D: *In other wo:rds several kilometres,*
Eli: useemman kilometrin,

In (5), the patient responds to a question about the amount of sugar she uses with an answer that denies excessive behavior. In so doing she treats her use of sugar as non-problematic and the mere denial as a sufficient answer. However, subsequently, in response to the doctor's silence, she (line 4) proceeds to elaborate her answer (cf. Stivers and Heritage 2001). In (6), the patient responds to a question about her exercise habits with an answer that provides a frequency and an unspecified amount of exercising. With the particle *kyllä* "definitely" and the stress on the element mentioning the amount (*jonkun* "some"), she portrays herself as somebody who does exercise and implies the non-problematic character of her exercising habits.

Health-oriented descriptions. When a general description of eating habits is invited by the doctor, the patients' no-problem-oriented answers often contain a health-oriented description:

(7) [5A2:6–7]

1 D: *What is your diet like.*
Minkäslainen se teiän ruokavalio on.
what.kind the your diet is
2 P: => *.mhh Well it's surely y'know like non-fat °heh he°*
.mhh Noh kyllähä se semmosta rasvatonta o °heh he°
well surely.y'know it such fatless is
3 D: *More,*
Enempi,

(8) [8A3:7–8]

1 D: *Yeah. .hhh hhhh Wha:t kind of diet do you have, h*
Joo. .hhh hhhh M:itenkäslaine ruokavalio teillä on, h
yeah what.kind diet you is
2 *In other words,hh what do you eat.*
Eli,hh mitä syöt:te.
in.other.words what eat.you
3 *(0.2)*
4 P: => *I have tried to eat in a balanced way so that,*
Aika monipuolisesti oon yrittänyt syödä että,
quite manysidedly have.I tried eat so
5 *(0.2)*
6 D: >*All kinds of food.*<
>Kaikenlaista.<
all.kinds

In (7) and (8), the patients have selected a description of a preferred type of diet advocated by health education ("non-fat"; "eat in balanced way"). By selecting these descriptions they display their knowledgeability of the recommendations and suggest that their eating habits are non-problematic.

Reception of no-problem answers

Talk about lifestyle usually continues for a while after the patient's initial no-problem answer. Only the flat-out rejections denying the existence of a given potentially harmful behaviour tend to be treated as sufficient answers; see example (3) above. In most other cases, the doctor receives the patient's answer with a request for specification, thereby treating the answer as insufficient for current purposes. The requests for specification do not, however, call into question the patients' initial proposal that the lifestyle is non-problematic.

Requests for specification take two main forms in our data. First, there are turns that prompt a specification of the answer without indicating the kind of specification requested, and second, there are follow-up questions or candidate understandings (Schegloff et al. 1977:368, 378–9) that focus on a particular part of the answer. The following example contains both an example of a prompt (line 4) and candidate understandings (lines 6, 10, and 12); the patient has come to see the doctor because of high blood pressure:

(9) [5A1:15–16]

1 D: *.Yes yes, What about exercising.*
.Joo joo, Mites liikunta.
2 P: *Quite good,*
Aika hyvä.
3 *(0.2) ((D gazes at P))*
4 D: => *Which means,*
Eli,
5 P: *I (.) walk around with my dog quite a lot and then,*
Mä (.) kuljen koiran kans aika paljo ja sitte,
I go.I dog with quite a.lot and then
6 D: => *Several kilometers a day?=*
Useita kilometrejä päivässä.=
7 P: *=Well (.) I don't walk quite every day (.) so awfully*
=No (.) en minä ny ihan päivittäin (.) kauheen
well not.I I now quite daily awfully
8 *many, kilometers but nevertheless I do some*
useita, kilometrejä mee mutta kyllä sitä ny jotain
several kilometers go but surely it now some
9 *(.) >get some< of it. .hhh [(exercise.)]*
verran (.) >jonkun verran< tulee. .hhh [(liikuntaa.)]
amount some amount comes [exercise]
10 D: => *[Three kilometers?]*
[Kolme kilometriä,]
11 P: *Well (.) I do even more than three °kilometers°,*
No (.) kyllä ylitteki tulee kolme °kilometriä°,
well surely over.even comes three kilometers
12 D: => *Dail[y.*
Päivit[täin.

13 P: [.*Yeah*
[.Nii
14 D: .*Yes*,
.Joo,

Here, after the patient has described his habit of exercising with a positive evaluation "Quite good," which treats his exercising as non-problematic, the doctor (line 4) produces a response, the particle *eli* ("Which means"; "in other words"), that invites the patient to specify his answer. The turn treats the entire answer as one to be specified. It also leaves it to the patient to specify the meaning of "Quite good" exercising. In line 5, the patient begins to detail his answer with a report of his everyday activity (walking his dog). He then goes on to project another piece of information to come ("and then"). During a break in the patient's talk, the doctor (line 6) produces a candidate understanding of the patient's report, and subsequently (lines 10 and 12) two further candidate understandings.

The candidate understandings in lines 6, 10, and 12 have two main aspects to them. First, they offer an understanding that specifies the patient's description in abstract terms, stripped of references to the patient's possible everyday activities (cf. Sacks 1992b:561–9; Heritage and Boyd this volume). Second, they portray the given conduct by the patient as favorably as possible, thereby aligning with the patient's prior answer.[3] In some parallel cases the doctors even offer understandings that turn out to be "too favorable" and not acceptable by the patient (cf. Haakana 1999:143–57).[4]

In sum, the no-problem orientation established in patients' initial answers is sustained by the doctors when receiving the answers. While a no-problem answer is often treated as in need of specification by the doctor, the kinds of specifications sought serve to get a description in terms of a numerical or otherwise abstract estimation. In asking and receiving the specifications, the doctors leave intact the no-problem thrust of the patient's initial answer.

[3] This might be a more general feature of turns incorporating a candidate answer (cf. Pomerantz 1988).

[4] Prompts and candidate understandings are found also following unspecified answers to questions about drinking. However, when talking about eating habits, the doctors respond to the patients' answers also by asking questions that introduce a new sub-area of diet: after having heard the patient's answers about, for example, fats, the doctor may ask about bread and thereafter about vegetables.

Exits from the discussions on a lifestyle issue in no-problem cases

After having heard the patient's initial no-problem answer and (in most cases) after having pursued specifications of it, the doctors drop the topic, typically without giving any evaluative comments or advice to the patients. By virtue of its non-evaluative character, the closure of the lifestyle topics also leaves intact the no-problem thrust of the patient's initial answers.

Doctors usually close a lifestyle topic in no-problem cases by simply producing a question that initiates a new topic and/or new activity. In some cases, before producing the question, the doctor may first separately acknowledge the patient's answer. In the following example, the doctor (line 1) initiates a discussion about the patient's diet. His subsequent questions in lines 9 and 13–14, move the discussion from one area of diet to another and then, in line 27, he moves to ask about drinking:

(10) [5A2:6–7]

1 D:-> *What is your diet like.*
Minkäslainen se teiän ruokavalio on.
what.kind the your diet is
2 P: *.mh Well it's surely y'know like non-fat °heh he°*
.mh Noh kyllähä se semmosta rasvatonta o °heh he°
well surely.y'know it such fatless is
3 D: *More,*
Enempi,
4 P: *Yeah,*
Nih,
5 D:-> *So that's the way it is,*
Et sillai,
so in.that.way
6 P: *.mhh hh I don't eat butter at all and (.) .hh [non-fat*
.mhh hh Voi:ta en syö ollenkaa ja (.) .hh [rasva]tonta
butter no.I eat at.all and [fatless
7 D:-> [*What*]
[Mites]
[how]
8 P: *sou:r milk °and°,=*
pii:mää °ja°,=
9 D:-> *=What about bread,*
=Mites leipää,
how bread

10 P: *.hhh Well the bread is like rye: bread. I've been eating*
.hhh No lei:pä on semmosta limp:pua. Oon syöny
well bread is such loaf have.I eaten
11 *these days.*
kyllä nykyää.
surely these.days
12 *(0.2)*
13 D:-> *What about then the:: (.) fruits and this kind of*
Mites sitte tää#:: (.) hedelmä ja tämmönen
how then this fruit and this.kind
14 -> *vegetable stuff.]*
vihannes[puoli#.]
15 P: [*.hhh*] *Well I do y'know get to eat them*
[.hhh] No ky:llähä niitäki tullee
[ ] well certainly those.also comes
16 *to some extent.*
syötyä jonku verra.
eat some. extent
17 *(1.0)*
18 D: *Regularly.*
Säännöllisesti.
19 *(0.8) ((D looking at the computer screen))*
20 P: *Yea[:h,]*
Nii[:,]
21 D:=> [*I see,*
[Jah]a,
22 P: *>I do get to eat them every day at least*
>Kyl (.) mel' (.) joka: päivä vähä ainaki
certainly almost every day a.little at.least
23 *a little of] those greens at*
tulee syö[tyä] ruuan kans nuita (0.2) .hhh
comes eat meal with those
24 D:=> [>*Yeah.*<
[>Joo.<]
25 P: *meals.h[h he (How do you put it).*
rehuja.h[h he (Miten 'tä] ny) sanoo.
greens [how it now says
26 D:=> [*Yeah.*]
[Joo.]
27 D:-> *What about alcohol use,*
Mites alkoholin käyttö,

In line 9, the doctor moves to ask about another aspect of the patient's diet, thereby treating the prior discussion about fats as sufficient. (Note also the first aborted effort to ask this question in line 7.) Similarly, in lines 13–14, he treats the prior talk as sufficient by asking a question about another area of diet.

The next move to a new area of lifestyle is managed in a slightly different fashion. In line 21, the doctor acknowledges the patient's confirmation with "I see." While the doctor produces this information receipt (cf. Heritage 1984b) only, the patient (line 22) proceeds to specify his prior response. Twice in the course of the specification, the doctor (lines 24 and 26) responds with an acknowledgment token. Through them, at the points where they are produced, the doctor claims to have understood what the patient has said and to treat the information offered as sufficient. When producing his response in line 26, the doctor turns towards his desk and begins to make a note. Thereafter, still oriented towards the desk, he (line 27) asks a question that initiates talk about alcohol. Thus, in this case, the doctor displayed his treatment of the information provided by the patient as sufficient before moving to a new activity with a question.

The type of acknowledgment tokens recurrently used by the doctors, most notably the response token *joo* ("yes"; "yeah") as above, treat the patient's description as understood and imply its sufficiency for the current purposes (cf. Sorjonen 2001), but they are indifferent as to how the patient's description should be evaluated: they do not address the issue whether it is problem-indicative or not. A non-evaluative way of receiving the patient's no-problem answer (by moving to a new question, preceded sometimes by a separate acknowledgment) is systematic when lifestyle is discussed for the first time. The absence of evaluation constitutes this phase of talk as part of information-gathering for doctor's diagnostic purposes. In later phases of consultation, possible places for an evaluation are ones where diagnosis is delivered, information is provided, and/or treatment is discussed. However, also within these phases, talk about lifestyle is systematically absent in no-problem cases in our data.

We now turn to discuss cases in which the patient's lifestyle gets treated as medically problematic.

Establishing lifestyle as problematic

In some cases, the patient's answer to the doctor's questions about lifestyle is distinctively different from what we have seen so far:

it indicates explicitly or implicitly that there is a problem. This orientation is usually taken up by doctors, and thereby the participants jointly establish an orientation to the patient's lifestyle as problematic.

As already mentioned, there is an association between the placement of the initial lifestyle question (see p. 342) and the tendency of the participants to treat the patient's lifestyle as problematic or non-problematic in our data. When the question is asked *further away* from the formulation of the medical problem (i.e., when the question is a part of a larger history-taking phase), the lifestyle is very rarely treated as problematic: we have only one case with a problem orientation in our collection of 26 sequences in such location; see example (11) below. However, when the question is asked *subsequent* to a formulation of a medical problem, an orientation to the lifestyle as problematic is established in more than half of the cases in our collection of 12 sequences in that location.[5]

The problem orientation can be either overtly or incipiently brought up in the patient's initial answer. In the former case, the patient explicitly treats his or her habits as problematic. When such an orientation is displayed in the initial answer, it strongly proposes that the doctor take up the problem orientation in his subsequent turns. An incipient problem orientation, by contrast, makes it interactionally possible for doctors to take up the problem orientation but does not constrain them in that direction. Thus, the incipient problem orientation can be consolidated in the subsequent talk.

When the question–answer sequence has brought up a problem orientation, the talk about an aspect of lifestyle regularly leads to advice-giving. In what follows, we will first examine ways in which the problem orientation is brought up in the patients' answers and doctors' follow-up questions to the answers. In the next section, we will then explore advice-giving sequences.

Overt problem orientation

In some cases, the patients overtly treat their habits as problematic in their initial answer to the doctor's question. In the following

[5] Within this set, the problem orientation is established especially in cases where the problem formulation takes the shape of an announcement of problem-indicative test results or findings of a physical exam.

example, the doctor asks questions about the use of sugar – data not shown, see example (1) – and the use of fats (line 18) after an announcement of a rise in cholesterol level. The patient's answer, starting in line 19, contains an explicit problem orientation, which then is maintained in the subsequent talk.

(11) [continuation of (1)]

17 P: *–but usually I don't (0.2) (like) (0.2) use*
–mut en mä yleensä (0.2) (siis et) (0.2) käytä
but not.I I usually so that use
18 *sugar.*
sokeria.
19 D: *°Yeah:.° What about fats.*
°Joo:.° Entäs rasvoja.
20 P: => *Well there are (.) there are perhaps too °much°. But now*
No niitä on (.) niitä n't ehkä lii°kaa°. Mut nyt
well they is they probably too.much but now
21 -> *I have tried for a week .hhh for two weeks I've been*
mä oon yrittäny s'tte viikon .hhh kaks mä oon nyt
I have tried then week two I have now
22 -> *now< (.) without heh as I started to look at those*
ollu sitte< (.) il:man heh ku mä rupesin kattoo noita
been then without as I started look those
23 -> *.hh[hh] symptoms and results there so,*
.hh[hh] oireita ja tuloksia tossa ni,
24 D: [*Yes,*]
[Nii,]
25 *(0.7)*
26 D: *Yeah:.*
Joo:.
27 P: *↑°(so)°*
↑°(ni)°
28 *(0.4)*
29 D: *Yes. What kind of >↑in what ways< .hhh have you tried*
Joo. Minkälais:ta >↑millä tavalla< .hhh te ootte
yes what.kind what way you have
30 *to decrease the fats.*
sitä rasvaa vähentäny.
the fat decrease

In line 20, the patient formulates her use of fats as problematic by a characterization "too much." She then (lines 21–23) continues her turn by reporting measures that she has already taken to change the diet. In this case then the patient both displays recognition of her behavior as problematic and reports efforts to change it.[6] In her follow-up question (lines 29–30), the doctor seeks a specification of the patient's efforts. After the patient's specification, the doctor (data not shown) shifts the topic. But somewhat later (again, data not shown), she takes up the issue again in terms of advice. Thus, in this case, by topicalizing – and in that way indicating the importance of the patient's efforts to change her behavior – and by giving advice, the doctor treats the patient's behavior as something that is in need of a change, thereby also aligning with the patient's initial characterization of her use of fats as problematic.

Consolidating an incipient problem orientation

In a number of cases, the patient's initial answer involves an incipient problem orientation, which then can (but need not) get consolidated in the subsequent discussion. Extract (12) below provides an example. It is also the only case in our data where a problem orientation is established in a discussion that takes place away from a medical problem formulation, as a part of a larger segment of history-taking. In this case, the patient with high blood pressure displays an incipient problem orientation in his initial answer to a question about drinking. In line 1, after having announced that he will take the patient's blood pressure, the doctor asks a question about the use of salt; and in line 8, he moves to ask about the patient's drinking habits:

(12) [12B1:5]

1	D:	*Do you use much salt.*
		Ootteko te ahkera suolankäyt°täjä°.
		are.you you diligent salt.user
2	P:	*Well< (.) not really and< (0.2) sugar at least*
		No< (.) e:m mää ny sillain oo ja< (0.2) tota sokeria
		well not I now in.such.way be and that sugar
3		*I have tried to avoid*
		mä oon nyt (.) ainaki (0.2) yrittäny välttää
		I have now at.least tried avoid

[6] Probably it would be face-threatening for patients to merely describe their habits as problematic, without referring to any efforts to change their behaviour. In our data, there are no such cases.

4 *so that I haven't put it in the coffee and*
sillai etten mä ain kahvinkaa oo laittanu °ja
such.way not I always coffee.with have put and
5 *the like,*
tollai ni°,
so
6 D: °*Yeah*°.
°Joo°.
7 *(0.2)*
8 D: -> *What about a:lcohol,*
Entäs al:koholia,
9 P: => *Well it is used som- now in the summer*
No sitä käy:tetään sem- nyt on kesällä tullu
well it is.used now has summer come
10 => *one has ended up using it a bit more (and) (.) we've*
käytettyä vähä runsaammin (ja) (.) °kaljaa on
use a.little more and beer has.been
11 => *had beer and,*
otettu ja°,
taken and
12 D: *Yes.*
Joo.
13 *(0.7) ((D gazing at P, then turning to his desk to reach for the stethoscope))*
14 D: -> *How much (.) is it approximately (.) so that one could*
Paljonko (.) suunnilleen sitä 'tä (.) että vois
much.how approximately it so that could
15 -> *then assess how much it affects (0.2)*
arvioida sitte vähä paljonko se vaikuttaa (0.2)
estimate then little much.how it affects
16 -> *the blood pressure.*
verenpai#neese[en#.
17 P: [*#Wonder how much it is# (0.2) perhaps*
[#Mitähän se on# (0.2) oiskohan se
[what.y'know it is is.y'know it
18 *it is (1.1) <twice> (0.2) a week at least beer and,*
(1.1) <kaks (0.2) kertaa> viikossa ainaki olutta ja,
two times week at.least beer and
19 *(0.2) ((D gazing at P and nodding))*
20 D: *Yes.*
Joo.
21 *(0.5) ((D gazing at P))*
22 D: *Is it one: bottle or more.*
Onks se yks: pullo vai useampi [pullo.

is it one bottle or more [bottle
23 P: *[It's more.*
[U:seampi pullo on.
[more bottle is
24 *(1.8) ((D turning to the blood pressure measurement equipment,*
then turning to set it on P))
25 D: -> *.mh It surely is one ((‘an amount’)) that can inc[rease]*
.mh Se on semmonen kyllä minkä voi vähän nos[taa]
it is such surely what can little raise
26 P: *[Mm.]*
27 D: -> *(0.2) °increase the blood pressure a bit°.*
°nostaa sitä verenpainetta°.
raise the blood.pressure
28 *(1.0) ((D making preparations for measuring the*
blood pressure))
29 D: *I gather the liver tests were not taken at any point or*
Maksa-arvoja ei taidettu ottaa missää vaiheessa vai
liver.values not take any stage or
30 *w- (.) were they.*
o- (.) otet°tiinko°.
take

In his answer in lines 9–11, the patient describes his drinking as having increased. Even though he portrays the change as possibly temporary by setting it within the frame of summer, the mere mentioning of the increase, together with the formulation *tullu käytettyä* “ended up using,” which implies that the drinking is beyond control, suggest that there may be a problem. He finishes his turn with a continuation-implicative “and” (line 11), which could imply a move to a mentioning of other kinds of alcohol. After an acknowledgment and a silence (lines 12–13), which provide space for the patient to elaborate on his answer, the doctor (line 14) poses a follow-up question. With his question the doctor explicitly treats the description of the amount of drinking as insufficient. This question is followed by a rationale for asking it, formulating the possibility that the drinking may be connected to the patient's medical problem. The patient responds in lines 17–18 by describing the frequency of drinking beer as “at least” twice a week, followed, again, by a continuation-implicative “and.” Again, the doctor provides space for the patient to continue (lines 19–21). No continuation forthcoming, he requests for a further specification of the amount of drinking (line 22), and then, in lines 25 and 27, provides an evaluation of the patient's drinking as something that may increase his blood pressure.

Notice here how the participants reach the specification of the amount of drinking. The doctor's follow-up question at line 22 seems to invite a response favoring a larger amount of drinking. In his question, the doctor offers the smallest possible amount of beer, a bottle (0.33 litre), as his starting point, and hence the subsequent alternative, the unspecified description "more" could be anything from two bottles of beer twice a week to any unspecified larger amount. Considering now that the patient has described his drinking as having increased, the selection of one bottle of beer as the starting point appears to work toward making it easier for the patient to admit a larger amount of beer. Furthermore, the selection of "more" works in the same direction: it makes it possible to leave the exact amount of drinking unstated. In his response (line 23), the patient accepts drinking more as a valid description. Thus the doctor's question design at line 22 appears to orient to a specific inferential framework here, one that leads to an understanding that the patient's drinking is problematic. This framework was invoked by the patient in his very first answer, when he reported an increase in drinking. The incipient problem orientation was sustained by the doctor in his account for the question and by the patient in his subsequent answer in lines 17–18, when he formulated the frequency of drinking as "at least" twice a week, followed by a continuation-implicative "and." The problem orientation was finally consolidated by the doctor through his evaluation in lines 25 and 27: the description "more" was enough for the doctor to provide the evaluation of the patient's drinking as problematic.

Example (13) below provides another case where the patient gives an answer with an incipient problem orientation, which then gets consolidated in the ensuing talk. In this case, the lifestyle question is asked subsequently to a medical problem formulation. Towards the end of this consultation, the patient introduced a new complaint – difficulties in moving her fingers, which she associates with stiffness in her neck and shoulders. In lines 1 and 3, the doctor closes a physical examination by reporting that she has found "these typical spots," which can be heard as referring to muscular tension. The question about lifestyle follows immediately after this announcement (lines 3 and 5).

(13) [21B2:16–18]

1 D: *(And) the typical spots can be found here.* [*( )*] (0.2)
(Ja) täältä löytyy nää tyypilliset kohdat. [( )]
and from.here found.is these typical spots
2 ?P: [.*Yea*]
[.Joo]
3 D: *they are tight. Do you go anywhere to do gym°work°.*
(0.2) kireet o. Käyttekö missään jum°passa°.
tight are go.you any gym work
4 *(1.0) ((D returns to his seat.))*
5 D: *Do you work out regularly at all.*
Onko mitää voimisteluharrastuk°sia°.
are.there any gymnastics.hobbies
6 *(0.6)*
7 P: *No I don't,*
Ei oo,
no are
8 *(0.4)*
9 P: *I haven't been going to the gym now for a little wh-*
Em mää nyt jumpassa o käyny vähään ai-
not I now gymnastics have visited little ?time
10 *>surely I have< been there but I haven't (.) haven't been going.*
>kyllä mä nyt< ollu oon mutta en (.) en o käyny.
surely I now been have but not.I not.I have visited
11 *(0.8)*
12 P: *now this autumn,*
nyt tänä syksynä,
13 *(2.5)*
14 D: *Earlier you have been going* [*anyway,*]
Ootte aikasemmin käyny [kuitenki,]
you.have earlier visited anyway
15 P: [*Earlier*] *I definitely*
[Aikasemm]in oon käyny
earlier have.I visited
16 *have been* [*going,*]
[kyllä,]
definitely
17 D: [*Yeah::,*] *.hh is it about to be dropped now*
[Joo::,] .hh onko se nyt jäämässä
yes is it now being. dropped
18 *for this winter.*
tältä talvelta.
19 *(0.4)*
20 P: *Well it shouldn't.*

No ei saisi.
well no should
21 *(0.6)*
22 P: *It shouldn't I ought to go to the swimming hall too,*
Ei saisi kyllä tohon uimahalliinkin täytys mennä,
no should surely that swimming.hall should go
23 D: *Yeah:,*
Nii:,
24 *(.)*
25 D: *.h As you thi[nk that there is wearing out in so*
.h Ku ajat[telee että on noi monessa nivelessä}
when thinks that is so many.in joint.in
26 P: *[Yeah,*
[Nii,
27 D: *many joints though and you have these problems so*
kuitenkin kulumaa ja näitä vaivoja ni
nevertheless wearing.out and these inconveniences so
28 *probably it would still be sensible,*
ehkä se olis sitte järkevää kuitenki,
possibly it would.be then reasonable however
29 *(0.4)*
30 P: *↑Yeah,*
↑Nii,
31 D: *try and go in spite of everything to go somewhere because –*
yrittää kaikesta huolimatta ni käydä jossaki koska
try everything in.spite.of go somewhere because

From her report of findings, the doctor (lines 3 and 5) moves to ask about the patient's exercising habits. The question focuses straight off on a specific type of exercise, "gym work," hearable as a possible treatment for the patient's problem. The patient's initial answer does not include components that would overtly be problem-oriented: in line 7, she gives a simple negative answer. However, as the question concerns a beneficial activity, this answer is hearable as incipiently problem-oriented (see also the delay in line 6). The subsequent discussion entails a stepwise consolidation of the problem orientation.

While the doctor remains silent, the patient (line 9) moves on to indicate that she has exercised earlier. Thereafter the doctor begins to pursue the need for exercising by follow-up questions (lines 14 and 17–18); in response to the latter question, the patient (lines 20 and 22) shifts into a prescriptive mode, stating that she needs to return to her earlier habits of exercising. By then, the participants have jointly consolidated an orientation to the patient's current behavior (no gym work) as problematic. Thereafter, the doctor moves to advice-giving.

To summarize, the patients' initial answers that display overt, as in example (11), or incipient, as in examples (12) and (13), problem orientation can give the ensuing discussion a direction that differs from the one in cases where the initial answer by the patient is no-problem-oriented. In example (12), as in the no-problem cases, the initial answer was followed by requests for specification of the patient's current behavior; but, unlike no-problem cases, here an explicit evaluation followed the question–answer sequence. In example (13), the doctor's follow-up questions pursued the need to exercise and led the patient to admit that she should exercise more; and in (11), the doctor's follow-up questions sought the specification of the patient's recent efforts to change her diet. Thus, in varying ways, the doctors took up the problem orientation expressed by the patients and the participants ended up jointly treating the lifestyle as problematic. The problem orientation gets its final confirmation as the doctor advises the patient to change his or her lifestyle.

Incipient problem orientation that is not consolidated

There is, however, no reason to suggest that the patient's initial answer would *determine* the direction of the ensuing interaction – the problem orientation is a joint achievement. Therefore it is remarkable that we do not have any cases where the participants, when discussing the patient's lifestyle for the first time, end up treating the patient's behavior as problematic, after the patient has initially given a no-problem-oriented answer. To put it simply, the thrust of the patient's initial no-problem orientation is never "turned down" by the doctors in our database. On the other hand, we do have a couple of cases where the patient's initial answer is designed in a way that is potentially hearable as displaying incipient problem orientation, but this orientation is not taken up by the doctor. One of them is presented below:

(14) [6B1:4–5]

1 D: *Do you have to use a lot of alcohol*
Joudutko sä (tuol) töitten puolest tai muute
have.to you there work because.of or otherwise
2 *because of your work or otherwise.*
alkoholii käyttää °paljo°.
alcohol use a.lot

3		*(0.2)*
4	P:	*I don't have to (bu-), (0.3) I do use it*
		E:n mä joudu (mu-), (0.3) ky'lä mä sitä käytä
		no.I I have.to ?but surely I it use
5		*(.) >approximately every week°end°<.*
		(.) >suurin piirtei joka viikon°loppu°<.
6		*(1.0)*
7	D:	*Beer,h*
		Olutta,h
8		*(0.2)*
9	P:	*Beer yeah::,*
		Olutta nii::,
10		*(8.5) ((D is preparing the blood pressure meter))*
11	D:	*Do you have many bottles,*
		Meneekö monta pulloo,
		go many bottle
12		*(1.6)*
13	P:	*Let's say four glasses .hh °haha Large ones°.*
		Sanotaa neljä tuoppia.hh °hehe Isoo°.
		say four glass large
15	D:	*°.Yes°,*
		°.Joo°,
16		*(24.0) ((D begins to measure the blood pressure and the topic is dropped.))*

The patient's initial answer (lines 4–5) has no minimizing or normalizing features that usually accompany the no-problem answers (see p. 348). Through his explicit rejection of the justification for drinking proposed by the doctor (line 2) and through the selection of a maximizing description of the frequency of drinking "every weekend," the patient on one hand describes his drinking as more than minimal, and adopts a somewhat defiant position vis-à-vis the doctor's initial inquiry on the other. This dual orientation comes to the surface again at line 13, in the patient's response to the doctor's follow-up inquiry. "Glass" is a standard measure of beer in Finnish bars which has two sizes: small (0.33 litre) and large (0.5 litre). By upgrading the measure and laughing along the delivery of the specification, the patient again defiantly chooses a maximizing description (cf. Haakana 1999:135–235 on unreciprocated patient laughter). The maximizing elements in his talk could be treated as incipiently problem-oriented. However, his defiance works toward the other direction, making it possible for the doctor not to take up the issue.

And that is the track followed by the doctor: the topic is dropped, with neither evaluation nor advice.[7]

Advice on lifestyle

In our database, discussions in which the patient's lifestyle is treated as problematic are invariably followed by advice on lifestyle. Advice-giving is in these cases the doctor's final confirmation of the interpretation of the patient's lifestyle as problematic: by giving advice, the doctor indicates that a change is needed in the patient's life. By contrast, in cases where the patient's lifestyle is described as non-problematic, regularly no advice is given, either. However, we also have some rare cases in which advice is given after a no-problem discussion; and in these individual cases moving to advice-giving provides the doctor with an opportunity to invoke a problem orientation.

In what follows, we will examine examples of advice in cases in which an orientation to the problematic character of lifestyle has been established earlier in the consultation. In these cases, advice can be located in three different places relative to the questions and answers through which information about lifestyle is gathered. Advice can be given within a distinct phase in which treatment is talked about, as separate from a segment of history-taking in which the lifestyle questions occur; it can be produced as the next activity after the lifestyle question–answer sequence; or it can take place without any prior questions and answers at all. We will first examine examples of advice in each of these three locations. Thereafter, we will take up a single case in which the doctor invokes a problem orientation through advice, even though the given aspect of lifestyle had been treated as non-problematic in the earlier talk.

[7] It should be noted that, unlike the other extracts examined in this chapter, this one is from a routine consultation: the patient has come to a checkup for his high blood pressure. Even though the design of the doctor's question does not indicate any orientation to prior discussions, the patient may have given accounts of his drinking to this or to another doctor during earlier visits. The fact that the patient constructs his description of drinking as one not to be taken up, and the fact the doctor does not in fact take it up, may be related to this.

Advice that is sequentially separated from the interview

We will first examine a case in which advice is given as a part of an activity that is marked as a distinct, concluding phase of the consultation. This consultation is the only one in our data where the doctor gives advice about aspects of lifestyle talked about as a part of a larger segment of history-taking, away from the formulation of the medical problem. In this example, a patient who has high blood pressure gets advice about diet, use of salt, and drinking – see example (12) above for questions and answers concerning drinking and use of salt within an earlier phase in this consultation. In line 1, the patient tries to recall the name of the blood pressure medicine taken by his wife:

(15) [12B1:8]

```
 1 P:          Kad- what Kadh (0.2) Kaddimunbeen or something
               Kad- mikä Kadh (0.2) Kaddimunbeen tai  joku
                    what              brand mark  or   some
 2             >like that<. Begins with K.=What is °(it)°,=
               >semmonen<. Koolla alkava.=Mikä se °(on)°,=
               such        K      begins   what it is
 3             (5.0) ((D writing))
 4 D:   ==>    .mhh >We do have to do so now
               .mhh >Kyllä meiän täytyy ny  sillä tavalla tehdä
                     surely we   must   now the way     do
 5      ==>    that we'll start the blood pressure °medication°.=
               että me alotetaan se verenpaine    °lää:kitys°.=
               that we start      the blood.pressure.medication
 6      1=>    =And let's continue trying to lose weight
               =Ja koetetaan edelleen sitä laihdutusta      ja
               and try       still    the getting.slimmer  and
 7      2=>    °.hh° and if you'd try to leave out even °( )-°
               °.hh°  ja  jos koettaisitte  jättää  vielä °a-°
                      and if would.try.you  leave   still  ?
 8      2=>    (0.4) even more salt and (0.2)
               (0.4) vielä tiukemmalle sen suola ja  (0.2)
                     still stricter     the salt and
 9      3=>    be- try to say even cut out alcohol
               o-  yrittäis   olla vaikka ilman  alkoholiaki
               ?be would.try  be   say    without alcohol.even
10      3=>    see if that #works out and#,
               jos vaa #onnistu-u ja#,
               if  just succeeds  and
```

11 *(0.2) ((D gazing at P))*
12 P: *Yeah.*
Joo.
13 *(0.4)*
14 D: *.tch And well let's see if we'd get it then*
.mt Ja tuota noin katottas jos me saatas sillä sitte
and well look if we get it.with then
15 *even go down with that so much that ((we)) could*
se °.hh° (0.2) vielä (0.3) laskeen niin paljo että vois
it still go.down so much that could
16 *imagine that (.) it could go down without blood*
kuvitella ettät (.) se vois laskee ilman
imagine that it could go.down without
17 *pressure (.) medicine °even°.*
verenpaine< (.) lääkkeitä°ki°.
blood.pressure medicine.even
18 P: *Mm:::,*

In line 4, the doctor begins to lay out the treatment of the patient's medical problem. He first announces the need for starting the medication. Without any gap he then moves on to give three pieces of advice. The three areas of lifestyle addressed by the doctor have each been talked about during the consultation. The doctor begins with advice about losing weight, which is something the patient has already made an effort toward. Thereafter, he gives advice on reducing salt – an area of lifestyle which the patient has reported to be unproblematic; see line 2 in example (12). (We will return to this advice on an "unproblematic issue" towards the end of this section.) Finally, the doctor takes up drinking, which is an area of lifestyle that the patient has implied as problematic.

In these three pieces of advice, the doctor proceeds from an utterance design that treats the patient's participation in the action proposed as self-evident or unproblematic to ones that formulate the compliance as more and more conditional. In the design of the advice about dieting and avoiding salt, the doctor displays an understanding that the patient has already taken measures toward the proposed direction, whereas the advice concerning drinking – the area of lifestyle that the participants have treated as problematic in this consultation – does not display such understanding. (For a more detailed discussion of the design of advice in this case, see Drew and Sorjonen 1997.)

Advice that is sequentially "next" after the history-taking

As pointed out above, in the consultation from which example (15) above was taken, the initial definition of the medical problem (high blood pressure), the questions about lifestyle, and the advice about lifestyle were all sequentially separated from one another. In contrast, when a question about lifestyle is asked subsequently to a formulation of a medical problem, the question–answer sequence is regularly followed by advice by the doctor. Hence, in these cases, the problem formulation, questions about lifestyle, and advice-giving form a tight sequence (cf. Heritage and Sefi 1992). The next example will show how the doctor moves into advice giving in the consultation from which extract (13) was taken. The patient's problem is stiffness of neck and shoulders. The doctor has asked the patient about her exercise habits. The patient first reports that she does not go to the gym but then adds having gone there earlier. The report is received by the doctor with the turn in line 17. This discussion leads to advice-giving in line 25.

(16) [continuation of 13]

14 D: *Earlier you have been going [anyway,*]
Ootte aikasemmin käyny [kuitenki,]
you.have earlier visited anyway
15 P: [*Earlier*] *I definitely*
[Aikasemm]in oon käyny
earlier have.I visited
16 *have been [going,]*
[kyllä,]
definitely
17 D: -> [*Yeah::,*] *.hh is it about to be dropped now*
[Joo::,] .hh onko se nyt jäämässä
yes is it now being,dropped
18 -> *for this winter.*
tältä talvelta.
19 *(0.4)*
20 P: *Well it shouldn't.*
No ei saisi.
well no should
21 *(0.6)*
22 P: *It shouldn't I ought to go to the swimming hall too,*
Ei saisi kyllä tohon uimahalliinkin täytys mennä,
no should surely that swimming.hall.too should go

23 D: *Yeah:,*
Nii:,
24 *(.)*
25 D: => *.h When you thi[nk that there is wearing out in so*
.h Ku ajat[telee että on noi monessa nivelessä}
when thinks that is so many.in joint.in
26 P: *[Yeah,*
[Nii,
27 D: => *many joints though and you have these problems so*
kuitenkin kulumaa ja näitä vaivoja ni
nevertheless wearing.out and these inconveniences so
28 => *probably it would still be sensible,*
ehkä se olis sitte järkevää kuitenki,
possibly it would.be then reasonable however
29 *(0.4)*
30 P: ↑*Yeah,*
↑Nii,
31 D: => *try and go in spite of everything to go somewhere*
yrittää kaikesta huolimatta ni käydä jossaki koska
try everything in.spite.of go somewhere because
32 *because the joints (.) have to be kept y'know in ↑motion*
kyllähä ne nivelet (.) pitää pitää ↑liikkeellä
surely.y'know the joints must keep move.in
33 *and .hh[hh a] nd well: (0.4) the muscles have to be*
ja .hh[hh j]a tuota: (0.4) vähä sitä: hh lihaksiaki
and and well a.little it muscles.too
34 P: *[Yeah,]*
[Joo,]
35 D: *strengthened a little.= .hh >and y'know often in these*
vahvis°taa°.= .hh >ja useihan näissä niska<vaivoissa
strengthen and often these.in neck.problems.in
36 *neck problems the very best thing is just .hh*
justiisa on hyvää tämmönen ihan .hh
exactly is good this.kind.of just
37 P: *(Yeah) (s[o) (just) (to)]*
(Juu) (e [ttä)(näin)(iha)]
38 D: *[gym] wo[rk.h*
[kuntovoi]mis[telu.h
39 P: *[Yeah,*
[Nii,

In line 25, after the patient has spelled out her need for exercise, the doctor begins to deliver advice. She begins her turn by offering the grounds for the advice, followed by the core of the advice in lines 28 and 31. Here, advice-giving is hearably a relevant next action after what has been done in the prior talk. In the immediately preceding question–answer sequence, the doctor (lines 14 and 17) pursues the need for exercise and the patient (lines 20 and 22) produces a prescriptively formatted response where she points out her "obligation" to exercise. Thus, the doctor's advice for the patient to "go somewhere" confirms the stance already expressed by the patient. Moreover, as we pointed out earlier, the sequence-initial question by the doctor – see line 3 in example (13) – can be heard as taking up a possible remedy for the patient's problem. As a treatment-oriented question, that utterance can be heard to anticipate the unpacking of the remedy in the form of advice.

Advice with no preceding interview

In most cases of advice-giving, a shared orientation to a need for change is established by the participants in a question–answer sequence prior to the advice proper. In the following case, however, the doctor delivers the advice as the next action following the announcement of test results (and a short intervening stretch of talk concerning the delay in getting other results).

(17) [1A3:1–2]

1 D: *You had tests in [the la] b.*
Siellä oli laboratorio[kokei]ta.
there were laboratory.tests
2 P: [*Yeah.*]
[Nii.]
3 P: *Yes.*
Joo.
4 D: *Yes. Let's see (there),*
Joo. Katsotaanpas (mitä tänne),
yes let.us.see what here
5 *(12.3)*
6 D: -> *Okay, (1.1) >blood sugar six point one:< it is*
No niin, (1.1) >veren sokeri kuus pilkku yks:< se on
7 -> *a bit higher than,*
pikkusen korkeempi ku mitä,
little higher than what

8 P: *I see and,*
Jaa ja,
and
9 D: *.hhh And the celiac an- erm antibodies were ↑taken*
.hhh Ja ne keliakia vas-, #öö# vasta-aineet on ↑tehty
and the celiac antibodies are done
10 *but there's (.) no results of that [yet*
mutta niistä (.) ei oo tullu vielä tulo[ksia.
but them.of not have come yet results
11 P: *[I see:. .I see they*
[Jaa:. .Jaa ne
12 *are so,*
on niin,
13 *(0.7)*
14 P: °°*Yes.*°°
°°Joo.°°
15 *(2.1)*
16 D: *Yes:.*
Joo:.
17 *(2.1)*
18 P: *It takes a long time then, as I thought that they would*
Kauan kestää sitte, ku mä luulin ne on ny jo
long lasts then as I thought they are now already
19 *already have arrived but they hadn't [then.*
jo tullu muttei ne sitte olluk[kaa.
already come but.not they then were
20 D: => *[.hhh Yes. .hhh*
[.hhh Joo. .hhh
21 => *Well m m at this point erm the blood sugar*
Tuota m m siihen pitäs: y tässä vaiheessa lähinnä
well it.to should this stage mostly
22 => *should be controlled mostly by (0.1)*
puuttua sillä tavalla tuohon (0.2) veren sokeriin
intervene the way that blood sugar
23 => *avoiding the use of real sug[ar.*
että (1.0) m oikeeta sokeria pitäs vält[tää.
that real sugar should avoid
24 P: *[Yes ( )*
[Joo ( )
25 *[( )*
26 D: => *[You should avoid (.) carbohydrates that get quickly*
[Nopeesti (.) imeytyviä hiilihydraatteja pitäs
quickly absorbing carbon.hydrates should
27 => *absorbed.*
välttää.

avoid
28 *(1.0)*
29 P: *Yes. Where do you have them then.*
Joo. Missäs niitä on sitte.
yes where they are then

In this case, the action expressed in the advice is treated as a necessity in terms of the patient's medical condition (lines 21–23 and 26–27). Through the design and location of her advice, the doctor indicates that the reason for the proposed change in the lifestyle is the rise in the level of the blood sugar identified through the test. The test result establishes objective evidence that blood sugar control is not as good as it should be, and that sets up the relevance of advice. The doctor, however, moves to the delivery of advice without seeking information concerning the patient's current behavior. In so doing, contrary to the two cases shown earlier, she does not open up a space where the patient could display his own understanding of the character of the problem before the delivery of the advice.

Invoking the problem orientation through advice

In the vast majority of cases of advice-giving in our collection, advice is preceded by actions which in one way or another display that there is a problem in the patient's lifestyle. This is the case in all our examples of advice-giving discussed above. By giving advice only on such lifestyle issues that have been demonstrated to be problematic, Finnish doctors treat advice on lifestyle as an activity that requires local intersubjective justification (on similar consideration in the delivery of diagnosis, see Peräkylä 1998, this volume).

There remain, however, two cases in the database where no such problem orientation is established prior to the advice-giving. In both cases, there are contingent factors that account for the relevancy of advice in spite of the lack of the problem orientation. These cases demonstrate the possibility of *converting the lifestyle into a problematic issue through advice-giving*. In terms of the overall structure of a medical consultation – consultation as a continuum of distinct phases, among which the discussion on treatment is the last one before termination (Byrne and Long 1976) – advice-giving provides the doctor with the *last* opportunity to treat an aspect of lifestyle as problematic.

The following example contains one of the above-mentioned instances. In it, advice on the use of salt is given to a patient with high blood pressure; advice-giving here has already been discussed as in example (15) above. As we pointed out there, the doctor in this case gave advice on an area of lifestyle that, earlier in the consultation, the patient had reported to be unproblematic (but which is generally considered as a central lifestyle factor causing hypertension). Below, we will present only the two fragments where the patient's use of salt is discussed and where the advice is given.

(18) [fragments of (12) and (15)]

1 D: *Do you use much salt.*
Ootteko te ahkera suolankäyt°täjä°.
are you diligent salt.user
2 P: -> *Well< (.) not really and< (0.2) sugar at least*
No< (.) e:m mää ny sillain oo ja< (0.2) tota sokeria
well not I now such.way are and that sugar
3 *I have tried to avoid so that*
mä oon nyt (.) ainaki (0.2) yrittäny välttää sillai
I have now at. least tried avoid such.way
4 *I haven't put it in the coffee and the like,*
etten mä ain kahvin kaa oo laittanu °ja tollai ni°,
not I always coffee with have put and so
5 D: *°Yeah°.*
°Joo°.
6 *(0.2)*
7 D: *What about a:lcohol,*
Entäs al:koholia,
---((3 pages omitted))---
8 D: *.mhh >We do have to do so now*
.mhh >Kyllä meiän täytyy ny sillä tavalla tehdä
surely we must now the way do
9 *that we'll start the blood pressure °medication°.=*
että me alotetaan se verenpaine° lää:kitys°.=
that we start the blood.pressure.medication
10 *=And let's continue trying to lose weight*
=Ja koetetaan edelleen sitä laihdutusta ja
and try still the getting.slimmer and
11 => *°.hh° and if you'd try to leave out even °( )-°*
°.hh° ja jos koettaisitte jättää vielä °a-°
and if would.try.you leave still ?
12 => *(0.4) even more salt and (0.2)*
(0.4) vielä tiukemmalle sen suola ja (0.2)
still stricter the salt and

13 *be- try to say even cut out alcohol*
o- yrittäis olla vaikka ilman alkoholiaki
?be would.try be say without alcohol.even
14 *see if that #works out and#,*
jos vaa #onnistuu ja#,
if just succeeds and
15 *(0.2) ((D gazing at p))*
16 P: *Yeah.*
Joo.

In line 2, as a response to the doctor's question, which is designed to prefer an affirmative answer, the patient denies excessive use of salt. After this rather minimal negative answer, he moves on to describe his efforts to reduce the intake of sugar. By this shift and through the design of his utterance ("at least") the patient implies that his conscious effort towards change has been targeted at sugar rather than at salt. The doctor then receives the patient's answer in line 5 with a neutral acknowledgment token; and in line 7, he moves on to ask about alcohol. Here, there may have been features of an incipient problem orientation in the patient's answer, but that orientation was not taken up by the doctor in the subsequent talk.

However, when the doctor some minutes later discusses the treatment with the patient, by giving advice on the use of salt he does treat this aspect of the patient's lifestyle as problematic. The status of the patient's behavior is thus converted from non-problematic to problematic. But this conversion is undertaken in a way that also aligns with the thrust of the patient's initial description of his use of salt: the advice is formulated so as to display an understanding that the patient has already taken measures towards the proposed direction and it only suggests an intensification of this effort ("leave out even even more salt"). Thus, even in this exceptional case, the doctor's advice on lifestyle was designed so as to accommodate the patient's definition of the status of his behavior.

There is still another important aspect in advice-giving. The advice given is typically restricted to utterances that indicate what the patient should do, as in example (15): the details of acting, for example, how to be able to cut down the use of salt, are not spelled out, neither is the patient informed about the specifics of the connection between his medical condition and the area of lifestyle talked about (e.g., the level at which use of salt or drinking has an impact on blood pressure). This kind of advice leaves it entirely up to the patient to seek ways in which the advice could in practice be followed. Sometimes, however, doctors do contextualize the advice, as in example (16), and in some other cases the patient asks about the details of the advice – see example (17).

Summary and conclusion

We began this chapter by pointing out that, in our sample of Finnish primary care consultations, lifestyle is discussed in a grossly similar fashion to that described in earlier Nordic research: doctors tend to ask questions rather than to give advice or information, and the discussions tend to remain on a rather shallow level of precision. Judging from previous studies, this pattern is different from what is found in North America, where doctors are more insistent on counseling the patients about better lifestyle. Thus the "medical gaze" (Foucault 1975) is probably less pervasive in Finland and other Nordic countries, as Nordic doctors (at least in acute consultations) tend to leave it to their patients to decide whether or not a change is needed in lifestyle.

We set as our task to analyze what kind of interactional dynamics lead to this state of affairs. In our analysis, we focused on the ways in which the participants define the patient's lifestyle either as problematic or as non-problematic. We then saw how patients in most cases give initial answers that treat their habits as non-problematic. This is particularly the case when the questions about lifestyle are asked as a part of a larger segment of history-taking and thus away from the formulation of a specific medical problem. Even though doctors usually seek specification to such answers, their follow-up questions do not call into question the non-problematic thrust of the patient's initial answer. These discussions are closed in a non-evaluative fashion, through a shift of topic or activity which may be preceded by neutral acknowledgment of the patient's answer.

We then showed how the patient's lifestyle in some cases is treated as problematic. We first pointed out that the likelihood of a problem orientation is much greater in those cases where the lifestyle question follows a formulation of a medical problem, especially one done by the doctor in the form of an announcement of test results or findings from a physical exam. We showed how the patient's initial answer can bring in an explicit problem orientation or how the problem orientation can be gradually consolidated after an initial answer which displays a merely incipient problem orientation. Finally, we showed how lifestyle discussions in problematic cases regularly lead to advice-giving by the doctor, but we also pointed out that doctors can, through advice-giving, also convert the patient's lifestyle from an issue that has been approached as a non-problematic one into an issue that is approached as problematic.

Promotion of a healthier lifestyle is widely considered as an integral part of the work of the primary care doctors. There is no reason to doubt that the doctors we have observed also share this sentiment. But our analysis suggests that the doctors also may orient themselves to certain interactional restrictions in accomplishing the health-promotional aspect of their work.

We could try and capture these restrictions into a putative norm of conduct that suggests that the doctor *should respect the integrity of the patient's evaluation of his or her lifestyle*. If the patient describes his or her behavior as non-problematic, the doctors following this putative norm do often acquire more details of his or her behavior, but they do not call into question the initially proposed non-problematic status of the behavior. A corollary of the norm suggests that the doctor should give advice only in such ways that align with the thrust of the patient's description of his or her behavior. Usually this means that they only give advice if the patient has described his or her behavior as problematic.

For the patient's part, one of the crucial considerations seems to be the location of the doctor's question. A question that is asked subsequently to a formulation of a medical problem seems to be interpreted as a more "serious" and "motivated" one than a question that is asked as a part of a larger segment of history-taking, away from any formulation of a medical problem. Such a question leads much more frequently to a problem-oriented description of the lifestyle. The fact that doctors sometimes pursue the problem orientation in their follow-up questions seems to indicate that, for the doctors, too, the questions that they ask subsequent to formulations of medical problems are the more serious ones.

The focus of this chapter has been on the practices of talking about lifestyle in one culture and cultural area – Nordic countries. In the introduction to this chapter, we reported results of some earlier studies that suggested that there may be considerable differences between the American and Nordic ways of discussing lifestyle in medical consultations. However, even though the Nordic discussions seem to differ from the American ones, the practices for introducing lifestyle issues – formulating them as problematic or non-problematic, responding to them, giving advice, etc. – might well be similar or general enough to occur at some times and places in America. In other words, it is possible that there are *generic practices for discussing lifestyle* issues which are made use of differently in different cultures. This, however, is a matter that should be settled through further empirical research.

13

Coordinating closings in primary care visits: producing continuity of care

Candace West

Introduction

One way of distinguishing social occasions from one another is by how free they are to vary in length (Clayman 1989). A casual conversation, for example, is an occasion whose length is quite free to vary; although demands outside a conversation (such as finishing a task or getting to work) may set upward limits on the amount of time available for talk, exactly when a conversation will be brought to a close must always be negotiated by participants (Sacks et al. 1974:701). A television news interview, by contrast, is an occasion whose length is rigidly restricted by broadcasting schedules; hence, regardless of what is to be talked about and by whom, a news interview must fill – but not spill over – boundaries that are set in advance (Clayman 1989:662–3). Between these two extremes lie most encounters that occur in institutional settings. College classes, for example, are usually assigned time slots of one to three hours; however, these often "run over" and sometimes "end early." Courtroom proceedings are scheduled to begin on particular days at particular times; but continuances routinely delay the onset of these proceedings by weeks or even months, thereby putting off any anticipated conclusions of them. And primary care visits are typically scheduled by appointment; yet the time allocated to an appointment does not determine just when or how such a visit will be brought to a close.

Despite the considerable attention researchers have paid to other phases of the primary care encounter (in this volume, for example, see Robinson, on openings; Heritage and Robinson, on establishing a reason for the visit; Boyd and Heritage, on history-taking; and Maynard and Frankel, on delivering diagnostic news), very few studies have addressed closing as a topic in its own right. As Jocelyn White, Wendy Levinson, and Debra Roter (1994) point out, doctors in training learn that there are distinct instrumental phases in a primary care visit: (1) opening, (2) history-taking, (3) physical examination, (4) education, and (5) closing.[1] Yet most claims about closings come from experts' opinions about what these should contain, rather than from systematic empirical studies of closings per se. Moreover, most claims have failed to distinguish between the "educational phase" – in which the doctor "informs the patient about the diagnosis and negotiates a treatment plan" – and the "closing phase" of the visit – "in which [doctors] should summarize the visit, clarify the plan of care, check for patient understanding, establish plans for interim contact, and demonstrate caring" (White et al. 1994:24).

The need for systematic study of closings in primary care visits is evident from doctors' recurring complaints about the "by the way syndrome" (see, for example, Barsky 1981; Byrne and Long 1976; White et al. 1994): patients afflicted with this "syndrome" frustrate their doctors by raising new, emotionally charged, and/or potentially life-threatening complaints in the final moments of their visits (when it is far too late to deal with those complaints without jeopardizing the rest of the doctor's schedule). But closings can present equally distressing maladies from patients' point of view: for example, having to leave a doctor without ever mentioning their chief concerns because the doctor ended the visit without ever affording them an opportunity to do so (cf. Korsch and Negrete 1972).

In this chapter, I examine the organization of closings in primary care visits (in family practice and internal medicine) in the United States. My study of these social occasions reveals systematic patterns with respect to who initiates closing and how they initiate it. Discussion of these patterns leads me to consider their connection to other interactionally relevant activities, such as constituting the primary care relationship as a "standing" one (Button 1991).

[1] The numbering and content of the phases apparently differs over time and place. In the United Kingdom, for example, Byrne and Long (1976) identified six phases: (1) relating to the patient, (2) discovering the reason for the visit, (3) conducting a verbal and/or physical examination, (4) considering the patient's condition, (5) detailing a treatment plan or plan for further investigation, and (6) terminating the visit.

Empirical studies of closings in primary care visits

In one of the (very rare) empirical studies of closings, White et al. (1994) describe how doctors and patients in the United States bring primary care visits to an end. Employing a form of Interaction Process Analysis (Bales 1950) known as the Roter Interactional Analysis System (Roter 2004), these researchers assigned coders to audiotapes of patient visits, having them sort doctors' and patients' phrases or complete thoughts into exhaustive and mutually exclusive categories. White and her colleagues (1994) found that, in patients' visits to doctors in family practice or general internal medicine, doctors were the ones who initiated the vast majority (86 percent) of closings. They also found that few patients (21 percent) raised previously unmentioned complaints during the closing phase of their visits, and that the only patient behavior that typified closure was "displaying agreement" with doctors (82 percent). To be sure, coders were the ones who identified instances of the phenomenon, operationally defining "closure" as sentences that, in their view, made the transition from "the educational phase" to "the closing phase" of the visit (e.g., "Okay, let's see you back in four or five months" or "If it's not better in a week, let me know"). So, while this study provides a sound description of primary care visit endings, it does not address the turn-by-turn organization of closings per se.

By contrast, Christian Heath (1986) employed Harvey Sacks, Emanuel Schegloff, and Gail Jefferson's (1974) model of turn-taking for conversation to study the sequential organization of leave-taking between doctors and patients in general practice consultations in the United Kingdom. As Heath explains (1986:128–9):

> In ending the consultation doctor and patient have to step from a state of mutual involvement and orientation and accomplish an inattention to each other's actions; they have to realign their responsibilities and obligations and rid their actions and activities of interactional consequence . . . The end also involves, as do many face-to-face encounters, the participants breaking each other's presence so that they are no longer interactionally or physically available. The process of taking leave is thoroughly bound up with the doctor's and the patient's movement out of the business of the consultation and a state of mutually coordinated talk.

Using transcripts and videotapes of interaction, Sacks et al.'s (1974) model of turn-taking, and Schegloff and Sacks' (1973) analysis of closing sequences in telephone talk, Heath advances a theoretically grounded approach to the problem of closing in primary care visits – an approach grounded in the study of talk-in-interaction (see Schegloff 1996a).

Like White et al. (1994), Heath found that doctors were the ones who initiated the majority of closing sequences and that patients rarely brought up new complaints during the final moments of a visit. But Heath raises sociological considerations that White et al. do not address. He notes, for example, that the general-practice consultation is a form of professional–client interaction and, like other forms of such interaction, "it is generally the patient who quits the doctor. The doctor remains seated whilst the patient stands and leaves the surgery" (1986:129). He observes, moreover, that the medical encounter is an interview: "In the medical consultation, as in other types of interview, it is the doctor, the interviewer, who typically initiates closure" (1986:138). Heath also remarks on "the monotopicality of medical encounters, an orientation to a single reason for a visit by both doctor and patient" (1986:143). Given that the patient is the one who quits the doctor, that the doctor and patient are engaged in an interview, and that the doctor and patient are both oriented to a single reason for the visit, it is understandable that doctors would initiate closings and patients would refrain from bringing up previously unmentioned complaints.

Studies of primary care visits in the United States strongly suggest that these are best described as interviews (Frankel 1990). Analyses of turn-taking (West 1984), opening segments (Beckman and Frankel 1984), and the organization of questions and answers (Frankel 1990; West 1983) show that primary care visits are constrained in special ways "with respect to what doctors and patients will treat as allowable contributions to the business at hand" (Drew and Heritage 1992:22; see also Levinson 1992). But at least two of the conditions that characterized Heath's (1986) general-practice consultations in the United Kingdom differ from those that prevail in primary care visits in the United States. First, while patients in the United Kingdom are usually the ones who depart from their doctors' presence (in the doctors' consulting rooms), doctors in the United States are typically the ones who depart from their patients' presence (in the doctors' examining rooms). Hence, if the sequences of activities involved in taking leave of a social occasion (Schegloff and Sacks 1973:323) are related to those involved in closing a conversation, variation in departure patterns may be associated with variation in closure patterns. Second, while doctors and patients in the United Kingdom may orient their actions toward a single reason for a visit, primary care doctors in the United States know that patients often come to see them for multiple reasons. Under these conditions, focusing prematurely on a first-mentioned problem can prevent patients from fully expressing their concerns (cf. Beckman and Frankel 1984).

There are reasons, then, for further study of the organization of closings in primary care visits. Of the few studies that have addressed this topic, one (White et al. 1994) did not address the turn-by-turn organization of closings as such. The other study (Heath 1986) focused on leave-taking, and thus addressed closing only in the context of this concern. Even so, White et al. (1994) offer a fine description of closing practices in one primary care environment, and Heath (1986) advances an excellent paradigm for analyzing the organization of closings in another. This paradigm is grounded in the methodology of conversation analysis and focuses on the sequential analysis of the problem of closing in conversation.

Closings in conversation

As Schegloff and Sacks observe, speakers who are trying to terminate a conversation face two basic problems.[2] First, they must conduct themselves in a way that will be seen as "closing" that conversation. Simply falling silent will not do this, because the turn-transition rule for conversation provides that silence may be heard as a lapse in – rather than as the end of – conversation (1973:293–5; see also Sacks et al. 1974). Thus, a current speaker who falls silent will encourage other participants to begin speaking themselves. To resolve this difficulty, a *terminal exchange* allows participants to collaboratively suspend the turn-transition rule for conversation, for example, by exchanging farewells:

[2] By "problem," Schegloff and Sacks (1973:290) don't mean something conversationalists consciously ponder over; rather, they mean an achievement – something that takes work to accomplish.

(1) (Schegloff and Sacks 1973:318)

B: *Bye* bye
C: Bye

– or by exchanging items like "OK," "See you," "Thank you," and "You're welcome." Second, speakers trying to terminate a conversation must provide an opportunity for all participants in that conversation to raise any not-yet-mentioned matters they might still want to talk about. Insofar as topical talk is organized turn by turn, one speaker's sudden initiation of a terminal exchange might leave others with no chance to introduce their "hitherto unmentioned mentionables" (1973:303). To address this problem, a properly initiated *closing section* provides each party with the opportunity to show that they do not choose to continue. One way of initiating a closing section is through an exchange of *possible preclosings*, for example, one in which each speaker passes the floor to another without contributing anything to topical development. A simple exchange of items such as "OK . . . ," "We-ell . . . ," or "So-oo . . . " (note the downward intonational contours) will serve this purpose:

(2) (Schegloff and Sacks 1973:304)

A: O.K.
B: O.K.
A: Bye bye.
B: Bye.

Just above, each "O.K." serves as a possible preclosing, through which speakers show each other that they have "nothing more" to talk about. Once both parties have completed the pre-closing sequence, they have established a warrant for treating the conversation as possibly closed.

Schegloff and Sacks (1973) contend that a properly designed closing section contains at least a possible preclosing and a terminal exchange. But it may contain much more. For example, the possibility of further talk in the wake of a possible preclosing is a very real contingency: in one two-party conversation Schegloff and Sacks examined, they found the first possible preclosing on page 20 of an eighty-five-page transcript. Moreover, given that *the proper place for a possible preclosing is at the analyzable end of a topic* (1973:304), possible preclosings may be found in the turn spaces following multiple (and sometimes quite elaborate) topic-closing techniques.

Bounding off and shutting down conversational topics[3]

Some conversational topics do not have analyzable ends, because speakers can move off a topic by adding refocused-but-related talk to a last topically relevant utterance (cf. Jefferson 1984c; Maynard 1980; Maynard and Zimmerman 1984). But speakers often undertake the collaborative bounding off and shutting down of a conversational topic, and when they do, their actions "may mark that topic as a possibly last one, that marking conferring upon the following conversational slot its distinctive relevance for possible preclosings" (Schegloff and Sacks 1973:306, n. 10).

One way participants may bound off and shut down a topic is by *summarizing* the topic-in-progress (Button 1991). Below, two parties collaboratively produce a summary through one party's characterization of a "lesson" or "moral" of the talk-so-far and the other party's affirmation of it (Button 1991; Schegloff and Sacks 1973):

(3) (Button 1991:255)

A:	-->	Yeah well, things uh always work out for the best
B:	-->	Oh, certainly. Alright, [Bea
A:		[Uh huh, okay,
B:		G'bye
A:		Goodnight

In this instance, the party who initiates the summarizing activity also provides for the possibility that talk on the topic-thus-far might be terminated. The party who acknowledges, confirms, or generally agrees with the summary thereby displays their orientation to the topic as possibly closed.

Another way to bound off and shut down a topic is by *making arrangements for future activities*; for example, to do something at a later date or meet someone at a later time (Schegloff and Sacks 1973; see also Button 1985, 1987, 1991). In the course of talk about arrangements, a party who proposes a future plan of action may provide a candidate resolution of those arrangements and, hence,

[3] In this section, I draw heavily from an earlier paper with Angela Garcia (West and Garcia 1988).

justification for treating talk about them as possibly concluded. A next speaker who affirms the resolution thereby agrees with that possibility and paves the way for a possible preclosing:

(4) (Button 1991:256–7)

A: She works in the after[noon, so that' that's out I guess.
B: [In the afternoon.
B: Mmhm, Yeah, [(Well that lets me out)]
A: [Uh huh
B: --> Well uh, I'll try an' get ahold of Dorothy,
A: Okay honey you uhm uh I'll I'll call 'er anyway so I c'n check er off, but I just thought maybe that if you had time you might ask 'er.
B: --> Yeah. uh-uh huh,
A: --> O[kay,
B: [Okay, okay well I will we'll see you,
A: Okay [dear
B: [Bye
A: Bye.

The making of arrangements is so strongly closing implicative that Schegloff and Sacks (1973; see also Houtkoop-Steenstra 1987: 134–5) describe it as a topic type that is independently "closing-relevant" (like "request-satisfaction topics" and "complaint-remedy topics"). Thus, parties may even bound off and shut down a current topic of talk by *reintroducing arrangements* made earlier in a conversation (Button 1991). With a preface such as "anyway," parties can mark such arrangements as previously agreed to, albeit not the current topic of talk:

(5) (Button 1991:259)

J: I mean there wz only Su:s'n who wz et the age sohrt of h .hh who'd of been left in the house [et (.) on 'er ow:n.
A: [Ye:s.
(0.3)
A: M *m*:,
(0.4)
A: [Yes,
J: --> [A::nyway. .hh:
A: --> [(Ah'll seh-)
J: --> [I'll see you inna few min[utes then.
A: [See you inna few min[utes.

J: [.hh
J: O[kay Ann Bu[h bye,
A: ['k a:y [*Bye:.*

Just above, "A::nyway" prefaces the reintroduction of a proposed time to meet ("inna few minutes"), and a closing section soon follows.

To be sure, closing sections may still be delayed by participants *holding over* closing implicative activities in their next turns at talk (Button 1991). Below, for example, Fran formulates a summary of her prior talk on lines 1–2, Ted affirms Fran's summary on lines 3–4, and both Fran and Ted hold over that affirmation on lines 5–6:

(6) (Button 1991:252–3)

Fran: Ah-ee- Well *th*at's why I *sa*id I'm not g'nnuh say
anything I'm not making any commen[ts about anybu:ddy.=
Ted: [mkhm
Ted: deh Ye::a::h [hhh
Fran: [Y:::[:a:::h.
Ted: [Yea::h.
Fran: .hhh *A::*lrighty. Well ah'll give yih call before we
decide tih come down. Oka:[y?
Ted: [Oka:y
Fran: *Aw*:::righty::.
Ted: Oka[y
Fran: [Wil- see y' then,
Ted: Oka[y
Fran: *Bye* b[ye
Ted: [Bye

But parties who "hold over" components of prior turns in their next turns are neither elaborating further on the topic nor providing one another with the resources for doing so; thus, they are still proposing that talk on the topic-in-progress be concluded and still preserving a warrant for topic closure.

Announcing closure

Closing down a topic of talk provides speakers with a warrant for ending their conversation just then – namely, that they have "nothing more" to talk about. There is nonetheless a way of initiating a possible preclosure without respect for topical boundaries, that is, by *announcing closure* (Schegloff and Sacks 1973:311–12). Declarations such as "I have to go" (or, over the phone, "I have to hang up now") can appear after topics that have been bounded off, but they can also be interjected in the middle of a topic-in-progress – or even in the middle of a current speaker's turn. The party who announces closure cannot in fact prevent further talk in the wake of such an announcement, but this possible preclosing technique does not invite it.

In short, *whenever* a conversational topic is shut down, a set of contingencies comes into play:

[Topic closure]
↓
Okay } Preclosing
Okay }
↓
Goodbye } Closing
Goodbye }
[End of conversation]

Topic closure normally must occur for the initiation of preclosing, preclosing contributions normally must be completed before closing can be initiated, and the terminal exchange normally must be finished before the conversation can be terminated. An archetypical example appears just below:

(7) (Button 1990b:94)

1	Emma:		And, u-uh I'm w- I'm with you,
2	Lottie:		Yeah,
3	Emma:	-->	Oright,
4	Lottie:	-->	Okay [honey,
5	Emma:	-->	[Bye, dear=
6	Lottie:	-->	=Bye.

– end call –

On lines 1 and 2, Emma provides a possible summing up of the topic-thus-far, and Lottie accepts the summary. On lines 3 and 4, Emma and Lottie generate a possible preclosing exchange and, on lines 5 and 6, they produce the terminal exchange of this conversation.

With these basic "building blocks," parties may produce closings to fit a wide variety of contexts; for example, television news interviews (Clayman 1989), 911 emergency calls (Whalen and Zimmerman 1987; Zimmerman 1992; Zimmerman and Wakin 1995), and telephone calls requesting permission to do survey interviews (Maynard and Schaeffer 2002). What is more, these basic building blocks allow parties to initiate closing sections at any particular time.[4] But alternative activities (extending, protracting, or moving out of closure) are possible at each step in the process, up to and including the first part of a terminal exchange (Button 1990b; see also Button 1987, 1991; Jefferson 1984c).

As Steven Clayman (1989:668) points out, one virtue of the closing format is its sensitivity to the complex contingencies of interaction: participants set about closing a conversation "only when each participant has shown a readiness to do so." Another virtue of this format is the opportunity it offers for participants to engage in further talk, thereby providing for "the flexible, locally negotiated timing of termination characteristic of informal conversational encounters" (1989:668).

Below, I look at how doctors and patients actually employed the closing format in the primary care visits I studied.[5]

Closings in primary care visits

Termination

Across the primary care visits I examined, talk ordinarily ended with a terminal exchange between doctor and patient, consisting

[4] For example, Schegloff and Sacks (1973:315) find that, on the telephone, preclosing offerings (e.g., "Are you busy?", "Are you done eating?") usually appear prior to the start of a topic, rather than at a topic's analyzable end. If accepted, such an offering can bring conversation to a close before a first topic of talk has even been initiated. Moreover, Heath (1986) finds that, face to face, a patient's acceptance of a preclosing offering co-occurs with his or her beginning to take leave of the doctor.

[5] The data I analyze below consist of 62 primary care visits: 20 visits to doctors in family medicine, and 42 visits to doctors in general internal medicine. Richard Frankel and Howard Beckman collected audiotapes of the visits to internists in the northeastern United States (for a detailed description of these data, see Beckman and Frankel [1984]). I collected videotapes of the visits to family practitioners in the southern United States (for a detailed description of these data, see West [1984]). Because staff members in the residency programs where these tapes were made sometimes turned off recording equipment prior to the projected actual end of a visit (e.g., when a visit was temporarily adjourned while the doctor left the room), 15 of these visits were not taped in their entirety. Even so, they illuminate the relationships among adjournments, possible preclosings, and doctors' and patients' orientations to monotopicality; I therefore include them in my analysis.

of farewells or, more often, items like "OK," "See you," "Thank you," or "You're welcome." Using a "thank you"-type closing – rather than a "bye-bye"-type closing – seemed to formulate the visit as a service encounter, rather than a visit among friends. Like participants in television news interviews (Clayman 1989), 911 emergency calls (Zimmerman and Wakin 1995), and telephone calls for survey interviews (Maynard and Schaeffer 2002), participants in primary care visits tend to employ closing items that display their standing as beneficiaries and providers:

(8) (Frankel and Beckman 109:15)

Doctor:		[Okay
Patient:	-->	[Wehl thank you.=
Doctor:	-->	=Yer welcome (0.9) Come on out this way:
Patient:		Okay
		((door opens, noises from hallway, end tape))

(9) (West 05:536)

Patient:	-->	O:kay, tha[nk you. ((she goes out the door))
Doctor:	-->	[O::key doke. ((he is at his desk writing))
		((end tape))

In excerpt (8), for example, the patient's "thank you" elicits a promptly timed "Yer welcome" from the doctor. In excerpt (9), the patient's "O:kay, thank you." calls forth an overlapping "O::key doke" from the doctor – one that even anticipates what the patient is about to say as she is in the process of saying it (Jefferson 1973).

In these data, as in Heath's (1986), participants in primary care visits ordinarily engage in a collaborative exchange to suspend the relevance of the turn-transition rule (Sacks et al. 1974) and terminate their state of talk. Very few visits appeared to end with a terminal utterance from only one of the participants:

(10) (Frankel and Beckman 106:21)

Patient:		Oka-ay
		(3.0)
		((door opens))
		(0.4)
Patient:	--->	°Thank you.°
		(4.3)
		((end of tape))

In excerpt (10), for example, the patient's final utterance ("°Thank you.°") is met with silence rather than a rejoinder by the doctor. In cases like this one, however, activities associated with leave-taking (e.g., door opening or displaying recipiency of door opening) may generate "post-terminal" final utterances.[6] A look further "upstream" revealed that doctors and patients were jointly involved in producing these closings.[7] Hence, albeit visits might end with a last utterance from the patient, they were not terminated unilaterally.

In fact, the absence of a terminal utterance from the patient seemed to be a *noticeable* absence:

[6] Videotape is not available in these cases, so there is no way to tell for sure. However, Heath's (1986) findings indicate that, once the first part of the terminal exchange has been produced, the process of leave-taking is so far along that doctor and patient are no longer visually monitoring one another.

[7] For example:

(10) (Frankel 106:21)

1			(0.9)
2	Doctor:		°Oka:y Mrs. Sims° (.) Mrs. V.//we'll have ah: (.5) we'll
3			have them schedule you to see D.S.=
4	Patient:		=Awri:ght then. (.) Uhm hm:.
5	Doctor:	->	°Good.° Do you have any other questions or pro:blems?
6	Patient:	->	N(h) o:: I (hh) – I (h) can't think of anymo(h)re
7			ah: [(.) Dr. T.
8	Doctor:		[°'kay.°
9	Doctor:	->	°↑Oka:y.°
10	Patient:	->	Ay:- (.) eh heh (hh) I ((voice quavering)) know befoahr I
11			(h) didn't fee(h)l it quite as bad as I di(h)d ((sniff))
12			you kno:w it's after I le:ft [you know well it wasn't
13	Doctor:		[Mm hmm
14	Patient:		immediately .hh but it look like as things kept ro(h)llin')
15			you [know
16	Doctor:		[Mm hmm
17	Doctor:		Ye(h)s. Ye(h)s.
18	Patient:		Mm hm
19	Patient:		Oka-ay
20			(3.0) ((door opens))
21			(0.4)
22	Patient:		°Thank you.°

Here, participants carefully bound off and shut down their topic-so-far (on lines 2–4) and the doctor explicitly asks the patient if she has "any other questions or pro:blems" (on line 5). When the patient says no, she "can't think of anymo(h)re", the doctor takes a passing turn ("°Oka:y.°") that again invites the patient to contribute any previously unmentioned mentionables (and this time she does so).

(11) (Frankel and Beckman 112:4)

1			(13.5)
2	Doctor:	-->	Fi:ne, see yuh the:n.
3		-->	(0.3)
4	Doctor:	-->	Awri:ght?
5	Patient:		°(Okay)

Above, for example, the doctor issues a possible terminal utterance on line 2. When a short silence occurs – rather than a terminal utterance from the patient – on line 3, the doctor issues a possible preclosing with interrogative intonation ("Awri:ght?"). It appears, then, that the preferred organization of closing includes a terminal exchange *between* doctor and patient. In this respect, primary care visits look more like ordinary conversations (Schegloff and Sacks 1973; Button 1987, 1990b, 1991) than other interview situations that have been systematically studied (cf. Clayman's [1989] analysis of closings in television news interviews and Zimmerman and Wakin's [1995] analysis of closings in emergency calls).

Preclosing

In each of the primary care visits I examined, the party who first initiated a possible preclosing was the doctor. This was true regardless of the doctor's specialty (family medicine or general internal medicine), the reason(s) for the visit (e.g., continuing problems or new ones), or the length of the relationship between doctor and patient (e.g., first meeting or last). Possible preclosings appeared at the analyzable (to participants) ends of topics (Schegloff and Sacks 1973:304), and in the wake of treatment proposals that patients agreed to (a point I discuss further in the next section).

Occasionally, doctors initiated possible preclosings through announcements of closure:

(12) (Frankel and Beckman 141:3)

Doctor:	-->	O:kay Bo:b. Well I think u::h (.) this is it fer me an' you. Okay?
Patient:		°Awright.

(13) (West 07:801)

Doctor: --> Okay. The *time* is getting *late* (an u:h), (.) I: have o:ther things tuh do a:n' (.) as well as you [have
Patient: --> [I app re:ciate [your ti:me.
Doctor: [Y'know (A lot to do:,)

Here, for instance, doctors announce that "this is it" in extract (12), and that "*time* is getting *late*" in extract (13), thereby providing explicit grounds for closing just then. But, whatever their incidence in casual conversations, preclosing announcements were few and far between in the primary care visits I examined: doctors used them in only 3 cases (of the 48 in which closure actually occurred) and only in the company of other preclosing techniques. Therefore, most primary care visits were not terminated simply by doctors' announcements of the need to end them.

As Jefferson (1984c) points out, showing attentiveness to others' interests is a general resource for managing topic shifts and closing, so it is quite common to find it in closing sections of conversation. However, by contrast to preclosing offerings that use the other party's interests as their warrant for initiating closing – on the telephone, for example, "Well I'll letchu go. I don't wanna tie up your phone" (Schegloff and Sacks 1973:310) – the doctor in excerpt (13) puts *the work of doctoring* ("I: have o:ther things tuh do") ahead of his patient's concerns ("a:n' (.) as well as you have")'. This doctor was not alone in placing his obligations as a doctor before the interests of any patient in particular. For example:

(14) (West 10:1073)

Doctor: Okay?
(0.4) ((patient puts the prescription into her purse))
Doctor: *Thi:s* ((doctor hands patient a sheet of paper that had been lying on the desk)) needs tuh go ba:ck tuh the *biz:*ness o:ffice, (0.2) *thi:s* needs tuh go *he:re* ((doctor slips another sheet of paper into the patient's chart)) ((Doctor rips up another sheet of paper and tosses it into the trash. Patient watches him as she slowly closes her purse.))
Doctor: --> An' then I: need tuh give you a *hu:g*, ((doctor rises))
--> 'cuz I've godda go see my nex' pa:tient.

Above, the doctor explains that he "needs" to give *this* patient a hug goodbye since he's "godda" go see his *next* patient. In so doing, he displays that his interest in this patient is curtailed by the responsibilities of doctoring itself. Unlike casual conversations, primary care visits were not brought to a close simply because parties to talk discovered that they had "nothing more" to say. For example, doctors rarely initiated possible preclosings with anything that looked like a passing turn (in only 4 of the 48 primary care visits in which closure actually occurred), and then they used them in conjunction with other preclosing technique(s). In a few cases, doctors initiated closing sections by explicitly asking patients if there was "anything else?" of concern to them:

(15) (Frankel and Beckman 109:15)

Doctor:	-->	Di- you . . . have any- any (other) questions or problems?
Patient:		Uh: no:, (I don't think so).
Doctor:		Great
Patient:		Okay=
Doctor:		[Okay
Patient:		[Wehl thank you.
Doctor:		=Yer welcome (0.9) Come on out this way:
Patient:		Okay ((door opens, noises from hallway, tape ends))

(16) (Frankel and Beckman 113:4)

Doctor:		Okay. Well let's go out an' make that appointment for
	-->	y'. Do you have anything else you wanna ask about?
Patient:		No: hh
Doctor:		Okay. That's re:al good.
		((end tape))

But this form was not favored as a preclosing technique, either: it appeared in only 4 of the 48 cases in which closure actually occurred.[8] Hence, most primary care visits did not end once doctors ascertained that patients had "nothing else" to talk about.

[8] Of course, doctors employed variants of "anything else?" to achieve a variety of different ends, such as eliciting patients' concerns at the start of a visit, and ensuring that patients' itemization of their concerns was complete. So, the mere occurrence of "anything else?" did not necessarily foreshadow a possible preclosing of a visit. But, *when this query appeared at the analyzable end of a topic* (Schegloff and Sacks 1973:304), and *when arrangements for treatment had already been proposed and accepted*, "anything else?" worked to elicit a warrant for treating the visit as possibly closed.

In the clear majority of primary care visits (37 out of 48), doctors initiated closing sections through the *making of arrangements* (for example, to do something at a later time or see someone at a later date):

(17) (West 02:569)

Doctor:		(°Oh=whad=Isay,) A w*ee*::k the:n, fer the stitches ou:t?
		(.)
Patient:		°Um-kay=
Doctor:	-->	=would make it *two*: weeks (.4) Jus' so we could get- what we need

(18) (West 04:570)

Doctor:	-->	.h Ah'll see yuh back in a couple months (1.0) OKay?
Patient:		Alright.

(19) (West 05:504)

Doctor:	-->	LE:Mme SEE yuh back on Thurs::day afternoo:n.
		[(Ah'll) be in the clinic.
Patient:		[OKay

(20) (Frankel and Beckman 104:5)

Doctor:	-->	°Okay. (1.0) well we'll get your mammogram (.) we'll do y- (.) your mammograms again in September
Patient:		[°°Uh huh

(21) (Frankel and Beckman 131:7)

Doctor:	-->	.Hhh Okay. We'll call (outside)
Patient:		Uh u(hh)m
Doctor:	-->	get ya the appointment (.) see if we c'n get ya in there ((rip)) tomorrow or Monday. (This'll give you) a few days supply of the medicine

One reason arrangements may be so prevalent in these movements into closings is that part of the business at hand in a primary care visit is "providing the patient with appropriate management for a particular complaint" (Heath 1986:270). Thus, in most visits, making arrangements to do something at a later time or see someone at a later date is necessary for managing particular complaints. In the case of the excerpts just above, however, the arrangements in question were *already* proposed by the doctors and agreed with by the patients earlier in these visits. Of the 37 visits in which doctors initiated preclosings through talk about arrangements, 32 consisted of *reinvocations of arrangements that had already been made.*

Participants in these visits talked about arrangements in more and less disciplined ways. Above, for example, doctors variously address the question of *when* patients should return to the clinic: at a particular time of a particular day ("Thurs::day afternoo:n"), on one day or another ("tomorrow or Monday") in a specific number of weeks ("t*wo*:"), in a designated month ("September"), and "in a couple months." Sometimes they specify *what* the patient should return for ("A w*ee::*k the:n, fer the stitches ou:t?," "we'll get your . . . mammograms again in September"); sometimes they don't ("t*wo:* weeks (0.4) Jus' so we could get- what we need," "LE:Mme SEE yuh back on Thurs::day afternoo:n."). Of course, different procedures involve different degrees of freedom with respect to scheduling and its contingencies: stitches should be removed within a designated number of days in order to avoid infection; mammograms should be repeated within a specified number of months (or years) in order to ensure early detection. One might therefore be tempted to attribute variations in the "tightness" and "looseness" (cf. Goffman 1963) of talk about arrangements to the nature of the activities being arranged. But examination of the contexts in which participants make arrangements shows that, regardless of the activities in question, participants reinvoke arrangements in less disciplined ways than they originally make them. Above, for example, the doctor in excerpt (17) may seem almost cavalier in asking "(°Oh=whad=Isay,) A w*ee::*k the:n, fer the stitches ou:t?" and almost offhand in alluding to "t*wo:* weeks (0.4) Jus' so we could get- what we need." In fact, he is reinvoking a set of arrangements that he and his patient made six pages earlier in this transcript – in step-by-step fashion and painstaking detail:

(22) (West 02:394)

Doctor: °mm: Let's see. (.4) .hh ((mumbling here)) godda completely finish examining you, but assuming thet there's no::thing special thet I heed to recheck: Uh::

1-> Let's (3.2) sa::y tuh see: me:: (1.0) come back in two weeks (0.2)
Patient: Okay.
2-> Doctor: I'm not gonna ex-ray- we: ll- lemme loo:k at the- the cocc-syx ((sing-song)) again in a liddle more detail, but uh:: jus' from what chew tell me uhh:: I think I'd be be:tter (1.2) to wait an' see: how that does:: rather thun expose yih duh ex-rays [cuz if it's frac::tured we'll
Patient: [Okay. Thet's fine.
Doctor: (Pro'ly) not gonna do anything with that right no::w anyway=
Patient: =Okay
.
.
((17 lines omitted))
Doctor: if it's a ma::jor problem in two:: weeks, then I::'ll lo::ok into tha:t in more detail.
Patient: O[kay:
3-> Doctor: [Uh:: As far [as the sti::tches, 's been no::t qui::te
Patient: ['T's fine
Doctor: a week, it'd be a goo::d ide::a tuh lea::ve them i::n, espesh'ly in the knee:, we'll leave it in another wee::k .hh where yuh pull on i::t an' ev'rything.
Patient: [Mm-hmm.
Doctor: [And' bout all you'd need tuh do:: would be duh
4-> come ba::ck (.) .hh early nex' week, Monday, Tuesday,
(.)
Patient: Al[ri:ght
Doctor: [Uh: jus'tuh see uh:: (.) San::dra, an' then she::c'n take ('em out) yuh wouldn' need duh see me=
Patient: =Okay=
Doctor: =But the::n uh see me th' nex' week=
Patient: =Alright. hehh -hh!

At arrow 1, the doctor specifies when the patient should come back to see him about her tailbone and, at arrow 2, he explains why she should see him then; at arrow 3, he explains what she should do about her stitches and, at arrow 4, he specifies when she should do that. The doctor advances each step of these arrangements as a proposal (e.g., "Let's sa::y" to come back in two weeks) and the patient agrees with each of them (e.g., "Okay") as it unfolds. By subsequently reinvoking these arrangements in the way he does ((°Oh=whad=Isay,) A w*ee*::k the:n, fer the stitches ou:t?"), the doctor evokes his patient's recognition that these are the arrangements they have already agreed to and her acknowledgment that closing is a relevant possibility ("°Um-kay=").

Preparing for preclosing

Because virtually all medicine involves requests for assistance, arrangements for furnishing that assistance are objects for which thanks are due as the appropriate response. Ergo, offers and arrangement-making may be ways of coercing thanks (not to mention ways of getting patients out of the examining room and off to the pharmacy, laboratory, X-ray department, or other treatment environment).

For example, recall excerpt (13), from a visit in which the doctor initiated a possible preclosing through announcement ("*time* is getting *late*" and "I: have o:ther things tuh do"). In the continuation of that visit below, note that, following the patient's expression of appreciation, the doctor offers his assistance – the possibility of "working on" the patient's problem in future visits:

(23) (West 07:801+)

801	Doctor:		Okay. The *time* is getting *late* (an u:h), (.) I: have o:ther
802			things tuh do a:n' (.) as well as you [have
803	Patient:	-->	[I
804		-->	app re:ciate [your ti:me.
805	Doctor:		[Y'know (A lot to do:,) .hh *uh:m*. (2.2)
806			My ow:n opinion i:s that (.) a person's thinking on those
807			issues: (0.8) *i:s* changeable. Under the right circumstances:.
808			(2.0) Uh:m (2.8) So:metimes it's hard duh fine the ri:ght
809		-->	circumstances. (2.0) My:: uh- (0.4) my o:ffering to you is
810		-->	thet u:h (1.0) if you'd like tuh *wor*:k on it (2.0) Ah'd be
811		-->	happy duh wor:k on it. With you alo:ne if yuh like? (0.6) Or
812		-->	with yuh bo:th ((the patient and her husband)) tuhge:ther.

At this point, having received the doctor's offer, the patient has the option of accepting it and thanking the doctor – and, thereby, agreeing on the relevance of closure. But, rather than accepting it (and thereby agreeing to move toward closure), the patient bypasses the offer and continues her troubles-telling:[9]

[9] I use "bypasses" rather than "ignores" or "doesn't hear" (the offer) due to the precision placement of the patient's sharp inbreath (".hh!") and continuation ("Fre::d.") at possible turn-transition relevant places (Jefferson 1973).

(24) (West 07:811+)

811	Doctor:		. . . With you alo:ne if yuh like? (0.6) Or
812			with yuh bo:th ((the patient and her husband)) tuhge:ther.
813	Patient:	-->	[It soun's like [.hh!
814	Doctor:		yih'd rather work alo:ne right no:w.=
815	Patient:	-->	=Fre::d. ((her husband)) hh-As far as I can te-hh-ll,
816		-->	ju::s' doesn' have it. ((continues, describing problems with Fred . . .))

Some time later, the doctor reiterates his offer, this time, phrasing it as a question (see arrow 1):

(25) (West 07:842+)

842	Patient:	*But* uh. I'm- I mean *ah'm okay*: every wh-hh-ere *else* but
843		there!
844		(.) ((doctor pulls the patient's chart on the desk toward
845		himself))
846	Patient:	((claps her hands together)) °engh-hengh-henh!
1-->847	Doctor:	Um kay. Would juh like tuh work on it?
849		(.)
2-->850	Patient:	((°sniff)) .h hhh Ye-hh ah! ((nodding)) hh I rilly
851		wou:ld=if yuh could stand all the te-hh-ars=.hh!
852		((simultaneously making little wiping gestures at the outer
3-->853		corners of her eyes with both hands)) Cuz aye don' have
854		anybody else! .hh! .h-.h-.h-.h! Tuh talk to about it!
855		((continues, describing her lack of friends))

This time, the patient accepts the doctor's offer (see arrow 2). However, she then moves in "stepwise" fashion to telling a further trouble (Jefferson 1984c); namely, she has no one to tell her troubles *to* (see arrow 3).

Later yet, the doctor reinvokes the arrangement they made through his offer and her acceptance of it:

(26) (West 07:867+)

867		(2.6) ((several hushed "sniffs" from the patient, as she dabs
868		at her nose with a tissue))
869	Doctor: --->	Wu'll talk more about all that kine a thi:ng nex' ti:me. (.)
870		An:d uh- y'know, after we've had some more time duh
871		ta:lk, (0.8) Uh:m. (1.0) Wu'll see whut else:: (.4) whut we
872		need duh do:
873		((continues, describing further details))

Although reinvoking this arrangement does not prevent the doctor from going on to elaborate on it (or prevent the patient from then introducing still more troubles), thirty or so lines later, the patient displays her own orientation to reinvoking their previously agreed-to arrangement as a means of moving into closing:

(27) (West 07:904+)

1->904	Patient:	.h *That's all ah'm goo:d for!*
905		(1.0)
906	Patient:	Seemingly.
907		(0.8)
908	Patient:	That's all ah'm good for.
909		(0.4)
910	Patient:	[A::n' uh-
2->911	Doctor:	[In yo:ur perception.
912		(.)
913	Patient:	H*unh*?
914	Doctor:	Yo:ur perception.
915		(1.0)
916	Patient:	Whu:t else- (.) Whu:t else *is* there? (.6) Tha::t- (0.8)
3->917		Wull=never=min'.=I won' even as- (.) *Ah'll* as' that *nex'*
918		time.
919		(.)
919	Doctor:	O:kay.

At arrow 1, the patient issues a possible summing up of the topic-in-progress through an assessment. Agreement with assessments ordinarily is preferred (Pomerantz 1984a) and closing implicative (Button 1987, 1990b, 1991); however, this assessment is a self-deprecation ("*That's all ah'm goo:d for!*"). Herein lies the conflict that perhaps accounts for the doctor's failure to disagree with the patient on lines 905, 907, and 909: agreement with negative self-assessments is dispreferred (Pomerantz 1984a) but *disagreeing* with the patient's negative self-assessment necessarily entails continuing to talk about the assessment itself. Finally (after three noticeable silences), the doctor offers a very weak disagreement with the patient's self-deprecation ("In yo:ur perception."). And, after posing and then withdrawing a question about the doctor's disagreement ("Whu:t else *is* there?"), the patient displays her own orientation toward closing ("*Ah'll* as' that *nex'* time.").

The moral of this story is as follows. In the context of the primary care visit, suggestions about doing something at a later time or seeing someone at a later date are necessary to advance a treatment proposal. The propositional character of these suggestions is evident from the conditional phrasing and interrogative intonation with which doctors put them forward – for example, "My:: uh- (0.4) my o:ffering to you is thet u:h (1.0) if you'd like tuh *wor:*k on it (2.0) Ah'd be happy duh wor:k on it. With you alo:ne if yuh like? (0.6) Or with yuh bo:th ((the patient and her husband)) tuhge:ther.," in excerpt (23). But, once a treatment proposal has been accepted (e.g., "Would juh like tuh work on it?" – "Ye-hh ah! ((nodding)) hh I rilly wou:ld"), the agreed-to arrangements can be reinvoked in upgraded form, that is, as *plans*, rather than proposals. In excerpts (26)–(27), for example, the doctor's "Would juh like tuh work on it?" is upgraded to "Wu'll talk more about all that kine a thi:ng nex' ti:me.," and the patient's "Ye-hh ah! ((nodding)) hh I rilly wou:ld" (excerpt [25]) is upgraded to "*Ah'll* as' that *nex'* time." (excerpt [27]).[10] It is this upgrading that distinguishes a treatment *proposal* from a treatment *plan*. And it is this upgrading that distinguishes what White et al. (1994:24) call the "educational phase" (in which the doctor "informs the patient about the diagnosis and negotiates a treatment plan") from the "closing phase" ("in which [doctors] should summarize the visit, clarify the plan of care, check for patient understanding, establish plans for interim contact, and demonstrate caring") of the visit.[11]

Responding to preclosing initiations

As I noted earlier, in casual conversations, the initiation of a possible preclosing exchange does not guarantee that closure will soon

[10] Some readers may find the doctor in excerpt (23) unusually attentive to this patient's "psychosocial" concerns (e.g., offering to work with her to change her thinking about those concerns – and to work with her alone, or with her husband as well). However, this doctor and another clinic staff member have held regular counseling sessions with the patient and her husband in the past. Moreover, the primary focus of this visit (the one that took up 32 of the 36 transcript pages) was the patient's difficulty in relating to her husband (including her tearful first-time admission of having being sexually molested as a child). Thus, what may look like an unusual attentiveness to "psychosocial" concerns was warranted by the fact that these comprised the primary business at hand.

[11] Here, there is an interesting convergence between White et al.'s (1994) coding (using the Roter Interactional Analysis System described earlier) and Schegloff and Sacks's (1973) argument: White et al.'s coders used things like "let's see you back in five months" as *indicators* of a move into closings; Schegloff and Sacks (1973) contend that the making of arrangements is a topic type virtually specialized for *doing* closings.

follow. Some initiations of preclosing (e.g., passing turns) actually invite any not-yet-mentioned mentionables in the turn-space following their use, and no preclosing device (even an announcement such as "I gotta go") can prevent this possibility (Schegloff and Sacks 1973:312). Among the primary care visits I analyze here, the initiation of a possible preclosing exchange did not ensure that closure soon followed, either. In some cases, patients promptly agreed with doctors' preclosing initiations and a terminal exchange indeed came next:

(28) (Frankel and Beckman 139:14)

Doctor:	-->	(So y') (why don't y') give me ca(h)ll in a week.
		(0.5)
Patient:	-->	Okay.
		(1.5)
		((below, patient and doctor sound distant, as if outside the exam room by this point))
Patient:	-->	Thank you:.=
Doctor:	-->	=Okay.
		((end tape))

(29) (West 15:947)

		((doctor makes a final note in the folder, puts his pen in his pocket, pushes his chair away from the desk, and picks up the folder as he stands up.))
Doctor:	-->	Well, I'm nod eg*za:ck*ly sure when (0.4) *when-* it wull be:,=
Patient:		((rising, pushing himself to his feet nearly solely through use of his arms))
Doctor:	-->	=bu:t. I have it dow:n for (0.4)
		((doctor hands the folder to the patient, who takes it))
Doctor:	-->	as soo:n as I have an *ope*:ning. hh
		(0.4)
Patient:	-->	((nods)) °Umka:y. (0.8) Tha:nk you ((as he turns and walks toward the door))
Doctor:	-->	((tch)) Nice tuh see yuh.
		((Doctor follows the patient to the door. Patient opens it, and the doctor holds it open as the patient leaves. Then the doctor walks back to the desk, sits down, and begins writing))
		((end tape))

Above, for example, patients issue agreement tokens ("Okay.", "°Umka:y.") in the turns following doctors' reinvocations of previously made arrangements ("give me ca(h)ll in a *we*ek," "as soo:n as I have an *ope*:ning"), and closing exchanges ("Thank you:." / "Okay." and "Tha:nk you" / "Nice tuh see yuh.") follow promptly.

In other cases, however, patients responded more equivocally to doctors' initiations of possible preclosings:

(30) (West 20:483)

Doctor:		O:kay. .hh An:ything el:se thut yuh'd like tuh do tuhday:? (0.2)
Patient:	→	°We:ll ((looking away)) hh (0.2) (°Nuhaw-) °Uh:m (1.2) hh-hh °No:::, not ri:lly, hh-hh

In excerpt (30), the patient's declination to add "anything else?" is prefaced with so many delays ("°We:ll," "hh," "Uh:m" (1.2), "hh-hh") and indications of reluctance (e.g., "((looking away))") that the patient herself sounds unconvinced of what she is in the process of saying (cf. Jefferson 1980b; Pomerantz 1984a). And, when the doctor probes more deeply, the patient reveals that there is indeed "something else":

(31) (West 20:485)

Patient:		°We:ll ((looking away)) hh (0.2) (°Nuhaw-) °Uh:m (1.2) hh-hh °No:::, not ri:lly, hh-hh (.)
Doctor:	-->	Not ri:lly? (0.6) We:ll ((tch)) (0.6) ((he glances at the folder and then back at her)) [Are yuh su::re?
Patient:	-->	[Bud aye- (0.8) ((patient is leaning forward now, reaching down toward her feet; her hand is obscured by the desk))
Patient:	-->	Um:-hmm. (0.6) Bud I hea::r some a the pro:blums .hh thad I ha:ve an' (I don' wan' 'em) put me through: y'know: (°lo:sen weight). (0.2) (°Lo:dda wei:ghts.)

In still other cases, even when patients agreed with doctors' initiations of possible preclosings, *doctors* went on to add something more:

(32) (West 18:335)

		(17.0) ((doctor is writing prescriptions, displaying great haste))
Doctor:		Now, don' jus' la::y *arou::n'* without that *hea::t* on it cuz' at rilly-hh (0.6) Ah cain' tell yuh how it duz:: it, but (.) it wi::ll (1.2) you'll gedda fee::lin' bedder *quicker*. h
		(0.2) ((doctor extends his hand with the slips in it over to the patient's side of his desk and drops them on the desk))
Patient:	-->	Ah: won't. hh
		(0.2)
Doctor:		Jis' give tha:t ((handing the folder over to the patient)) to 'um at the fron' desk=you: hold o::n duh those:
		(0.8) ((as the patient picks up the folder, he rises, picking up his hat with his other hand))
Doctor:		slips there:.
		(1.0) ((the doctor arranges the slips sitting on the desk; the patient dons his hat))
Doctor:	-->	Get o:n theah with that as:prun?
		(.)
Patient:	-->	Uh-[huh ((as he picks up the slips from the desk))
Doctor:	-->	[Throw some HEA:T on it!
		(0.2)
Patient:	-->	Al *ri:ght*.

Above, the patient affirms the doctor's reinvocation of arrangements they agreed to considerably earlier in the visit. Yet, even after the patient has donned his hat, the doctor goes on to reinvoke still more previously made arrangements – now upgraded from suggestions to recommendations.

It is probable, of course, that the leave-taking preparations shown in excerpt (32) – on the doctor's part, passing the patient prescriptions, handing the patient a folder, and arranging the slips on the desk, and, on the patient's part, picking up the folder, rising, and donning his hat – are implicated by the considerable prolongation of this closing section (see, for example, Heath's [1986] analysis of how taking leave is finely fitted to movement out of the business of the primary care visit and out of a state of talk). But *the way* this closing section is prolonged is familiar by now: through the doctor's expression of concern for and attention to his patient's interests. What is possible here is that, even though doctors are the ones who must hurry things along (by initiating preclosings), they nevertheless show that they are attentive to the interests of their patients, and therefore on top of doctoring them. Through the display of other-attentiveness that, in ordinary conversation, allows speakers to shift topics or close down a state of talk (Jefferson 1984c), these doctors not only shift topics and close down states of talk but, simultaneously, display their doctoring.

"By the way . . ."

Among the primary care visits I examined, there were no instances of patients responding to doctors' initiations of closure by raising new, emotionally charged and/or potentially life-threatening complaints in the final moments of their visits (exhibiting what doctors have called the "by the way syndrome"). Instead, when patients declined their doctors' possible preclosings, their next turns focused backward on the doctors' last turns, indicating some problem with the preclosing initiations themselves. For example, some initiations of possible preclosings were followed by requests for repair (Schegloff et al. 1977) rather than by agreements to close, as shown in an extended version of excerpt (11):

(33) (Frankel and Beckman 112:4)

		(1.5)
Doctor:	-->	°So (it's) in February huh (sixteenth)
		(2.1) ((background voices and noises audible))
Patient:	-->	((zipper sound)) You said Ma:rch
Doctor:		Oh: Ma:rch (.) hheh (.5) (°)
		(13.5) ((background voices and noises audible))
Doctor:		Fi:ne, see yuh the:n. (.3) Awri:ght?
		(0.5)
Patient:		°(Okay)
Doctor:		(*Hm*m see you hhh)

Above, the doctor's reinvocation of a plan to have the patient come back for a complete physical examination (discussed earlier in the visit) prompts the patient's query about when they agreed she should return ("in February," as he originally proposed, or in "Ma:rch," as she originally counterproposed).

In 2 visits (out of the 48 in which closure occurred), patients did raise new or emotionally charged concerns in the final moments of their visits but only in response to doctors' invitations to say "something more." For example, in one case, the patient ventured a possible joke in response to the doctor's initiation of preclosing:

(34) (Frankel and Beckman 126:9)

1	Doctor:	-->	Awright why don't we do tha::t and ah:: keep up with
2			the ga[rgling.
3	Patient:	-->	[(Then c'n we ah-) (0.2) pu:nch me: ou:t if I don't
4			'ave a voice on Mo:nday
5			(0.3)
6	Doctor:	-->	Punch you ou:t? Y'mean [y'know come insi:de
7	Patient:		[um-hmm
8	Doctor:		an' punch ou:t
9	Patient:	-->	eh-heh huhm. hhh go::tta do so:mething if I don't
10			'ave a voice by Mo:nda:y

Here, the doctor uses a rhetorical question ("why don't we do tha::t") to invoke earlier-made arrangements for managing his patient's sore throat on the job. In response, the patient answers the rhetorical question (offering a presumably funny alternative if those arrangements don't work – the doctor can "punch him out" if his voice doesn't return by Monday, thereby excusing him from work). In the other case, the patient raised a new and possibly emotionally charged concern in the wake of the *doctor's reopening* of a just-initiated closing section:

(35) (Frankel and Beckman 133:7)

1	(3.1)		
2	((sound of paper being ripped from a pad))		
3	(3.3)		
4	Doctor:	-->	Oka:y. .Hhhhh Awright. Lemme give y' th' sa:mples:
5		-->	an::' oh I: fill this out too? ((rattling sound))
6	Patient:		Yeah we:ll so:metime they send money (don't they) [doctor
7	Doctor:		[That's
8			ri:ght.
9			(0.3)
10	Doctor:		They'll hafta give ya the: (.) fill out the number up
11			fro:nt.
12			(0.4)
13	Patient:		An' this is gonna help my hea:dache (.) also?
14	Doctor:		[The- the A::ctifed will. Yeah.
15	Patient:		[(This one here-)
16	Patient:	-->	(We:ll) (Yea:h) whichever o::ne. (Lemme) (I wanna) ask
17			you a que:stio::n. [Uhm

18 Doctor: [°Sure
19 Patient: I plan on havin' ki::ds in about say three yea:rs.
20 Doctor: Yeah.
21 Patient: --> Would I ha:ve any pro:blem with havin' a tilted wo::mb?

On line 5, the doctor displaces the possible preclosing he has just advanced (his reinvocation of their earlier agreed-upon arrangement to give the patient samples of penicillin) with a change-of-state token (Heritage 1984b) appended to an additional concern ("oh I: fill this out too?"). Only after this (and after the patient's reinvocation of another earlier agreed-upon arrangement) does the patient raise her new and potentially emotionally charged concern ("Would I ha:ve any pro:blem with havin' a tilted wo::mb?").[12]

By contrast to these cases – and in stark contrast to prevailing complaints about patients' "by the way syndrome" – there were two visits in which *doctors* raised new/possibly emotionally charged concerns after possible closing sections had been completed. In one case, the doctor re-entered the examining room to "talk about something real brief that [he] forgot ta mention" (line 21 below) after already taking leave of the patient and her friend:

(36) (Frankel and Beckman 108:7)

1 Doctor: so: in about three months (0.4) give us a call.
2 Patient: Uh huh=
3 Doctor: =When- whenever you wanna come in
4 (0.4)
5 Patient: O:kay::=
6 Doctor: =Good
7 Patient: O:Kay::
8 Doctor: Until then take care now.
9 (0.2)
10 Patient: Aw[right
11 Friend: [will
12 (.)
13 Patient: Thank you
14 Friend: Thank y[ou
15 Doctor: [Good bye
16 Friend: Thank you:
17 Patient): Thank you-

[12] For an analysis of the "preliminaries to preliminaries" involved in the patient's preface to her new concern – "(Lemme) (I wanna) ask you a que:stio::n." – see Schegloff (1980).

18 ((door closes, doctor leaves; noises from machinery, thumps
19 and bangs; door slams open))
->20 Doctor: Uh- I just wanted to talk about something real brief that
21 I fo[rgot ta mention.
22 Patient: [Okay
23 (0.6)
->24 Doctor: Yo- you know Missez Ginet that (0.5) that you have heart
25 valves (.) that (.) aren't working correctly
26 (0.7)
27 Doctor: Okay (0.3) you have heart murmurs . . .

The doctor involved in excerpt (36) went on to explain that the patient's heart valves could become infected if any bacteria ever got into her bloodstream; therefore, she should take antibiotics before any dental work or medical procedure that might involve a risk of this happening. In the other case – (37), focused primarily on "psychosocial" concerns – the doctor raised a not-yet-mentioned physical ailment after the patient rose to leave the examining room:

(37) (West 07:935)

Patient: ((zips purse closed)) hhh! Well. ((putting purse over her
shoulder)) I appreciate your time. hh ((getting up)) (0.2)
Doctor: Tha's o:Kay. ((he points to a sheet on his desk for her to
---> take, the patient takes it)) As fa:r as- by the way, as far as the
me:dicine, did it wor:k?

The patient involved in extract (37) replied that the medicine did indeed work ("I don' have any more i:tching there's- no discharge"), but then, she went on to introduce a previously unmentioned concern of her own (".hh! so:mething stra:nge *did* happen about . . . a wee:k ago" – she excreted a very clear, very thick sort of mucus from her vagina). Thus, even though the patient was ready to walk out the door, the doctor's addition of his previously unmentioned mentionable made way for the patient's introduction of hers – in what otherwise might have been the final moments of their visit.[13]

[13] This transcript actually continues for three more pages. On the last one, the doctor and patient are walking out of the examining room together, as the patient raises *yet another new concern* (".hh An' *al*so I nodiced . . . Ten days buhfore my period, I get quite a bit a ba:ck ache . . ."). In every case, however, the introduction of a new concern is marked to display the speaker's orientation to a closing section as "not a place for new materials" (Schegloff and Sacks 1973:319–20): the doctor cuts short his introduction of a new concern to preface it with a misplacement

Discussion

In this study of primary care visits, I find – like Heath (1986) and White et al. (1994) – that doctors are the ones who initiate closings. I also find (again, like Heath [1986] and White et al. [1994]) that patients rarely bring up new complaints during the final moments of a visit. Recall my earlier discussion of two factors that distinguish general-practice consultations in the United Kingdom (which Heath [1986] studied) from many primary care visits in the United States: (1) patients in United Kingdom are usually the ones who depart from their doctors (in the doctors' consulting rooms); and (2) doctors and patients in the United Kingdom orient their actions in relation to a single reason for a visit. In the primary care visits I analyzed, these factors do not account for the patterns of closing I observed. For example, while doctors initiated closing in all the visits I examined, patients departed from their doctors in 10 visits; doctors departed from their patients in 6 visits, and the two departed together from examining rooms in 11 visits (of the 27 visits in which departure patterns were evident).[14] Moreover, doctors and/or patients routinely displayed their orientation to the possibility of multiple reasons for their visits (in 38 of the 48 cases in which closure occurred). Doctors displayed this orientation through their routine (and, often, repeated) use of "anything else?" in eliciting patients' concerns; patients displayed this orientation through frequent serial prefaces to what was troubling them (e.g., "First," "And another thing," "The other thing is").

Managing termination and producing continuity of care

Beyond patterns that are similar to Heath's (1986) and White et al.'s (1994), I found that closings in primary visits were routinely initiated through the making of arrangements (for example, to do something at a later time or see someone at a later date). To be sure (and as I noted earlier), part of the business at hand in a primary care visit is

marker ("As fa:r as by the way, as far as the me:dicine, did it wor:k?) and the patient prefaces her introduction of new concerns by prefacing them with contrast markers ("so:mething stra:nge *did* happen about . . . a wee:k ago" and "An' *al* so I nodiced . . .").

14 In twenty-one visits, the transcript of the audiotape did not clearly indicate who departed from whom.

"providing the patient with appropriate management for a particular complaint" (Heath 1986:270); thus, making arrangements to do something at a later time or see someone at a later date is usually necessary for the management of patients' complaints. Yet, even after talk about arrangements has been demonstrably concluded, physicians tend to reintroduce arrangements (or arrangement tokens – see Button 1991) to initiate closings. Insofar as there are a variety of mechanisms for initiating closure of a state of talk – some of which appear in addition to the making of arrangements – the problem I raise here is: *why do doctors use this mechanism in particular*? As Schegloff and Sacks (1973:312) note,

> [i]nvestigation of this problem can be expected to show that such a selected item operates not only to initiate or invite the initiation of the closing of a conversation (which any of the other available components might do also, and which therefore will not account for the use of the particular component employed), but accomplishes other interactionally relevant activities as well.

One possible explanation for doctors' reinvocations of arrangements comes from Heritage and Lindström's (1992) analysis of health visitors' interactions with new mothers in the United Kingdom. Heritage found that mothers were often reluctant to acknowledge the advice they received from health visitors, since such acknowledgment would belie their competence as mothers. But, without mothers' acknowledgments, health visitors could not terminate sequences of advice-giving. Heritage shows how health visitors frequently secured mothers' acknowledgments by building offers onto the advice they dispensed (e.g., "and if that doesn't work, call me at home."). When mothers acknowledged the health visitors' offers, they implicitly accepted the advice and thus terminated the advice-giving sequences. Like the health visitors who used offers in Heritage and Lindström's (1992) study, doctors in these primary care visits may use previously agreed-to arrangements as a resource for "terminating the interminable": patients who may be loath to end their visits will nonetheless confirm the arrangements they previously agreed to and, in the process, accept doctors' proposals to close.

A second possible explanation for doctors' reinvocations of arrangements comes from Button's (1991) contention regarding the significance of arrangement-making for closing casual conversations:

> In using arrangements to place conversation on a closing track, participants may, in providing for some future conversation, and thereby providing for the present conversation as a conversation-in-a-series, testify to, elaborate upon and invoke as relevant a relationship between them that is "*standing.*" (1991:272; emphasis in original)

Here, Button does not mean "a standing relationship" in the abstract – something that is always relevant and organizes how parties interact with one another. Nor does he mean that parties whose relationship might be described as "standing" use arrangement-making to close their conversations with one another (cf. Goffman 1967:41). Instead, he argues that, by using this technique to achieve closure, parties "constitute at that juncture of their interaction a sense of what a 'standing' relationship might be for them; they elaborate upon it and constitute it as relevant for their talk and conduct, *in* their talk and conduct" (Button 1991:272; emphasis in original).

In the primary care visits I examined, the evidence suggests that, by using arrangements to put primary care visits on a closing track, doctors and patients attest to the relevance of their relationships as "standing" (Button 1991) and thereby *produce a continuity of care in their primary care relationships*. For example, although doctors rarely used announcements to launch possible preclosings (in 3 cases of the 48 in which closure occurred), they always used these components to initiate temporary adjournments of primary care visits (i.e., in 100 percent of the cases of adjournment):

(38) (West 17:725)

Doctor:	-->	(I'm) jus' gonna ((doctor pulls the curtain open)) get 'ts
		all- open for yuh- jus' hold o:n fer a sekkin'=.h you cun
		put cher trou:zers o::n. (0.4) In the *mean*time. ((doctor
		pulls curtains around examining table area)) (.2) O*ka:y?*
		(1.0) .h An' ah'll be ri:ght ba:ck.
		((doctor goes out the door))

Just above, the doctor announces that he's just going to open the curtain around the examining table – in the meantime, the patient can put his trousers on. Note that, in this case (as in the case of all but one of adjournments I observed), the doctor's pre-adjournment announcement includes a reference to when he will see the patient again ("ah'll be ri:ght ba:ck"). In fact, when doctors did *not* include such references in their pre-adjournment announcements, patients treated the missing references as accountably absent (Levinson 1983:306):

(39) (Frankel and Beckman 126:8)

Doctor: .Hhh okay very good. Awrigh' lemme: have the lady come in fer a blood test an' we'll look at the resu:lts uhm (.) see wha' sort of de:cisions we c'n make. .Hhh
Patient: --> An' that mea:ns y're gonna come ba:ck in ri::ght?
Doctor: Yeah. [Right
Patient: [Heh-hhheh Jus' che::cki:ng.

Hence, the organization of adjournment sequences indicates that, even in the case of brief temporary separations, doctors and patients work to "testify to, elaborate upon and invoke as relevant a relationship between them that is '*standing*'" (Button 1991:272; emphasis in original).

Consider further the organization of closing sections in primary care visits where doctors and patients are meeting for the first time. Under these conditions, doctor and patient are also parting for the first time, with no prior relationship between them:

(40) (West 11:740)

Doctor: O *Ka:y*!
(0.6)
Patient: °O:Kay.
(0.6)
Doctor: --> We:ll, I've enjoy:ed *mee*:ting you! hh
(0.2)
Patient: --> I ha:ve too::. En joy:ed meeting you:. cuz I've nev- .hh
(0.6) Nev:uh *ha:d* a fe:male docktuh befoah!-hunh-
hunh-hunh-hunh!-.hh [-.hh-.hh!-.hh!
Doctor: [*New*: *exper*:ience! HU::h?=
Patient: --> Ye:ah! cuz jus' lahk uh: (0.4) when they furs' tole me,
they=say=yer=gonna=have=a=fe:male=dockuh=Ah say,
O:h my goo:'ness! Ah dunno how ah'm gon' li:ke tha:t . . .

Beyond their displays of enthusiasm in lines 5–13, this doctor and patient go on to show extensive appreciation of their newly formed relationship with one another for three more pages before the transcript of their first visit comes to an end.

Finally, consider the organization of closing sections when doctors and patients are meeting for the *last* time. In the visit that also contained excerpt (14), the doctor originally initiated a possible preclosing through a passing turn:

(41) (West 10:772)

Doctor:	-->	*O ka::y!* hh ((as the doctor says this, the patient reaches out to put her hand on his shoulder. As the patient does this, the doctor extends his hands and places them on her hips))
		(0.4)
Doctor:		But n[ow:
Patient:	-->	[Yer the be::s' docktur ah ever ha:d!= ((as the patient says this, she leans over to hug him, and the doctor rises, patting the patient's shoulder with one hand and holding her other hand))
Doctor:	-->	=We:ll, (1.0) ((patting the patient's shoulder)) Thank yuh so: much! ((doctor presses his cheek against the patient's. The patient turns and kisses his cheek once))
		(0.6)
Doctor:		Yer a swee:theart.
		(1.2) ((the doctor audibly pats the patient on the shoulder five times))
Patient:	-->	An' ah'll love yuh alweez, more than anybody in thuh wor:ld

More lavish displays of appreciation followed, before the doctor again initiated preclosing through the reinvocation of arrangements he and the patient previously agreed to:

(42) (West 10:924)

	(1.2)
Doctor:	.h *No:w, let's do thi:s.* .h *E:llie*, if yer ar:m gets better (0.4) with ((looking up from his writing)) the combinations of the injeckshuns an' the Mowtrun, .h then ah think (0.4) ah would suggest that you come see Doctor Kre:ss ((the new doc, who will replace him)) (.) .h in about a *mon*th 'r six *wee*:ks.

The original initiation of preclosing appeared on page 29 of this transcript; the reinvocation of previously made arrangements appeared on page 35. But the doctor's and patient's extensive exchanges of appreciation contribute to *ten more pages of transcript* before the following sequence of turns brought the visit to a close:

(43) (West 10:1158)

Doctor: Take ca:re, Ellie.
(0.2)
Patient: Ye:ah,
(1.0) ((patient and doctor are now out of range of the video monitor, but audio picks up the patient coming to a halt on their way out of the room))
Doctor: Bye-bye:. (.) O[ka:y?
Patient: [You'll *al*:weez be my ba:by.
(.)
Doctor: .h Ah'll thi:nk about cha. O[kay?
Patient: [Ah'll al:weez love yuh.
Um-hmm. ((patient's steps continue for 8.0 seconds, then the door closes))

In this visit, of course, the doctor (who is in his early thirties) and the patient (who is in her early eighties) display considerable affection. But prolonged and extensive exchanges of appreciation also appeared in the closing sections of last visits where the doctor and patient were less overtly affectionate. Hence, these protracted closing sections seem to convey doctors' and patients' *regard for the standing relationship between them*, quite apart from their actual feelings about one another. Like invoking the name of the practitioner who will succeed him ("Doctor Kre:ss"), the doctor's prolongation of the preclosing – despite his presumably busy schedule – affirms the continuity of care implicit in their relationship. As Schegloff and Sacks (1973:323) put it, "The sectional organization of closings thus provides a resource for managing the articulation between the conversation and the interaction in which it occurs."

Closing

Less than a decade into the twenty-first century, the United States faces an escalated crisis in health care. It is spending more than twice as much on its health care system as is the average developed nation, yet 41 million of its people are uninsured and still more are underinsured (Physicians' Working Group for Single-Payer National Health Insurance 2003). The costs of Medicare have increased by billions of dollars, yet prenatal care and immunizations cannot be guaranteed. For physicians who work in its market-driven system, "the gratifications of healing [are giving] way to anger and alienation [with] sick people [being treated] as commodities and physicians as investors' tools" (Physicians' Working Group for Single-Payer National Health Insurance 2003:798). In the context of these developments, support is growing for fundamental changes in the US system of health care delivery – for example, expansion of eligibility for Medicaid benefits; defined contribution programs for employed persons; or a national health insurance program.

What are the implications of such changes for the patterns of closing reported in this chapter? If any new health care delivery system were still predicated on *continuity of care* between physician and patient, I would predict that patterns of closure in primary care visits would continue to look like those I describe here. By contrast, if a system were to eliminate continuity of care in the relationship between physician and patient, I would predict that patterns of closure between physicians and patients would look less like ordinary conversations (Schegloff and Sacks 1973; Button 1987, 1990b, 1991) and more like other interview situations (cf. Clayman 1989; Zimmerman and Wakin 1995).

14

Misalignments in "after-hours" calls to a British GP's practice: a study in telephone medicine

Paul Drew

Introduction: after-hours calls as a form of telephone medicine

A significant proportion of the contacts which medical practitioners have with their patients occurs over the telephone. One study reports that approximately 15 percent of all ambulatory medical contacts in the US are made over the telephone (Curtis and Evens 1995:187). It is widely recognized that there are particular problems associated with telephone medicine, which arise from a variety of factors including the different communicative patterns over the telephone as compared with face-to-face interactions with patients, and the physician's reliance on the descriptions of diagnostic symptoms given by patients or carers calling on their behalf. The evidence from a number of studies seems to suggest that, for these and other reasons, telephone medicine is less satisfactory than face-to-face consultations, at least from the physician's point of view.[1] But the precise nature of the communicative patterns associated with diagnostic questioning over the telephone – including the ways in

The research for this chapter was conducted in preparation for a conference, "Dialogue in the Heart of Europe," Czech Language Institute of the Czech Academy of Sciences, Prague, April 1996, my participation in which was funded by the British Academy. The chapter was written whilst I was visiting the Department of Sociology, University of Lund, Sweden. I am grateful to the organizers of the Prague conference for providing the occasion for completing this research; to the British Academy for its financial support; and especially to Professor Ann-Mari Sellerberg and the Department of Sociology at Lund for their generous hospitality, which gave me the opportunity to write up this research.

[1] For an overview of the special conditions associated with telephone medicine, and the difficulties which these can engender, and evidence that as a consequence "physicians are less effective when using the telephone for medical care than they are in face-to-face encounters," see Curtis and Evens (1995). More particularly, on the matter of physicians' perceptions of the validity of after-hours calls, see John and Curtis (1988). See also Virji (1992).

which callers describe symptoms, how doctors manage giving advice about treatment, and so forth[2] – is little understood. This chapter focuses on the patterns of interaction between doctor and callers in one particular kind of telephone medicine; namely, "after-hours" calls. Such calls predominantly concern urgent medical problems – 92 percent of these calls concern clinical problems, compared with only approximately 50 percent of those calls made during office hours (Curtis and Evens 1995:188).[3]

The after-hours telephone calls which are the subject of this investigation were made to a British GP's practice. According to the terms of service in the British National Health Service (NHS), a GP – a general practitioner is a physician who has no particular clinical specialization – is responsible for the medical care of his or her patients round the clock.[4] This includes the condition that they should visit patients in their own homes if, in the doctor's opinion, the patient's condition demands it. Patients who feel too unwell to visit the practice, or feel that their problem is sufficiently urgent that they cannot wait until the practice is next open (referred to in Britain as "surgery hours," and in the US as "office hours"), may telephone to request the doctor visit them in their home. Thus, generally, after-hours telephone calls are made by patients, or by someone on their behalf, when they are concerned with some deterioration in the state of their health which seems sufficiently serious to be treated as an urgent matter, possibly requiring the doctor to visit them (Clyne 1961). Doctors have to decide, on the basis of the information supplied

[2] Curtis and Evens point out that "One of the distinguishing features of a telephone encounter is the emphasis on management rather than on diagnosis" (1995:191).

[3] The relatively small proportion of after-hours calls made about administrative matters, or to renew prescriptions, etc. indicates that callers treat the matter of making a call after or out of hours as quite different from calling during office hours – suggesting that they restrict such calls to ailments which they regard as urgent or emergencies, even though physicians may take a different view (John and Curtis 1988).

[4] However, studies of GPs' attitudes towards their terms and conditions show that, over the past twenty-five years, and coinciding with a rising demand among patients for after-hours care (Williams 1993), a majority of GPs have come to regard the principle of full (twenty-four-hour) responsibility for their patients as outdated. The latest evidence suggests that most would prefer a more limited contractual commitment, or the choice of opting out. For a review, see Hallam (1994:249–50). For a study of organizational changes in the provision of after-hours care under the British NHS, designed to accommodate the rising demand from patients and growing disaffection among providers, see Hallam and Cragg (1994). See also O'Dowd and Sinclair 1994.

during the telephone conversation/"examination," whether a home visit is necessary – or whether instead the caller's problem can be managed without a visit, for instance by reassuring the patient that the condition is not serious and therefore not a cause for alarm, offering advice about treatment, and perhaps advising the patient to visit the practice at some suitable later time.[5]

This study is based on an investigation of a corpus of recordings of after-hours calls made to a GP in a large town in the (English) Midlands. The purpose of the research reported here was not to evaluate the effectiveness of doctors' techniques for eliciting relevant diagnostic information in after-hours telephone calls, nor to assess the decisions they make about whether or not to make a home visit. The aim was solely to investigate and document some of the interactional or communicative patterns which seem evident in such calls. A word of caution should be given about the representativeness of the findings reported here about these patterns. The database is a quite restricted one: the corpus consists of approximately sixty calls made to one practice, and which were answered by one (male) doctor who was "on call" during the short period in which the data were recorded. The demographic characteristics of the patients who were the subjects of these calls appear to be congruent with what is known, statistically, about such calls more generally, at least in Britain.[6] Nevertheless there are no scientific grounds for claiming that this corpus is representative, in terms either of the kinds of after-hours calls made generally across all NHS authorities, or the manner in which doctors typically manage such calls (including the matter of how they arrive at decisions about whether or not to make a home visit). Hence the findings reported here should be treated as

[5] This aspect of the service which GPs provide in the NHS is controversial for a number of interrelated reasons, such as its cost, the real (medical) necessity of many of the calls made, the difficulties associated with making accurate diagnoses over the telephone, and whether in certain cases a doctor was justified in deciding not to visit the patient at home (e.g., in circumstances where, it later transpired, the patient was seriously ill, or even died; the charge of "failure to visit" is, apparently, one of the most common formal complaints made against GPs). Thus it has been proposed that "Doctors may well need a record of such consultations to show that they have made reasonable attempts at eliciting the history" (O'Dowd and Sinclair 1994).

[6] Majeed et al. (1995). For a study of the distribution of calls during the night, and the relationships between temporal distributions, demographic characteristics of patients, and associated trends of home visits, see Salisbury (1993). For studies of the demographic characteristics of those making after-hours calls in the US, and the morbidity profiles of patients who are the subjects of such calls, see Evens et al. (1985) and John and Curtis (1988).

provisional. Whilst the patterns reported demonstrably hold for this particular corpus, these findings can only suggest that such patterns might be found elsewhere in calls in other health service authorities or to other practitioners. More broadly, though, the analysis here suggests that associated with the patterns identified are some *misalignments* between callers and the doctor which, whilst they do not amount to anything like communicational failures, do reveal differences in the perspective or orientation of each to the doctor's diagnostic questioning. These differences, and misalignments, may inhabit after-hours calls more widely, and they may be associated with, and in part responsible for, the kinds of problems which various studies have suggested are encountered in telephone medicine (Curtis and Evens 1995).

The doctor's decision about whether to make home visits, in response to after-hours calls

A preliminary inspection of the data corpus revealed a clear pattern as regards the doctor's decision about whether to make a home visit. Extract (1) is typical of those cases in which the doctor agreed subsequently to visit the patient at home. The caller (Clr) is, as is usual for these calls, a carer, calling on behalf of the patient – in this case, a mother calling about her child.[7] After a characteristically brief opening (and an apologetic disclaimer, which will not be considered further here), the patient's mother begins to report the matter which she considers to be a cause for concern – that, although her daughter has had her nightly dose of Ventolin, she is still experiencing difficulty breathing.

#1 [1:1:10]

Doc: Hello:,
Clr: Hello, I'm sorry tuh trouble yuh,<my daughter has Ventolin:
e: :hm one spoonful at night,<˙hh I gave her some about an hour
ago<I kept (it late) with it being so hot but sh[e still=
Doc: [Yes,
Clr: =can't brea:th very easily, ˙hh Can I give her another
teaspoonful?
Doc: Wull shall I pop round and have a l:ook,

[7] Only 7 out of the 60 calls in the corpus were made by the patients themselves.

In constructing her report this way, the caller conveys something of her daughter's medical history, "my daughter has Ventolin:" (line 2), thereby indicating that she is an asthma sufferer, for which condition Ventolin is her regular (prescribed) treatment. She also reports the symptoms which are the cause of her present concern – that her daughter took the medicine an hour ago and yet is still having trouble breathing. These represent perhaps the two most general features of such opening reports by callers of the trouble which is the reason for calling, i.e., outlining or adumbrating in some fashion the patient's relevant medical history, and giving an account of the symptoms indicating some recent-and-current deterioration in the patient's condition. In combination, these two features work to portray the patient's condition as a medical problem, as a cause for concern or alarm and as a potentially urgent matter, hence warranting (perhaps even "justifying") this out-of-hours call.

In response to the caller's request for advice (lines 6–7), the doctor offers to visit the patient at home (line 8). His manner of doing so is typical of such offers in these calls, insofar as the expression "pop round" is characteristically casual. In this way the doctor offers to visit, but without giving any further indication that there might be anything seriously amiss about the patient's health. The key point to notice about his offer to visit is, however, that it is made immediately in response to the caller's opening report of the patient's condition; and his decision is made solely on the basis of that report. It may happen in such cases that the doctor goes on to ask about certain other details; for example, in the call from which example (1) was taken, the doctor subsequently asks the age of the child. But the significant point here is that he asks for further information only after he has already indicated that he will visit. So in these and similar cases in the corpus, the doctor makes a decision to visit the patient on the basis of the caller's opening report, and without asking for further diagnostic information before reaching that decision.

However, in the majority of cases the doctor does not so promptly indicate that he will visit the patient at home. The more usual trajectory of these calls is that, after the caller's opening report of the patient's trouble, the doctor begins to ask some diagnostic questions, as happens in the following two examples.

#2 [1:1:1]

1	Doc:		Hello:,
2			(0.4)
3	Clr:		Hello is that the duty doctor for ((name)),
4	Doc:		Yes, that’s right, doctor ((name)) speakinghh=
5	Clr:		=Oh:.˙hh U:m my name’s ((name)) my daughter’s: uh
6			((name)) she’s age four:,
7	Doc:		Ye:[s,
8	Clr:		[A:nd u:m (.) she’s been sick sri- six times this evening,
9	Doc:		Mm hm:,
10	Clr:	1->	A:nd then she’s just started wi:th diarrhea and it smells
11		1->	dis[gusting.
12	Doc:		[˙hhh
13	Doc:	2->	Rhi:ghht. ˙hh At’s why wi- u:m (.) uw- i- at-what was your
14			name again?<((name))
15	Doc:		Ri:ght. eYou’re doctor: ((name)) doctor na- nu-uh sorry
16			(tu-)[yeah,
17	Clr:		[([ )
18	Doc:	2->	[˙hh Fine. ˙h So: ho:w ho:w: this was: all just
19			started tonight, is it?

#3 [1:2:3]

1	Doc:		˙hh Hello:, Doctor ((name))
2	Clr:		Hello.<Um:, sorry to disturb you.<I(t)’s M’ssis ((name))
3	Clr:		I’ve got- a little gi:rl of nineteen months.
4	Doc:		R:ight,
5	Clr:		An’ I’ve just noticed in’ er mouth. that she’s got
6			˙hhhh at least three: quite bad ulcers on’ er tongue. (.) that
7			weren’t there: (d-) like two hours ago.
8			(1.0)
9	Doc:		Ri:ght,
10	Clr:		She did have (1.1) about two months ago she had um- (0.9) uh
11			cold sor:es in ’er mouth <the: herpes simplex in’er mouth.
12	Doc:		Mm hm,
13	Clr:		An’ she was on antibiotics for it. An’ um (0.3) she seem(s)
14		1->	t’have a temperature as well an’ I don’t know whether (1.0)
15		1->	yihknow what should i-ih
16	Doc:	2->	Ri:ght, sorry. ˙hh So- so how old didju’ say- you say your
17			daughter was,
18	Clr:		She’s nineteen months.<just.=
19	Doc:	2->	=Luh- ri:ght. ˙hh An’ how is she: in herself:.

Recall that in extract (1) the doctor indicated his decision to visit right after completion of the caller’s opening report. At the same position in extracts (2) and (3), the doctor instead begins to ask a series of diagnostic questions. The completions of the caller's initial reports are shown by arrow 1: these completions may be done through a dramatic account of the patient's current state, as in example (2), "A:nd then she's just started wi:th diarrhea and it smells disgusting."; or, following an account of the problem, an implicit or explicit request for advice about what to do, as the caller begins to do, but does not complete, in extract (3), "an' I don't know whether (1.0) yihknow what should I-ih."

Thus the doctor treats the completion of the caller's initial account of the problem as the place in which either he may decide to visit (on the basis of the information the caller has given), as in example (1); or alternatively he may choose to ask for more diagnostic information, as in extracts (2) and (3). In the majority of cases in the corpus – in 51 of the 59 cases – he does the latter. Moreover, it is clear that in the majority of cases in which the doctor embarks on diagnostic questioning – that is, in contrast to cases such as example (1) – the doctor does not agree to visit the patient at home. Only in approximately one third of cases in which the doctor engages in some verbal examination does he end up agreeing to visit (in 18 of the 51 such cases). In at least 7 of these 18 cases, the doctor treats the problem as not serious, partly through his indicating that he will be making some visits in the vicinity of the patient's home later that day/evening, and will "pop in" when he's over that way, often mentioning a period of two to three hours before he's likely to visit. In some of the 18 cases, it is fairly clear that the doctor agrees to visit not because there is anything especially urgent about the patient's condition, but because of the circumstances in which the patient is living, and in order to reassure the patient. So, for instance, he agrees to visit a young mother living alone with her very young children, not because her condition is urgent (she has a cold or flu), but because, it seems, she has no support, and no one to get her medication. These might be considered "special cases" in which the doctor's decision is taken not on strictly medical grounds, but with a view to the patient's welfare. The point is that in only a very small minority of cases does it appear that the doctor learns something during the diagnostic questioning which causes him to decide that he should visit the patient at home. In most cases the doctor ends the call by giving advice about treatment (possibly with the suggestion that "if things don't improve call me back"); and/or with the advice that the patient should come into the surgery when it is next open ("in the morning," "on Monday").

So the pattern which emerged in the data corpus as a whole is that if the doctor agrees to make a home visit, he generally does so immediately after the caller's opening report of the patient's condition, as illustrated in example (1). If, however, at that point the doctor embarks on diagnostic questioning, then in most cases he will conclude with a different disposition, involving his giving advice about treatment by the carer. Only very rarely does he decide, on the basis of information which emerges during diagnostic questioning, that the case is potentially urgent and that a home visit is warranted on medical grounds. A picture is beginning to emerge, which is somewhat consistent with the findings in some studies, that "physicians tend to jump to a diagnostic conclusion early in the conversation" (Curtis and Evens 1995:190).

A misalignment between caller and doctor

We have seen that there appears to be an association between the doctor embarking on diagnostic questioning (rather than deciding, just on the basis of the initial information that the caller has given, to visit the patient), and the likelihood that as a result of the information elicited through that questioning he will decide not to make a home visit. This is the background for what appears to be a kind of misalignment between the caller and doctor during this phase of diagnostic questioning. "Misalignment" is meant here in a quite technical sense: it does not imply any lack of affiliation between them, or tension or friction or lack of empathy – or indeed any other such evaluative description which might suggest anything like a schism in their interaction. This misalignment might be regarded as a form of asymmetry of perspective between them regarding the questions which the doctor asks.

Put very briefly, it appears that callers treat the doctor's asking them in more detail about their or the patient's condition as an opportunity to embellish their initial accounts, in order to convince the doctor of the seriousness or urgency of the condition – perhaps in an effort to persuade him to visit. The doctor, on the other hand, appears to ask the caller a series of diagnostic questions in order to check out what they by now suspect – that most likely there is nothing seriously or urgently wrong, and that therefore no visit is necessary. In various ways their questions appear to be built to presume "no trouble," which if correct – and of course the information given by callers in this phase may yet reveal something unanticipated and untoward – leaves him with the task simply to reassure the carer or patient and check he or she is doing the right things, and administer suitable advice about care and treatment. In a sense this amounts to each participant having a different orientation to questioning in this phase. The callers, alarmed by the apparent seriousness of the symptoms, and suspecting therefore that the patient might be in need of urgent treatment, orients to the questions as seeking information about that possible or likely seriousness. The doctor, however, seems oriented to the questions as means to elicit information which will confirm his initial impression that the case is "routine" and non-urgent: hence his questions are only "double-checking" what he suspects on the basis of the caller's initial report.

The evidence for there being this kind of misalignment between the orientations of doctor and callers during the phase of diagnostic questioning in these calls is not manifest in any overt misunderstanding or difficulty between the participants.[8] Instead, it is manifest in a more circumstantial fashion, in the regular occurrence in these calls of three patterns, in which it is evident that the caller's descriptions and the doctor's responses are going in different directions – the caller's, in the direction of serious, urgent, alarming; the doctor's, in the direction of routine, unproblematic, non-urgent.

The patterns in these calls which manifest a certain misalignment between caller and doctor during the diagnostic questioning involve, in outline, the following:

- Callers pursue a *dramatic detailing* of the patient's symptoms, often in answer to questions which did not ask about the particular symptoms which they describe.
- Caller and doctor display a *different sense of the diagnostic significance of certain symptoms*, in terms of what they convey about the potential seriousness of the patient's condition.

[8] For an example of a misalignment that is manifest in a difficulty which occurs overtly and regularly between participants, in the context of calls to the emergency services, see Jefferson and Lee (1992).

- The different sense which each has about the significance of the patient's reported symptoms applies also to the *diagnostic hypotheses* which it turns out callers sometimes have about the condition (ailment) from which the patient is suffering.

In the remainder of this chapter, each of these patterns will be reviewed.

Callers pursue dramatic detailing of patients' symptoms

When the doctor embarks on diagnostic questioning, he performs a verbal examination of the patient by proxy, and in circumstances where he cannot see for himself how the patient looks. Therefore he is having to rely on the caller's account of the patient's symptoms, and in particular his or her descriptions of the appearance, severity, etc. of those symptoms. Equally, the caller is attempting to convey the nature of the patient's condition, and why it is a cause for concern, in circumstances in which he or she cannot rely on the doctor seeing for himself how alarming the symptoms are. At any rate, the verbal examination in telephone medicine is unsupported by the kind of visual evidence which is available to the doctor, and to the caller/carer, in face-to-face consultations.

When, in the phase of the calls after a caller has given an initial report of the patient's condition, the doctor asks diagnostic questions, it is apparent that there is a pattern of response by callers to those questions. Their responses are characterized by a number of features, the first being that callers often do not restrict themselves to answering only the point which the doctor asked about. Instead, they add other details concerning the patient's symptoms – and in this way treat the question as providing an opportunity to report other aspects of the patient's condition which are cause for alarm. The following is a case in point.

#4 [1:1:8:1:28–39]

```
1  Doc:   She's ten, did you say?
2         (0.8)
3   Clr:  [Yea:(s),
4  Doc:   [Te-
5  Doc:   Ten years old.
6   Clr:  Yeah,=
```

7 Doc: =Yes, ˙hh[h
8 Clr: --> [She's gone ever so thin, she's like a skeleton,
9 Doc: Is she? [˙hh
10 Clr: --> [(do it) and she's keep[s cryin' because she's hungry,=
11 Doc: [p!
12 Clr: =but she can't eat anything,

The question with which the doctor opens his diagnostic questioning in this call is the one shown in the extract (line 1), and concerns the child's age (he repeats his confirmation check about her age in line 5, probably because of the slight hiatus arising from the delay in the caller's initial confirmation in lines 2–3, her audible uncertainty, and the overlap which results in lines 3–4). The caller (mother) repeats her confirmation of her daughter's age (line 6), and then goes on to describe aspects of her condition (lines 8–12) in terms which are not directly responsive to the doctor's question, that is, which do not concern the patient's age. So one feature of this pattern of answering diagnostic questions is that, in her response, the caller goes beyond what was asked about in the doctor's question and describes other alarming symptoms of the patient.

Two other features of this example are worth noting, because they are fairly recurrent. The first is that the caller's description of these "additional" symptoms takes quite a dramatic form: "She's gone ever so thin, she's like a skeleton, (do it) and she's keeps cryin' because she's hungry, but she can't eat anything." Indeed her descriptions resemble the kinds of "extreme case formulations" which Pomerantz (1986) notes are frequently used in circumstances in which the teller is trying to convince the recipient of something: "like a skeleton" and "can't eat anything" are particularly clear instances of the construction of "extreme case formulations" with which to describe the patient's not eating.

The second feature is that, having initially answered the doctor's question, the caller begins her continuation (of these other alarming symptoms, which he had not asked about) in overlap with the doctor.

[from extract (4)]

Doc: Ten YEars Old.
Clr: Yeah,=
Doc: =Yes, ˙hh[h
Clr: --> [She's gone ever so thin, she's like a skeleton,

The overlap seems only slight, involving as it does her overlapping with his inbreath. However, this overlap is significant in so far as it is quite audible from the intonation of his "Yes," together with his inbreath, that the doctor was starting up to speak, and presumably to ask a next question. In this respect the caller is *pursuing* her dramatic detailing of the patient's alarming symptoms, not only by not restricting herself to answering only what the doctor asked but also by continuing at a point where the doctor was in the course of starting up to say something (the inbreath), and may have been about to have asked a next question.

The following are some further cases, which share many of the features exhibited by example (4).

#5 [1:2:8:2]

```
 1Doc: --> Any problems with' er breathing,=
 2Doc:     =°(m[m,) n[o? no?
 3 Clr: -->        [No:, [no she's alright she's' er eyes are very red.<'Er
 4         eyes are extremely bloodshot,
 5Doc:     Mm hm,
 6 Clr: --> U:m: a::nd she's su- sayin' ow! all the ti:me, ehm sort'u
 7         holdin' 'er stomach an' 'er head is very hot (an') 'er
 8         ˙hhh like a back an' (uh) (uh) chest (an' uh)(˙hh[h)
 9Doc:                                                   [Ri:gh[t,
10 Clr: -->                                                      [An' then
11         she's (sit) dozy now,
```

#6 [1:1:3:2:19–30]

```
 1 Doc: --> Ri:ght, uw::and how' bout the headache. Is that settled,
 2          or [is (uh)
 3  Clr: -->   [That's settled but she's runnin' a high temp- well I think
 4          she's runnin' a temprature.
 5 Doc:     Yeah,
 6          (0.3)
 7 Doc:     Yeah,
 8  Clr: --> [Yihknow, she gets ver]y ho[t (       ) she's been sick,
 9 Doc:     [˙h h ˙h h ˙h h h h]          [kmhh! ((cough))
10 Doc:     ((swallow)) Right, ˙hh[h
11  Clr: -->                      [She's just completely exhausted I
12          think,
```

#7 [1:1:3:2:37–42]

Doc: --> She's not vomiting blood or anything¿
Clr: No,=
Doc: =No, it's jus[t-
Clr: --> [No it's j[ust fl u i]d a[:nd brown stu[ff.
Doc: [clear, is it?] [Yeah, [˙hh
Doc: And brown stuff [>is it¿<
Clr: [Mm(hm),
(0.9)
Doc: pt Du-ah:m: ˙hhh [Ri:ght,
Clr: --> [(See) yesterday she was tellin' me that
'cause normally I do manuals, ...

In these instances, too, callers pursue their accounts of the alarming condition of the patients by reporting symptoms which had not specifically been asked about by the doctor in his prior question. So in extract (5) the caller (mother) briefly answers the doctor's question about the patient's breathing, and then goes on to describe the state of her eyes ("er eyes are very red.<'Er eyes are extremely bloodshot,"), the pain she appears to be in ("she's su- sayin' ow! all the ti:me, ehm sort'u holdin' 'er stomach an' 'er head is very hot"), and finally her current drowsy state ("she's (sit) dozy now,"). In example (6), having confirmed that the patient's headache has settled, the caller then continues to detail other symptoms, namely the patient's temperature, her vomiting, and exhaustion. Then in extract (7), having answered the question about whether the patient has been vomiting blood, the caller goes on to report some further diagnostic information concerning something the day before (her daughter's request to do "her manuals"), which might have indicated the trouble was beginning then.

As in extract (4), callers proceed to give quite dramatic versions of the diagnostic details which they report. Furthermore, there is evidence of their embarking on these "continuations" often at points where it seems the doctor is speaking or is audibly starting up to do so, and may be about to ask a next question.

[from #5]

Doc: Ri:gh[t,
Clr: --> [An' then she's (sit) dozy now,

[from #6]

Doc: ((swallow)) Right, ˙hh[h
Clr: --> [She's just completely exhausted I think,

[from #7]

Doc: =No, it's jus[t-
Clr: --> [No it's j[ust fl u i]d a[:nd brown stu[ff.
Doc: [clear, is it?] [Yeah, [˙hh
Doc: And brown stuff [>is it¿<
Clr: [Mm(hm),
(0.9)
Doc: pt Du-ah:m: ˙hhh [Ri:ght,
Clr: --> [(See) yesterday she was tellin' me that 'cause normally I do manuals, ...

#8 [1:1:4:1:21–29]

Clr: [(was) sick again,
Doc: [Right,
Doc: Ri:ght, ˙hh[h
Clr: --> [She's eaten no:thing. at all today,

It is noticeable also in cases such as extracts (4)–(7) that the callers pursue their detailing of the patients' symptoms in answer to questions about diagnostic signs/symptoms which as it happens are *not* present. That is, in each of extracts (4)–(7), the doctor inquires about diagnostic signs (diarrhea, problems breathing, headaches, vomiting blood, etc.). Just parenthetically, one can notice that the doctor usually frames these questions in terms of a presumption that these pathological signs will not be present (e.g., "She's not vomiting blood or anything¿" – rather than the open form of the question "Is she vomiting blood?").[9] But in each case the caller responds by indicating or confirming that this sign is not present, that is, that the patient is not having problems breathing, has not been vomiting blood, etc. Each of the doctor's questions, of course, is designed to check on fairly standard diagnostic signs which would indicate whether things are as they should be, are "normal"

[9] The doctor's question in extract (5) comes closest to being formed as an open question; but there is the possibility here that he is very ready with the negative answer to his question (and is therefore asking about what he takes to be a null symptom). His continuation in line 2 is latched to his question in line 1.

(e.g., that there is nothing untoward about the patient's vomit or diarrhea, these being "normal" for someone who simply has gastroenteritis, or a virus, etc.); or whether there is something unusual, and therefore potentially urgent, about the case – such standard indications being, for example, evidence of blood in the vomit or feces. Hence "negative" answers to such questions, such as confirming in extract (7) that the patient is not vomiting blood, indicates that in some respects (at least in respect of the symptom about which the doctor has just asked) there is "nothing wrong," nothing especially untoward, unusual, or alarming. It seems, then, in such cases as these – when callers respond to questions concerning some particular null symptom – that by continuing to report other symptoms which the patient is experiencing, the caller is reporting something else which is amiss or alarming. It is as though the further detailing is designed to negate the implication conveyed in the (negative) answer to the question which the doctor asked, that implication being that the patient is "normal" (that is, "normally unwell").[10]

#5 [1:2:8:2]

Doc: Any problems with 'er breathing,=
Doc: =°(m[m,) n[o? no?
Clr: [No:, [no she's alright . . .

As a result it is not entirely clear whether his "no? no?" in line 2 is responding to the caller's "No:, no" in line 3, or was produced independently of her answer. It almost lies between these, giving the impression that this was the answer he expected and had ready.

[10] It might seem that example (4) is unlike the other cases, in one respect at least. Whilst the caller pursues her dramatic detailing of her daughter's symptoms, she does so in response to a question which, unlike the questions in each of the other cases in extracts (5)–(7) and (9), appears not to ask specifically about a diagnostic sign or symptom. The doctor has asked only "She's ten, did you say?," this being the opening of his questioning after the caller's initial report. However, the mother has reported that her daughter is suffering from diarrhea and sickness, and has been for the past three days. In this context, the matter of how old the child is can matter greatly. A very young child – for instance, one who is ten months old – is potentially much more vulnerable (especially to dehydration) than an older child. The mother had begun her report by saying, "My little girl, she's ten,"; therefore, when the doctor asks subsequently, "She's ten, did you say?," he might be heard to be checking whether the mother meant ten years or ten months. That in turn can be heard to be medically relevant, not exactly to the diagnosis (the child is suffering from gastroenteritis however old she is), but to an assessment of the "severity" of the ailment and the potential risk to the child. Hence the mother may be responding to this question as though her child's age is a diagnostically relevant factor or sign, much as other signs or symptoms are.

Thus, although the answer to the question which the doctor has asked might indicate that the patient's condition is not especially alarming, the callers pursue their sense of the possible urgency of the case by reporting other dramatic or worrying symptoms. This pattern is rather well illustrated in the following instance.

#9 [1:1:3:1:48–18]

Doc: ˙hh Ri:ght, and this: i-she was a really f: quite well up until
about fou:r,
(.)
Clr: Yea[h,
Doc: [˙h tiday,
Clr: [°Yeah,
Doc: [˙hh=
Clr: --> =She'd complained of a headache,
Doc: [Mm hm,
Clr: [(and)
(.)
Clr: --> A:n:d then nearly fell asleep in 'er wheelchai:r,
(.)
Doc: uRi:ght,
Clr: An' then she started ti! (1.0) well I noticed when she's lying
--> on the bed that- there was diarrhea a:ll up her back.
(0.7)
Doc: Ri:g[ht,
Clr: --> [(And) then she's been vomitin' as well and she keeps
complainin' (a') severe (0.6) stomach pains,

The doctor's question "she was a really f: quite well up until about fou:r," (lines 1–2), might suggest that the patient has only been unwell for a short time, and therefore it might be too early to tell whether anything is really amiss. The caller agrees to that (hence to a "negative" symptom), but then again continues by adding further details (note the doctor's inbreath in line 7, and the immediate incoming and continuation by the caller in line 8, where she begins her detailing of the "positive" symptoms; that is, the symptoms which have been present since four o'clock). In this way she pursues a very different and more alarming account of the patient's condition.

In this pattern, then, it appears that the two participants are misaligned, or even going in different directions. The questions concern diagnostic signs or symptoms which are *not* present – from which the patient is not suffering: indeed, generally the questions are framed in a fashion which conveys that the doctor expects or presumes that the patient is not experiencing them – e.g., in extract (7), "She's not vomiting blood or anything¿"; the precise nature of this framing varies in each case. So the import of the questions, and the answers to the questions (in each case the answer confirms that the patient has not experienced that symptom, or is no longer doing so), is that, in that respect at least, there is nothing particularly untoward or abnormal about the patient's health. By not restricting themselves to answering only the question asked, but continuing and describing – generally in very dramatic terms – other signs or symptoms from which the patient is suffering, callers appear to attempt to counter the optimistic implications of the questions, by providing details which are alarming and suggest a more pessimistic view of the illness. Furthermore there is a real sense in which they *pursue* portraying the patient's symptoms in this more pessimistic light; they continue their detailing of these other symptoms at just those points at which the doctor is gearing up to speak, to continue his questioning. In order not to leave the matter on an optimistic, "no-problem" note, the caller seems to take the opportunity, before the doctor has actually begun his question, to step in and detail other more alarming symptoms from which the patient is suffering. A similar sense of their pulling in different directions is evident in the second pattern found in these telephone calls to the doctor.

Caller and doctor display a different assessment of the significance of certain diagnostic signs or symptoms

We have seen that callers describe patients' symptoms in quite dramatic terms, conveying their alarm at the patient's condition. Plainly, a caller's account of the patient's symptoms is related to his or her *construction* and *sense* of the seriousness of the problem, and therefore of the urgency of the case – hence justifying this after-hours call, and possibly also a home visit by the doctor. In most cases it is apparent that the doctor does not attribute to those symptoms the same (alarming) significance as they evidently have for the callers. For example, the caller in example (2) reports that her four-year-old daughter vomited six times that evening and has just begun having diarrhea that "smells disgusting," the combination of which is evidently sufficiently alarming to have prompted her to call the doctor. He, however, treats these as signs of a quite "normal" case of gastroenteritis which, with suitable treatment, will run its usual course until the child recovers – as is clear from the doctor's subsequent diagnosis and advice about treatment.

#10 [1:1:1:3:3–9] ((This extract is taken from the call 2 minutes. 15 seconds after extract [2]))

Doc: . . . . . ˙hh I mean: it- it sounds a little bit (jus')
like'a a touch a' gastroenteritis posh word really for
diarrhea and v(h)omiting i(h)sn't i(h)t? [˙hh You don't really=
Clr: [Yes,
Doc: =need me tuh- ˙hh ta tell ya that but u::m I mean what we
normally do: is if you can just (.) encourages (.) fluids. (.)
and not bother abou:t (.) e:m solids,

The difference between the caller's view of the alarming nature of these symptoms, and the "normal" diagnostic significance which the doctor attributes to the symptoms she has described, is rather diffuse in this call. That is, the doctor's attribution of normality or non-seriousness to these symptoms only emerges later in his diagnosis (lines 1–3 in example [10]) and his advice about treatment (lines 6–7). Frequently the different and non-alarming significance which the doctor attributes to the patient's symptoms is *embedded in* his subsequent diagnosis and advice about treatment: the difference does not rise to the interactional surface of the talk in any *exposed* way (for this distinction, see Jefferson 1987). Briefly, there is some interactional distance between the caller's descriptions of how alarming the symptoms appear to be, and the doctor's "normalization" of those symptoms, and therefore the patient's condition generally.

However, this difference between the caller and doctor in their assessment of the significance of the patient's symptoms is frequently more locally manifest, and hence more exposed or explicit. This often occurs when callers report how long some alarming symptom has been present. Very frequently, indeed in almost every case, callers not only describe symptoms; they also indicate when those symptoms began or how long they have been present. Callers thereby construct the symptoms as alarming, in part, by virtue of their persistence "through the evening," "all morning," "for two hours now," etc.

#11 [1:1:1:3]

1 Clr: 1-> Well this is (.) sort've been since quarter
2 1-> past seven, an'it's nearly quarter past nine now.
3 Doc: et!Yeah! Yeah. ·h No I mean often you find
4 2-> that thu- things do: (.) just settle with a bit'a ti:me,
5 [·hh
6 Clr: [Mmh[m
7 Doc: [U::m, (0.4) so I-ud- (.) give' er a bit
8 a Calpol now,

#12 [1:1:14:1–2]

1 Clr: She's just been really s:(yuhknow), sick bad, you know, ·hh
2 but she's not in l- yuhknow she hasn't any labor pains er
3 anything,
4 Doc: She hasn't. [·hh
5 Clr: [No. hh[h
6 Doc: [And when did this all sta:rt,
7 (0.4)
8 Clr: 1-> She's been like this fer abu- uh: 'bout an hour now,
9 Doc: 2-> Just an hour,
10 Clr: Yeah, [h h h h h h h h]
11 Doc: [·hhh A:um when you say] sick, I mean
12 [(0.4) just vomit]ing.
13 Clr: [h h h h h h h h]
14 Clr: Yes,
15 Doc: That right?
16 .
17 . ((34 lines omitted))
18 .
19 Doc: 2-> ·hhh A:hm (0.8) (b-) it's: I mean it- she's only just started
20 to be sick,

#13 [1:2:8:1]

1 Clr: She's been tryin' clingin' to: me,<>an' then this is sort'u<
2 come to a head. ·hhh I dunno whether she's got mumps or noth'n I
3 j's sor- my husband just said ta phone ya because I'bi-·hh
4 1-> 'cause I se-if [I give 'er Calpo:l, ·h[h u:m
5 Doc: [Yes [You've given her

6 some, have you.
7 Clr: That's right.<we given 'er a dose 'a Calpol and uh .hh
8 Doc: Wh[en did yu-
9 Clr: [tryin'a get drinks down 'er,
10 Doc: >Right.<
11 Clr: A[:n':
12 Doc: [Wu- when did you give 'er some: Calpol.
13 (0.4)
14 Clr: 1-> E:hm: tu- m-well. About a half an hour ago,
15 [(Some'in like) that,
16 Doc: [Righ-
17 Doc: 2-> Ri:ght. So you only just recently given it.

In these examples the callers have constructed accounts of the length of time the patients have been experiencing certain symptoms, in such a way as to convey the possible seriousness of the condition indicated by that length of time (see the first arrowed turns). So in extract (11) the caller constructs an account indicating that her daughter's vomiting and diarrhea have been persisting for nearly two hours (lines 1–2); in example (12), that the patient has been "sick bad . . . fer abu- uh: 'bout an hour now,"; and in excerpt (13), the mother reports administering medication ("Calpo:l," line 4) "half an hour ago," (line 14), without it having had any apparent beneficial effect. In each case, the doctor's response (second arrowed turns) is specifically to downgrade the diagnostic significance of the length of time which the caller reports the symptoms having lasted, succinctly illustrated in this example.

[from example (12)]

Doc: [And when did this all sta:rt,
(0.4)
Clr: 1-> She's been like this fer abu- uh: 'bout an hour now,
Doc: 2-> Just an hour,

The doctor manifestly takes a different view than the caller concerning the diagnostic significance to be attributed to the symptoms the caller reports (or, more precisely, the length of time those symptoms have persisted), this being evident in the downgraded version which he gives in his next turn.

There are other instances which resemble the pattern illustrated in examples (11)–(13): following the caller's report of some alarming symptom, the doctor's response appears to play down the significance which may be attached to that symptom. But, whereas in the previous cases the doctor plays down that significance overtly, through downgrading the time descriptions, in these other cases that is managed much more implicitly – through the doctor citing another symptom, and one which is, in contrast, positive or more optimistic. Here are two examples.

#14 [1:2:13:2]

Clr: ˙h Well, just I should think about half an hour ago. (Um)
they've only let me know within the last few minutes, an' ˙hh
1-> she (had) been very sick before I got there and she has been
1-> vomiting since. ˙hh No blood, (0.2) but-
Doc: R:[ight,
Clr: [You know, she just has (been) sick.
Doc: 2-> R:ight. ˙hh U:m: but otherwise she's been quite well mosta
th'day,

#15 [1:1:8] ((continuation from extract [4]))

Clr: 1-> . . . and she's keeps cryin' because she's hungry, but she
can't eat anything,
Doc: 2-> 'N: is she drinking plenty?
Clr: Yes, she's drinkin' plenty, but it's just goin' straight
through 'er.<As soon as she drinks it

In response to the callers' reports (first arrowed turns) of their daughter vomiting in extract (14) and cries of hunger in example (15), the doctor checks that the patient has been well most of the day, and that she is drinking plenty, respectively (second arrowed turns). These questions focus on what are plainly more optimistic aspects of the patient's condition.[11] Thus the sense that the doctor does not attribute the same (alarming) diagnostic significance to certain symptoms as does the caller is conveyed in his asking a question which *implicitly mitigates* the alarming character of the symptom

[11] It was noted in the previous section, but it is particularly salient here, that the questions are formed to make the optimistic version quite explicit, rather than being asked as an open question – for example, "How has she been during the rest of the day?" or "Is she drinking?," in the case of extract (15). It should be noted also that in confirming that optimistic version in example (15), the caller goes on to counter that optimism by citing another worrying symptom, in the manner discussed in the previous section.

reported by the caller, by juxtaposing that symptom with other more optimistic signs about the patient's condition.

In this section instances have been reviewed of the misalignment between caller and doctor concerning the diagnostic significance (that is to say, seriousness) to be attributed to the symptoms which the caller reports. This misalignment is manifest in the ways in which the doctor, either explicitly or implicitly, gives a downgraded – and hence much less alarming – version of the symptom which the caller reported in his or her prior turn.

Callers' diagnostic hypotheses

The final pattern exhibiting a misalignment between doctor and callers is associated with the hypotheses which callers sometimes have about the ailment from which the patient is suffering. It becomes apparent in some calls that a caller may have a tentative "diagnosis" in mind, an idea, suspicion, or fear about what might be wrong with the patient. However, they do not mention any such hypotheses in their opening reports (that is, before the phase of diagnostic questioning), and usually they do not articulate this suspicion or fear in the earlier stages of his or her questioning. It seems, therefore, that callers may fear that the symptoms may be those of a more serious condition than they are willing to admit outright – and hence they tend to mention those suspicions only later, and in particular circumstances. The following is an instance.

#16 [2:1:2:2]

Doc: .hhh an' this 'as really been going on:: in::
th'las::'- <f'th'las:'> ^week[(you said.)
Clr: [well re:ally.
<I mean the:y- he-'e> seemed alri:ght during th'week,
but then::, (.) as I say yesterday (.) it all came
back again:.=<(an') 'e said I thought this:-> (0.2)
was only s'posed t'() la:st me for twenty four
hours 'e said. .hhh an' I said well u:sually it
does.='e says well my- (.) my p- tummy's still
ever so so:re.
(.)
Doc: hm:. .hhhh hmm, (.) well it doesn't sou:nd I

think- (.) too exci:ting but-=
Clr: --> =no[: . I don't <think of it maybe a> grum:blin'
Doc: [.hhh mm,
Clr: --> appen:dix or: som:ethi:ng. y'kno:w, hh
Doc: *mm* ye:h- well there isn't really such a thi:ng as
a grum:bling appen:di:x,

Some time into this call (1 minute 25 seconds) the caller mentions her hypothesis about what may be causing her son's persistently troubling symptoms; namely, that it might be a "grum'blin' appen:dix" (lines 14 and 16). There are two features of this instance which are characteristic of the manner and circumstances in which callers may articulate such hypotheses. First, the caller refers to the possibility of it being a grumbling appendix in a hedged or qualified manner, prefacing it with "maybe," and concluding with "or: som:ethi:ng.", which has the effect almost of diminishing her suggestion. Second, the caller introduces her hypothesis in response to the doctor having explicitly indicated that he thinks there is nothing much wrong with the patient, "well it doesn't sou:nd I think- (.) too exci:ting" (lines 12–13).[12] The caller has described, and has been asked about, the patient's various worrying symptoms; nevertheless, it is evident in his unspecific but "nothing especially worrying" diagnosis in lines 12–13 that the doctor is moving to a "no-problem," routine disposition of the case. The caller appears to attempt to counter that move by mentioning her concern that it might be a "grumbling appendix"; that is, she proffers her diagnostic hypothesis. Here, as in all such cases in the data, the doctor immediately rejects her hypothesis (lines 17–18), which raises a doubt about a claim made in the research literature that doctors may be more easily misled over the telephone into accepting the patient's self-diagnosis.[13]

[12] "Nothing very exciting" is a standard British idiom – at least among doctors, especially when speaking to patients – for there being nothing seriously amiss.

[13] This is claimed in Curtis and Evens (1995:190). It should be acknowledged that they are referring to the likelihood that physicians might miss the possibility that the patient is suffering from something more serious than the patient thinks might be wrong: "The caller's certainty that he has 'food poisoning' or that she has 'menstrual cramps' may mask a more threatening medical situation, which the physician fails to uncover because he or she accepts the caller's assessment of the problem" (1995:190). Doctors may indeed from time to time misdiagnose a patient's condition from the details reported by the caller, and in particular miss the possibility that the condition is more serious than the patient believes or is indicating. But the evidence from the corpus analyzed here is that doctors are not misled into accepting the caller's diagnosis, specifically.

The misalignment here, then, is associated with the doctor having proposed that the patient's condition is nothing especially to worry about, or presents "no (urgent) problem." In response, the caller immediately (not in overlap, but taking over in line 14 at a point where the doctor had been going to continue)[14] introduces her hypothesis of what might be wrong – one which suggests a rather more serious diagnosis than anything implied in the doctor's prior turn. The position in which this caller introduces her hypothesis is thus one in which the doctor's prior turn is a summary "diagnostic" turn, "it doesn't sou:nd I think- (.) too exci:ting . .". Here then he is completing the phase of diagnostic questioning and moving to a disposition of the case – a disposition in the sense of his giving a diagnosis and advice about treatment. Hence the caller introduces her hypothesis not quite during the diagnostic questioning, but at a point where the doctor appears to be bringing that questioning to an end, without seeming to share the caller's sense of the possible gravity of the case, and in a manner which suggests he is going to advise continued treatment by the caller, without his making a home visit.

There is, then, a sense in which the caller only introduces her hypothesis, perhaps even her "worst fears," about what might be wrong with her child as a *last resort*. She does so only after her previous attempts to convey the possible seriousness of his condition, through describing his symptoms (in the manner outlined on the section on pp. 428–9), have apparently failed to convince the doctor that there is anything particularly the matter with the child. The following, example (17), suggests that introducing a suspicion or hypothesis about what is wrong may indeed be oriented to by callers as a practice of last resort. We have seen in extract (16) that the caller proffers her hypothesis at exactly the point where, from the doctor's summary assessment in lines 12–13, it appears that he may be drawing the questioning to a close without having treated the case as anything more than a "normal," non-urgent case. However, in extract (17) there is evidence that the caller *only* mentions her suspicion at this (possibly final) position. This example suggests

[14] That the doctor had been going to continue is particularly evident from the conjunction at the end of line 13. This "but" only confirms that the turn-thus-far is incomplete: this is only prefatory to his giving his assessment of the case, and possibly also advice about what the caller should do.

that callers may defer introducing such hypotheses until the point at which they see the doctor may be concluding his questioning with a diagnosis of "no special problem." To show this, it is necessary to include in the extract a segment from somewhat earlier in the diagnostic questioning.

#17 [1:1:1]

1	Doc:		Uh: is-was she eating <right today?>
2			up until: lunchtimeish or
3	Clr:		Yeah she ju- she had hu- um: half a cheese sandwich at
4			lunchtime, [( )
5	Doc:		[Right
6	Clr:		an ice cream in a cone and that was it.
7	Doc:	-->	Yeah.˙hh Anyone else:: in the family with: (.) tummy bug or
8			anything?
9	Clr:	-->	No one el[se, touch wood [everyone seems to be okay at the=
10	Doc:		[No, [˙hhh
11	Clr:		m(h)om(h)enth[h
12	Doc:	-->	[Right.<She doesn't go to any' um: play groups
13			or anyni- no- y[ou-
14	Clr:	-->	[No, [she's broken [up now=
15	Doc:		[No, [˙hhh
16	Doc:		Ah: right. ˙hh E:m:, ˙hhh and she's- is she feverish? didju
17			say?

.
. ((91 lines omitted))
.

109	Doc:		I mean often you find that thu- things do: (.) just settle
110			with a bit'a ti:me,
111			[˙hh
112	Clr:		[Mmh[m
113	Doc:		[U::m, (0.4) so I-ud- (.) give 'er a bit
114			a Calpol now, yeah, she's four you say, [˙hh
115	Clr:		[Mm hm,
116	Doc:		So you can give her the maximum (.) dose for a four year old
117			which I think should b[e
118	Clr:		[Two,=
119	Doc:		=Two, yeah. [˙hhh
120	Clr:		[Two five mils,
121	Doc:		Two five mils, that's ri:ght, ˙hh A:um: a:nd in fact I mean
122			if she's not interested in drinking it doesn't matterh. ˙hh

.
. ((6 lines omitted))
.

Doc: Oh i-it< often is a little bit- id it takes a little while
just ta: (0.3) ta settle down.<Normally the vomiting
stops ·h a:h before the diarrhea I mean the diarrhea can
last a couple'a days. If it's just a tummy bug. ·hhhhhmt!
Doc: U[:m
Clr: --> [(well) 'at's the only reason why I was sort of a
--> bit conce[rned, because my nephew's had salmonella,
Doc: [Yeah,
Doc: Ye:s,=
Clr: --> =And um: I do child mindin 'an' an' the mother had salmonella
--> an' she was off work for nine weeks, with it, you know,
Doc: Ri:ght,

The final segment of this extract (see lines 129–140) occurs when the doctor is advising the caller about how best to treat the patient, having diagnosed the child's illness as gastroenteritis, shown as extract (10 above). The caller has, in ways which it is not necessary to consider here, succeeded in "reopening" the questioning and information-giving; but in lines 109–110 the doctor again proffers a summary, "I mean often you find that thu- things do: (.) just settle with a bit'a ti:me," implying there is nothing special to worry about. He continues by giving advice about treatment (lines 113–122), again drawing to a close without having shared the caller's sense of the possible urgency of the case. Then, following his advice about treatment, the doctor gives a further summary assessment, a kind of final prognosis of the case (lines 129–132). The caller can anticipate from this that the doctor might be going to bring the call to a close. At this point she introduces her hypothesis about what she suspects her child might be suffering – salmonella (line 135). Note that in summarizing his assessment of the case, the doctor repeats his earlier assessment that things settle down with time (lines 109–110 and 129–130), and concludes this summary with a repetition of his diagnosis, "If it's just a tummy bug." It is this – and specifically his having constructed that diagnosis in the conditional mood (line 132) – which provides the caller with the opportunity to introduce her hypothesis. She manages this as a kind of "adding to" his diagnosis: she constructs her turn, in such a way as to mention salmonella but without contrasting with or otherwise disputing the doctor's diagnosis (a construction which is assisted by the possibility that salmonella can be considered a form of "tummy bug").

What is clear from the first segment reproduced in this extract (lines 1–17) is that the caller had an earlier opportunity to mention her suspicion that her child might be suffering from something he has contracted from her nephew, namely salmonella. The doctor asks specifically whether anyone else in the family has a tummy bug (lines 7–8); his further question about whether she goes to a play group (lines 12–13) might perhaps have given her a further opportunity (perhaps, "No, but she's been playing with her cousin who's had salmonella . . . "). These were clear opportunities to have mentioned her concern about salmonella at an earlier point during the diagnostic question. The fact of her not doing so here, but instead only when it appears that the doctor may be about to close, continuing to assess the case as something quite normal (". . *just* a tummy bug"), is evidence for her introducing her hypothesis only as a last resort, when it appears that the doctor may be about to close, without having accepted her view about the possible seriousness of the case, without having addressed what really concerns her might be wrong, and without having agreed to visit the patient at home.

Therefore in this third pattern of misalignment between caller and doctor, the caller anticipates that the doctor is about to close by treating the patient's condition as non-urgent (no special cause for alarm), and without offering to make a home visit. The caller responds by making a "last resort" attempt to convey the possible seriousness or urgency of the patient's condition. This is done by abandoning describing of the patient's particular and alarming symptoms, and instead mentioning (albeit tentatively) the suspicions that he or she has about what might be wrong. Thus the caller articulates his or her hypothesis about what the patient may be suffering from – an hypothesis which may have been the organizing frame for interpreting the symptoms as alarming or a cause for special concern. In other words, it may be that it is not so much the symptoms in themselves which are alarming to callers; rather, it may be their suspicions/hypotheses about what the symptoms signify – what they are possibly symptoms of – that are the cause of their concern. That is a rather speculative point for the present. Nevertheless, the pattern of misalignment between the doctor's treatment of the cases as non-urgent, and the caller's continued concern that the case may be more serious than the doctor seems prepared to allow, is manifest in the kind of instances shown in this section, in which callers respond to and counter the doctor's closing-relevant and "normalizing" (optimistic) summaries by introducing their more alarming diagnostic hypotheses.

Conclusion

There is a general sense in which there is a misalignment between the perceptions of physicians, and those making after-hours calls for emergency care (e.g., a home visit), concerning the "abnormality" and hence urgency of a patient's condition. Callers make the decision to telephone the doctor after hours (and sometimes at "unsocial" hours in the middle of the night) specifically because they are alarmed by the patient's condition, and feel that the matter may be urgent and cannot wait until the clinic/surgery is next open.[15] However, those symptoms which are regarded by callers as abnormal and therefore alarming are quite likely to be viewed by a doctor as "normal" signs of a "normal" ailment, which needs only regular treatment by the carer in order for the patient to recover according to the usual course taken by such an ailment. This misalignment between callers and doctors regarding what are "normal" and "abnormal" symptoms is manifest both in the statistical (in)frequency with which doctors decide to make a home visit (in this corpus, but also reported in studies more widely), and in the proportion of calls which physicians regard as having been made unnecessarily (John and Curtis 1988).

However, the three patterns exhibited in, and which appear to be characteristic of, the interactions between callers and doctor during the phase of diagnostic questioning in after-hours calls indicate that the misalignment between them is salient in the interactions between them over the telephone. These patterns of misalignment do not become salient in the sense of generating misunderstandings or overt conflicts between them (though, of course, misunderstandings

[15] For a useful analysis of the accounts which callers give for making after-hours calls in the British system, see Hopton et al. (1996). They make the point that "decisions to seek medical help are based on ideas about normal and abnormal illness" (1996:994), and that callers' ideas about abnormality of a patient's condition need to be understood in the context of the medical history of the patient ("past frights"), their previous attempts to manage the problem, awareness of specific illnesses and their possibly innocuous symptoms (e.g., meningitis), and their previous experiences of health services and health professionals.

do commonly occur).[16] Nor is this to make any claim that these patterns have any bearing on the extent to which callers/patients are satisfied with the service which doctors provide over the telephone – and specifically their possible dissatisfaction with doctors' decisions not to make a home visit.[17] These patterns are salient only in so far as they manifest different perceptions of the "abnormality" and "normality" of symptoms described by callers, and ways in which each (that is, caller and doctor) resists – albeit implicitly, and perhaps passively – the other's apparent assessment of the seriousness or urgency of the ailment/condition which those symptoms may betoken.

[16] For a review of aspects of misunderstandings in medical consultations see West and Frankel (1991).

[17] Most studies report generally high levels of caller satisfaction with the care provided by physicians in after-hours calls: for details, including comparisons of patient satisfaction when dealt with by their own doctors and deputizing doctors, see McKinley et al. (1997a, 1997b), Hopton et al. (1996), Evens et al. (1985), and Hallam (1994).

References

Abbott, Andrew (1988). *The System of Professions: An Essay on the Division of Expert Labor*. Chicago and London: University of Chicago Press.

Angell, M. (1994). "The doctor as double agent." *Kennedy Institute for Ethics Journal* 3:279–86.

Arborelius, E., Bremberg, S., and Timpka, T. (1991). "What is going on when the general practitioner doesn't grasp the situation?" *Family Practice* 8:3–9.

Armstrong, D. (1983). *The Political Anatomy of the Body: Medical Knowledge in Britain in the Twentieth Century*. Cambridge: Cambridge University Press.

Arney, W. R. and Bergen, B. J. (1984). *Medicine and the Management of Living*. Chicago: University of Chicago Press.

Atkinson, J. Maxwell (1982). "Understanding formality: notes on the categorisation and production of 'formal' interaction." *British Journal of Sociology* 33:86–117.

Atkinson, J. Maxwell and Drew, Paul (1979). *Order in Court: The Organisation of Verbal Interaction in Judicial Settings*. London: Macmillan.

Atkinson, J. Maxwell and Heritage, John (1984). *Structures of Social Action: Studies in Conversation Analysis*. Cambridge: Cambridge University Press.

Atkinson, Paul (1995). *Medical Talk and Medical Work*. London: Sage.

Atkinson, Paul (1999). "Medical discourse, evidentiality and the construction of professional responsibility." In Srikant Sarangi and Celia Roberts (eds.) *Talk, Work and Institutional Order: Discourse in Medical, Mediation and Management Settings*. Berlin: Mouton De Gruyter, pp. 75–107.

Bakeman, R. and Gottman, J. M. (1986). *Observing Interaction: An Introduction to Sequential Analysis*. Cambridge: Cambridge University Press.

Bales, R. F. (1950). *Interaction Process Analysis: A Method for the Study of Small Groups*. Reading, MA: Addison-Wesley.

Balint, Michael (1957). *The Doctor, His Patient and the Illness*. London: Pitman.

Baquero, F., Baquero-Artigao, G., Canton, R., and Garcia-Rey, C. (2002). "Antibiotic consumption and resistance selection in Streptococcus pneumoniae." *Journal of Antimicrobial Chemotherapy* 50 (Supplement C):27–38.

Barden, L. S., Dowell, S. F., Schwartz, B., and Lackey, C. (1998). "Current attitudes regarding use of antimicrobial agents: results from physicians' and parents' focus group discussions." *Clinical Pediatrics* 37:665–72.

Barsky, A. J. (1981). "Hidden reasons some patients visit doctors." *Annals of Internal Medicine* 94:492–8.

Bates, Barbara, Bickley, Lynn S., and Hoekelman, Robert A. (1995). *Physical Examination and History Taking*, 6th edition. Philadelphia, PA: J. B. Lippincott Company.

Beach, Wayne A. (1993). "Transitional regularities for casual 'okay' usages." *Journal of Pragmatics* 19:325–52.

Beach, Wayne A. (1995). "Preserving and constraining options: 'okays' and 'official' priorities in medical interviews." In Bud Morris and Ron Chenail (eds.) *Talk of the Clinic*. Hillsdale, NJ: Lawrence Erlbaum.

Becker, G., Janson-Bjerklie, S., Benner, P., Slobin, K., and Ferketich, S. (1993). "The dilemma of seeking urgent care: asthma episodes and emergency service use." *Social Science and Medicine* 37(3):305–13.

Becker, Howard S., Geer, Blanche, Strauss, Anselm L., and Hughes, Everett C. (1961). *Boys in White: Student Culture in Medical School*. Chicago: University of Chicago Press.

Beckman, Howard and Frankel, Richard M. (1984). "The effect of physician behavior on the collection of data." *Annals of Internal Medicine* 101:692–6.

Bergh, K. D. (1998). "The patient's differential diagnosis: unpredictable concerns in visits for acute cough." *Journal of Family Practice* 46(2):153–8.

Bergmann, Jorg (1992). "Veiled morality: notes on discretion in psychiatry." In P. Drew and J. Heritage (eds.) *Talk at Work: Interaction in Institutional Settings*. Cambridge: Cambridge University Press, pp. 137–62.

Bergmann, Jorg (1993). *Discreet Indiscretions: The Social Organization of Gossip*. Hawthorne, NY: Aldine De Gruyter.

Billig, Michael, Condor, Susan, Edwards, Derek, Gane, Mike, Middleton, David, and Radley, Alan (1988). *Ideological Dilemmas: The Sociology of Everyday Thinking*. London: Sage.

Billings, J. A. and Stoeckle, J. D. (1989). *The Clinical Encounter: A Guide to the Medical Interview and Case Presentation*. Chicago, IL: Year Book Medical Publishers.

Blanchard, C. G., Labrecque, M. S., Ruckdeschel, J. C., and Blanchard, E. B. (1988). "Information and decision-making preferences of hospitalized adult cancer patients." *Social Science and Medicine* 27(11):1139–45.

Bloor, Michael (1976). "Bishop Berkeley and the adeno-tonsillectomy enigma: an exploration of variation in the social construction of medical diagnosis." *Sociology* 10:43–61.

Bloor, Michael (1997). *Selected Writings in Medical Sociological Research*. Aldershot: Ashgate.

Bloor, Michael and Horobin, Gordon (1975). "Conflict and conflict resolution in doctor-patient interactions." In C. Cox and A. Mead (eds.) *A Sociology of Medical Practice*. London: Collier Macmillan, pp. 271–85.

Borzo, G. (1997). "Consumer drug ads booming: FDA reviews restrictions." *American Medical News* 40(6):1, 37.

Bosk, Charles L. (1979). *Forgive and Remember: Managing Medical Failure*. Chicago: University of Chicago Press.

Boyd, Elizabeth (1998). "Bureaucratic authority in the 'company of equals': the interactional management of medical peer review." *American Sociological Review* 63(2):200–24.

Braddock, C. H., Edwards, K. A., Hasenberg, N. M., Laidley, T. L., and Levinson, W. (1999). "Informed decision making in outpatient practice: time to get back to basics." *Journal of the American Medical Association*, 282(24):2313–20.

Bradley, C. P. (1992). "Uncomfortable prescribing decisions: a critical incident study." *British Medical Journal* 304:294–6.

Bredmar, Margareta and Linell, Per (1999). "Reconfirming normality: the constitution of reassurance in talks between midwives and expectant mothers." In Srikant Sarangi and Celia Roberts (eds.) *Talk, Work and Institutional Order: Discourse in Medical, Mediation and Management Settings*. Berlin: Mouton De Gruyter, pp. 237–70.

Bresler, D. E. (1979). *Free Yourself from Pain*. New York: Simon and Schuster.

Brody, D. S. (1980). "The patient's role in clinical decision-making." *Annals of Internal Medicine* 93:718–22.

Brody, D. S., Miller, S. M., Lerman, C. E., Smith, D. G., Lazaro, C. G., and Blum, M. J. (1989). "The relationship between patients' satisfaction with their physicians and perceptions about interventions they desired and received." *Medical Care* 27(11):1027–35.

Brody, D. S., Miller, S. M., Lerman, C., Smith, M. D., and Caputo, C. (1989). "Patient perception of involvement in medical care: relationship to illness attitudes and outcomes." *Journal of General Internal Medicine* 4:506–11.

Brody, H. (1987). *Stories of Sickness*. New Haven, CN: Yale University Press.

Brown, C. S., Wright, R. G., and Christensen, D. B. (1987). "Association between type of medication instruction and patients' knowledge, side effects and compliance." *Hospital and Community Psychiatry* 38:55–60.

Brown, Judith Belle, Stewart, Moira, and Ryan, Bridget L. (2003). "Outcomes of patient–provider interaction." In T. Thompson, A. Dorsey, K. Miller, and R. Parrott (eds.) *Handbook of Health Communication*. Mahwah, NJ: Lawrence Erlbaum.

Brown, Penelope and Levinson, Stephen (1987). *Politeness: Some Universals in Language Usage*. Cambridge: Cambridge University Press.

Brown, Phil (1995). "Naming and framing: the social construction of diagnosis and illness." *Journal of Health and Social Behavior* 35 (extra issue):34–52.

Buckman, Robert (1984). "Breaking bad news: why is it still so difficult?" *British Medical Journal* 288:1597–9.

Butler, C. C., Kinnersley, P., Prout, H., Rollnick, S., Edwards, A., and Elwyn, G. (2001). "Antibiotics and shared decision making in primary care." *Journal of Antimicrobial Chemotherapy* 48:435–40.

Butler, C. C., Rollnick, S., Pill, R., Maggs-Rapport, F., and Stott, N. (1998). "Understanding the culture of prescribing: qualitative study of general practitioners' and patients' perceptions of antibiotics for sore throats." *British Medical Journal* 317:637–42.

Button, Graham (1985). "End of an award report: the social organization of topic closure in naturally occurring conversation." G00230092. London: Economic and Social Research Council.

Button, Graham (1987). "Moving out of closings." In G. Button and J. R. E. Lee (eds.) *Talk and Social Organisation*. Clevedon, England: Multilingual Matters, pp. 101–51.

Button, Graham (1990a). "On members' time." In B. Conein, M. de Fornel, and L. Quere (eds.) *Les Formes de la Conversation*, vol. I. Paris: CNET, pp. 161–82.

Button, Graham (1990b). "On varieties of closings." In G. Psathas (ed.) *Interaction Competence*. Lanham, MD: International Institute for Ethnomethodology and Conversation Analysis University Press of America, pp. 93–148.

Button, Graham (1991). "Conversation-in-a-series." In D. Boden and D. H. Zimmerman (eds.) *Talk and Social Structure*. Berkeley: University of California Press, pp. 251–77.

Button, Graham and Casey, Neil (1984). "Generating topic: the use of topic initial elicitors." In J. M. Atkinson and J. Heritage (eds.) *Structures of Social Action: Studies in Conversation Analysis*. Cambridge: Cambridge University Press, pp. 167–90.

Button, Graham and Casey, Neil (1985). "Topic nomination and topic pursuit." *Human Studies* 8(3):3–55.

Button, Graham and Lee, John R. E. (eds.) (1987). *Talk and Social Organisation*. Clevedon: Multilingual Matters.

Byrne, Patrick S. and Long, Barrie E. L. (1976). *Doctors Talking to Patients: A Study of the Verbal Behaviours of Doctors in the Consultation.* London: Her Majesty's Stationery Office.

Carroll, J. Gregory (1995). "Evaluation of medical interviewing: concepts and principles." In Mack Lipkin, Samuel Putnam, and Aaron Lazare (eds.) *The Medical Interview: Clinical Care, Education and Research.* New York, Springer Verlag, pp. 451–9.

Cassell, Eric J. (1985a). *Talking with Patients,* vol. I, *The Theory of Doctor-Patient Communication.* Cambridge, MA: MIT Press.

Cassell, Eric J. (1985b). *Talking with Patients,* vol. II, *Clinical Technique.* Cambridge, MA: MIT Press.

Cassell, Eric J. (1991). *The Nature of Suffering and the Goals of Medicine.* New York: Oxford University Press.

Cassell, Eric J. (1997). *Doctoring: The Nature of Primary Care in Medicine.* New York: Oxford University Press.

Cassileth, B. R., Zupkis, R. V., Sutton-Smith, K., and March, V. (1980). "Information and participation preferences among cancer patients." *Annals of Internal Medicine* 92:832–6.

Chafe, W. (1986). "Evidentiality in English conversation and academic writing." In W. Chafe and J. Nichols (eds.) *Evidentiality: The Linguistic Coding of Epistemology.* Norwood, NJ: Ablex, pp. 261–72.

Chafe, W. and J. Nichols (eds.) (1986). *Evidentiality: The Linguistic Coding of Epistemology.* Norwood, NJ: Ablex.

Charon, Rita, Greene, Michele J., and Adelman, Ronald D. (1994). "Multidimensional interaction analysis: a collaborative approach to the study of medical discourse." *Social Science and Medicine* 39(7): 955–65.

Cicourel, Aaron (1983). "Hearing is not believing: language and the structure of belief in medical communication." In S. Fisher and A. Todd (eds.) *The Social Organization of Doctor–Patient Communication.* Washington, DC: Center for Applied Linguistics, pp. 221–39.

Clair, Jeffrey M. and Allman, Richard M. (1993). *Sociomedical Perspectives on Patient Care.* Lexington: University of Kentucky Press.

Clayman, Steven (1989). "The production of punctuality: social interaction, temporal organization, and social structure." *American Journal of Sociology* 95(3):659–91.

Clayman, Steven and Gill, Virginia Teas (2004). "Conversation analysis." In A. Byman and M. Hardy (eds.) *Handbook of Data Analysis.* Beverly Hills: Sage, pp. 589–606.

Clayman, Steven E. and Heritage, John (2002a). *The News Interview: Journalists and Public Figures on the Air.* Cambridge: Cambridge University Press.

Clayman, Steven E. and Heritage, John (2002b). "Questioning presidents: journalistic deference and adversarialness in the press conferences of Eisenhower and Reagan." *Journal of Communication* 52(4):749–75.

Clyne, M. (1961). *Night Calls: A Study in General Practice*. London: Tavistock.

Cohen-Cole, Steven A. (1991). *The Medical Interview: The Three Function Approach*. St. Louis, MO: Mosby Year Book.

Cohen-Cole, Steven A., and Bird, Julian (1991). "Function 3: education, negotiation, and motivation." In Steven A. Cohen-Cole, *The Medical Interview: The Three Function Approach*. St. Louis, MO: Mosby Year Book, Chapter 5.

Conrad, Peter (1988). "Learning to doctor: reflections on recent accounts of the medical school years." *Journal of Health and Social Behavior* 29:323–32.

Conrad, Peter and Schneider, Joseph W. (1992). *Deviance and Medicalization*. Philadelphia: Temple University Press.

Converse, Jean M. (1987). *Survey Research in the United States: Roots and Emergence 1890–1960*. Berkeley: University of California Press.

Coulehan, John L. and Block, Marian (1987). *The Medical Interview: A Primer for Students of the Art*. Philadelphia: F. A. Davis Company.

Coupland, J., Robinson, J., and Coupland, N. (1994). "Frame negotiation in doctor–elderly patient consultations." *Discourse and Society* 5(1): 89–124.

Cragg, D. K., McKinley, R. K., Roland, M. O., Campbell, S. M., Van, F., Hastings, A. M., French, D. P., Mankn Scott, T. K., and Roberts, C. (1997). "Comparison of out of hours care provided by patients' own general practioners and commercial deputising services: a randomised controlled trial. I: the process of care," *British Medical Journal* 314:187–9.

Cristino, J. M. (1999). "Correlation between consumption of antimicrobials in humans and development of resistance in bacteria." *International Journal of Antimicrobial Agents* 12(3):199–202.

Curtis, P. and Evens, S. (1995). "The telephone interview." In M. Lipkin, S. M. Putnam, and A. Lazare (eds.) *The Medical Interview: Clinical Care, Education, and Research*. New York: Springer-Verlag, pp. 187–95.

Darwin, C. (1979). *The Expressions of Emotions in Man and Animals*. London: Julian Freidman. First published 1872.

Davidson, J. A. (1984). "Subsequent versions of invitations, offers, requests and proposals dealing with potential or actual rejection." In J. M. Atkinson and J. C. Heritage (eds.) *Structures of Social Action: Studies in Conversation Analysis*. Cambridge: Cambridge University Press, pp. 102–28.

Davis, Fred (1963). *Passage Through Crisis: Polio Victims and Their Families*. Indianapolis: Bobbs-Merrill.

Deber, R. B. (1994). "Physicians in health care management: the patient-physician partnership: decision making, problem solving and the desire to participate." *Canadian Medical Association Journal* 151(4):423–7.

Deeks, S. L., Palacio, R., Ruvinsky, R., Kertesz, D. A., Hortal, M., Rossi, A., Spika, J. S., and DiFabio, J. L. (1999). "Risk factors and course of illness among children with invasive penicillin-resistant Streptococcus pneumoniae: the Streptococcus pneumoniae working group." *Pediatrics* 103(2):409–13.

Drew, Paul (1984). "Speakers' reportings in invitation sequences." In J. M. Atkinson and J. Heritage (eds.) *Structures of Social Action: Studies in Conversation Analysis.* Cambridge: Cambridge University Press, pp. 129–51.

Drew, Paul (1991). "Asymmetries of knowledge in conversational interactions." In I. Markova and K. Foppa (eds.) *Asymmetries in Dialogue.* Hemel Hempstead, UK: Harvester Wheatsheaf, pp. 21–48.

Drew, Paul (1992). "Contested evidence in a courtroom cross-examination: the case of a trial for rape." In P. Drew and J. Heritage (eds.) *Talk at Work: Interaction in Institutional Settings.* Cambridge: Cambridge University Press, pp. 470–520.

Drew, Paul (1997). "'Open' class repair initiators in response to sequential sources of trouble in conversation." *Journal of Pragmatics* 28:69–101.

Drew, Paul (2002). "Out of context: an intersection between life and the workplace, as contexts for (business) talk." *Language and Communication* 22:477–94.

Drew, Paul and Heritage, John (1992). "Analyzing talk at work: an introduction." In P. Drew and J. Heritage (eds.) *Talk at Work: Interaction in Institutional Settings.* Cambridge: Cambridge University Press, pp. 3–65.

Drew, Paul and Holt, Elizabeth (1988). "Complainable matters: the use of idiomatic expressions in making complaints." *Social Problems* 35:398–417.

Drew, Paul and Holt, Elizabeth (1998). "Figures of speech: idomatic expressions and the management of topic transition in conversation." *Language in Society* 27(4):495–523.

Drew, Paul and Sorjonen, Marja-Leena (1997). "Institutional dialogue." In T. A. van Dijk (ed.) *Discourse: A Multidisciplinary Introduction.* London: Sage, pp. 92–118.

Dreyfus, Hubert L. and Rabinow, Paul (1982). *Michel Foucault: Beyond Structuralism and Hermeneutics.* Chicago: University of Chicago Press.

Drummund, Kent and Hopper, Robert (1993). "Backchannels revisited: acknowledgment tokens and speakership incipiency." *Research on Language and Social Interaction* 26:157–77.

du Pré, A. (2000). *Communicating about Health: Current Issues and Perspectives.* Mountain View, CA: Mayfield.

Elwyn, G., Edwards, A., and Kinnersley, P. (1999). "Shared decision-making in primary care: the neglected second half of the consultation." *British Journal of General Practice* 49:477–82.

Emanuel, E. J. and Emanuel, L. L. (1992). "Four models of the physician-patient relationship." Journal of the American Medical Association 267:2221–6.

Emerson, Joan (1970). "Behaviour in private places: sustaining definitions of reality in gynaecological examinations." In H. P. Dreitzel (ed.) *Recent Sociology*. New York: Macmillan, pp. 73–100.

Emerson, C. (1983). "Bakhtin and Vygotsky on internalization in language." *Quarterly Newsletter of the Laboratory of Comparative Human Cognition* 5(1):9–13.

Ende, J., Kazis, L., Ash, A., and Moskowitz, M. A. (1989). "Measuring patients' desire for autonomy: decision making and information-seeking preferences among medical patients." *Journal of General Internal Medicine* 4:23–30.

Engel, George L. (1997). "The need for a new medical model: a challenge for biomedicine." *Science* 196:129–36.

Engeström, Y., Engeström, R., Helenius, J., Koistinen, K., Rekola, J., and Saarelma, O. (1989). *Terveyskeskuslääkäreiden työn kehittämistutkimus* (*Developmental Research Project on the Work of Health Centre Physicians*). LEVIKE-projektin tutkimushankkeen III väliraportti. Lääkärinvastaanottojen analysointia. Espoo: Espoon kaupungin terveysvirasto.

Erickson, Frederick (1999). "Appropriation of voice and presentation of self as a fellow physician: aspects of a discourse of apprenticeship in medicine." In Srikant Sarangi and Celia Roberts (eds.) *Talk, Work and Institutional Order: Discourse in Medical, Mediation and Management Settings*. Berlin: Mouton De Gruyter, pp. 109–44.

Evans, B. J., Kiellerup, F. D., Stanley, R. O., Burrows, G. D., and Sweet, B. (1987). "A communications skills programme for increasing patients' satisfaction with general practice consultations." *British Journal of Medical Psychology* 60:373–8.

Evens, S., Curtis, P., Talbot, A., and Smart, A. (1985). "Characteristics and perceptions of after-hours callers." *Family Practice* 2:10–16.

Faden, R. R., Becker, C., Lewis, C., Freeman, J., and Faden, A. I. (1981). "Disclosure of information to patients in medical care." *Medical Care* 19:718–33.

Fallowfield, Lesley (1991). *Breast Cancer*. London: Tavistock/Routledge.

Fallowfield, L., Hall, A., Maguire, G. P., and Baum, M. (1990). "Psychological outcomes of different treatment policies in women with early breast cancer outside a clinical trial." *British Medical Journal* 301:575–80.

Fallowfield, Lesley J. and Lipkin, Mack (1995). "Delivering sad or bad news." In Mack Lipkin, Samuel Putnam, and Aaron Lazare (eds.) *The Medical Interview: Clinical Care, Education, and Research*. New York: Springer-Verlag, pp. 316–23.

Fisher, Sue (1984). "Doctor-patient communication: a social and micro-political performance." *Sociology of Health and Illness* 6:1–27.

Fisher, Sue (1986). *In the Patients' Best Interest: Women and the Politics of Medical Decisions*. New Brunswick, NJ: Rutgers University Press.

Fisher, Sue (1991). "A discourse of the social: medical talk/power talk/oppositional talk?" *Discourse and Society* 2(2):157–82.

Fisher, Sue and Groce, Stephen (1990). "Accounting practices in medical interviews." *Language in Society* 19:225–50.

Fisher, Sue and Todd, Alexandre (eds.) (1993). *The Social Organization of Doctor-Patient Communication*. Norwood, NJ: Ablex.

Fitzpatrick, Ray (1996). "Telling patients there is nothing wrong." *British Medical Journal* 313:311–12.

Fitzpatrick, R. and Hopkins, A. (1981). "Referrals to neurologists for headaches not due to structural disease." *Journal of Neurology, Neurosurgery, and Psychiatry* 44:1061–7.

Foucault, M. (1972). *The Archaeology of Knowledge*. New York: Harper Colophon.

Foucault, M. (1975). *The Birth of the Clinic: An Archaeology of Medical Perception*. New York: Vintage Books.

Fox, Renee C. (1957). "Training for uncertainty." In R. Merton, G. Reeder, and P. Kendall (eds.) *The Student-Physician*. Cambridge: Harvard University Press, 207–41.

Fox, Renee C. (1963). "Training for 'detached concern' in medical students." In H. I. Lief, V. F. Lief, and N. R. Lief (eds.) *The Psychological Basis of Medical Practice*. New York: Harper and Row, pp. 12–35.

Fox, Renee C. (1989). *The Sociology of Medicine: A Participant Observer's View*. Englewood Cliffs, NJ: Prentice Hall.

Francis, V., Korsch, B. M., and Morris, M. J. (1969). "Gaps in doctor-patient communication: patients' response to medical advice." *New England Journal of Medicine* 280:535–40.

Frankel, Richard M. (1984a). "From sentence to sequence: understanding the medical encounter through microinteractional analysis." *Discourse Processes* 7:135–70.

Frankel, Richard M. (1984b). "The laying on of hands: aspects of organisation of gaze, touch and talk in a medical encounter." In S. Fisher and A. D. Todd (eds.) *The Social Organization of Doctor–Patient Communication*. Washington: Centre for Applied Linguistics, pp. 19–54.

Frankel, Richard M. (1990). "Talking in interviews: a dispreference for patient initiated questions in physician-patient encounters." In G. Psathas (ed.) *Interaction Competence: Studies in Ethnomethodology and Conversational Analysis*. Lanham, MD: University Press of America, pp. 231–62.

Frankel, Richard M. (1994). "Communicating bad news to patients and families." *Physician's Quarterly* 9:1–3.

Frankel, Richard M. (1995a). "Emotion and the physician-patient relationship." *Motivation and Emotion* 19:163–73.

Frankel, Richard M. (1995b). "Some answers about questions in clinical interviews." In G. H. Morris and R. J. Chenail (eds.) *The Talk of the Clinic: Explorations in the Analysis of Medical and Therapeutic Discourse*. Hillsdale, NJ: Lawrence Erlbaum, pp. 223–57.

Frankel, Richard M. (1996). "Asymmetry in the doctor-patient relationship: are we looking in all the right places?" In B. Nordberg (ed.) *Samspel och variation*. Institutionen for nordiska sprak: Uppsala universitet, pp. 121–30.

Frankel, Richard M., Quill, Timothy E., and McDaniel, Susan H. (eds.) (2003). *The Biopsychosocial Approach: Past, Present, Future*. Rochester, NY: University of Rochester Press.

Freeman, S. H. (1987). "Health promotion talk in family practice encounters." *Social Science and Medicine* 25(8):961–6.

Freemon, B., Negrete, V., Davis, M., and Korsch, B. (1971). "Gaps in doctor-patient communication: doctor-patient interaction analysis." *Pediatric Research* 5:298–311.

Freese, Jeremy and Maynard, Douglas W. (1998). "Prosodic features of bad news and good news in conversation." *Language in Society* 27:195–219.

Freidson, Eliot (1970a). *Profession of Medicine: A Study of the Sociology of Applied Knowledge*. Chicago: University of Chicago Press.

Freidson, Eliot (1970b). *Professional Dominance*. Chicago: Aldine.

Freidson, Eliot (1975a). "Dilemmas in the doctor/patient relationship." In Caroline Cox and Adrianne Mead (eds.) *A Sociology of Medical Practice*. London: Collier-MacMillan.

Freidson, Eliot (1975b). *Doctoring Together: A Study of Professional Social Control*. Chicago: University of Chicago Press.

Freidson, Eliot (1986). *Professional Powers: A Study of the Institutionalization of Formal Knowledge*. Chicago: University of Chicago Press.

Freidson, Eliot (1988). "Afterword." In Elliot Freidson (ed.) *Profession of Medicine: A Study of the Sociology of Applied Knowledge*. Chicago: University of Chicago Press.

Frosch, Dominick L. and Kaplan, Robert M. (1999). "Shared decision making in clinical medicine: past research and future directions." *American Journal of Preventive Medicine* 27(11):1139–45.

Gardner, R. (1997). "The conversation object Mm: a weak and variable acknowledging token." *Research on Language and Social Interaction* 30(2):131–56.

Garfinkel, Harold (1967). *Studies in Ethnomethodology*. Englewood Cliffs, NJ: Prentice Hall.

Garfinkel, H. and Sacks, H. (1970). "On formal structures of practical actions." In J. C. McKinney and E. A. Tiryakian (eds.) *Theoretical Sociology*. New York, NY: Appleton-Century-Crofts, pp. 338–66.

Gill, Virginia Teas (1995). "The organization of patients' explanations and doctors' responses in clinical interaction." Unpublished dissertation, University of Wisconsin-Madison.

Gill, Virginia Teas (1998a). "Doing attributions in medical interactions: patients' explanations for illness and doctors' responses." *Social Psychology Quarterly* 61(4):342–60.

Gill, Virginia Teas (1998b). "The interactional construction of lay and professional roles: patients' candidate explanations for illness and doctors' responses." Paper presented at the Netherlands Institute for Primary Health Care conference on Communication in Health Care, June 1998.

Gill, Virginia Teas, Halkowski, Timothy, and Roberts, Felicia (2001). "Accomplishing a request without making one: a single case analysis of a primary care visit." *Text* 21:55–81.

Girgis, Afaf and Sanson-Fisher, Rob W. (1995). "Breaking bad news: consensus guidelines for medical practitioners." *Journal of Clinical Oncology* 13:2449–56.

Gladwin, T. (1964). "Culture and logical process." In W. H. Goodenough (ed.), *Explorations in Cultural Anthropology: Essays in Honor of George Peter Mudock*. New York: McGraw Hill, pp. 167–77.

Goffman, Erving (1955). "On face work: an analysis of ritual elements in social interaction." *Psychiatry* 18(3):213–31.

Goffman, Erving (1956). "Embarrassment and social organisation." *American Journal of Sociology* 62:264–74.

Goffman, Erving (1961). Encounters: Two Studies in the Sociology of Interaction. New York: Bobbs-Merrill Press.

Goffman, Erving (1963). *Behaviour in Public Places*. New York: The Free Press.

Goffman, Erving (1967). *Interaction Ritual*. Garden City, NY: Anchor/ Doubleday.

Goffman, Erving (1978). "Response cries." *Language* 54:787–815.

Goffman, Erving (1981). *Forms of Talk*. Oxford: Blackwell.

Goffman, Erving (1983). "The interaction order." *American Sociological Review* 48:1–17.

Golin, Carol E., DiMatteo, M. Robin, and Gelberg, Lillian (1996). "The role of patient participation in the doctor visit: implications for diabetes care." *Diabetes Care* 19(10):1153–64.

Gomez, J., Banos, V., Ruiz Gomez, J., Herrero, F., Nunez, M. L., Canteras, M., and Valdez, M. (1995). "Clinical significance of pneumococcal bacteraemias in a general hospital: a prospective study 1989–1993." *Journal of Antimicrobial Chemotherapy* 36(6):1021–30.

Goodwin, Charles (1979). "The interactive construction of a sentence in natural conversation." In George Psathas (ed.) *Everyday Language: Studies in Ethnomethodology*. New York: Irvington Publishers, pp. 97–121.

Goodwin, Charles (1981). *Conversational organization: Interaction Between Speakers and Hearers*. New York: Academic Press.

Goodwin, Charles (1986). "Between and within: alternative sequential treatments of continuers and assessments." *Human Studies* 9:205–17.

Goodwin, Charles (1994). "Professional vision." *American Anthropologist* 96:606–33.

Goodwin, Charles (1996). "Transparent vision." In E. Ochs, E. A. Schegloff, and S. A. Thompson (eds.) *Interaction and Grammar*. Cambridge: Cambridge University Press, pp. 370–404.

Goodwin, Charles and Heritage, John (1990). "Conversation analysis." *Annual Review of Anthropology* 19:283–307.

Goold, Susan Dorr and Lipkin, Mack (1999). "The doctor-patient relationship: challenges, opportunities, and strategies." *Journal of General Internal Medicine* 14:S26–S33.

Gray, Bradford H. (1991). *The Profit Motive and Patient Care: The Changing Accountability of Doctors and Hospitals*. Cambridge, MA: Harvard University Press.

Greatbatch, D., Heath, C. C., Campion, P., and Luff, P. (1995a). "How do desk-top computers affect the doctor-patient interaction?" *Family Practice* 12(1):32–6.

Greatbatch, D., Heath, C. C., Luff, P., and Campion, P. (1995b). "Conversation analysis: human-computer interaction and the general practice consultation." In A. Monk and N. Gilbert (eds.) *Perspectives on Human-Computer Interaction*. London: Academic Press, pp. 199–222.

Greatbatch, D., Luff, P., Heath, C., and Campion, P. (1993). "Interpersonal communication and human-computer interaction: an examination of the use of computers in medical consultations." *Interacting with Computers* 5(2):193–216.

Greenberger, Norton J., and Hinthorn, Daniel R. (1993). *History Taking and Physical Examination: Essentials and Clinical Correlates*. St. Louis, MO: Mosby Year Book.

Greenfield, S. H., Kaplan, S., and Ware, J. E. (1985). "Expanding patient involvement in care: effects on patient outcomes." *Annals of Internal Medicine* 102:520–8.

Greenfield, S., Kaplan, S. H., Ware, J. E., Yano, E., and Frank, J. L. H. (1988). "Patients' participation in medical care: effects on blood sugar control and quality of life in diabetes." *Journal of General Internal Medicine* 3:448–57.

Guthrie, Anna (1997). "On the systematic deployment of okay and mmhmm in academic advising sessions." *Pragmatics* 7(3):397–415.

Haakana, Markku (1999). "Laughing matters: a conversation analytic study of laughter in doctor-patient interaction." Unpublished doctoral dissertation, University of Helsinki.

Haakana, Markku (2001). "Laughter as a patient's resource: dealing with delicate aspects of medical interaction." *Text* 21(1/2):187–220.

Hafferty, Fred (1991). *Into the Valley: Death and the Socialization of Medical Students*. New Haven: Yale University Press.

Hafferty, Frederick W. and Light, Donald W. (1995). "Professional dynamics and the changing nature of medical work." *Journal of Health and Social Behavior* 35 (extra issue):132–53.

Halkowski, Timothy (1998). "Patients' smoking counts: implications of quantification practices." *Journal of General Internal Medicine* 13(supplement 1):107.

Halkowski, Timothy (1999). "The achieved coherence of aphasic narrative." In J. Holstein and G. Miller (eds.) *Perspectives on Social Problems*, vol. II. Stamford, CN: JAI Press, Inc, pp. 261–76.

Hall, Judith A. (1995). "Affective and nonverbal aspects of the medical visit. In Mack Lipkin, Samuel Putnam, and Aaron Lazare (eds.) *The Medical Interview: Clinical Care, Education, and Research*. New York: Springer-Verlag, pp. 495–503.

Hall, Judith A., Irish, Julie T., Roter, Debra L., Ehrlich, Carol M., and Miller, Lucy H. (1994a). "Gender in medical encounters: an analysis of physician and patient communication in a primary care setting." *Health Psychology* 13(5):384–92.

Hall, Judith A., Irish, Julie T., Roter, Debra L., Ehrlich, Carol M., and Miller, Lucy H. (1994b). "Satisfaction, gender and communication in medical visits." *Medical Care* 32(12):1216–31.

Hallam, L. (1994). "Primary medical care outside normal working hours: review of published work." *British Medical Journal* 308:249–53.

Hallam, L. and Cragg, D. (1994). "Organization of primary care service outside normal working hours." *British Medical Journal* 309: 1621–3.

Harre, R. (1991). *Physical Being: A Theory for a Corporeal Psychology.* Oxford: Blackwell.

Hass, Robert (1996). *Sun Under Wood*. Hopewell, NJ: Ecco Press.

Haynes, R. B. (1979). "Strategies to improve compliance with referrals, appointments and prescribed medical regimens." In R. B. Hayes, D. W. Taylor, and D. L. Sackett (eds.) *Compliance in Health Care*. Baltimore: John Hopkins.

Heath, Christian (1981). "The opening sequence in doctor-patient interaction. In P. Atkinson and C. Heath (eds.) *Medical Work: Realities and Routines*. Aldershot: Gower, pp. 71–90.

Heath, Christian (1982a). "The display of recipiency: an instance of sequential relationship between speech and body movement." *Semiotica* 42:147–67.

Heath, Christian (1982b). "Preserving the consultation: medical record cards and professional conduct." *Sociology of Health and Illness* 4: 56–74.

Heath, Christian (1986). *Body Movement and Speech in Medical Interaction*. Cambridge: Cambridge University Press.

Heath, Christian (1992). "The delivery and reception of diagnosis in the general-practice consultation." In Paul Drew and John Heritage (ed.) *Talk at Work: Interaction in Institutional Settings*. Cambridge: Cambridge University Press, pp. 235–267.

Heath, Christian, Sanchez Srensson, Marcus, Hindmarsh, Jon, Luff, Paul, and vom Lehn, D. (2002). "Configuring awareness." *Computer-Supported Cooperative Work* 11:317–47.

Helman, Cecil (1992). *Culture, Health and Illness*. Oxford: Butterworth.

Henderson, L. J. (1935). Physician and patient as a social system. *New England Journal of Medicine* 212(2):819–23.

Heritage, John (1984a). *Garfinkel and Ethnomethodology*. Cambridge: Polity Press.

Heritage, John (1984b). "A change-of-state token and aspects of its sequential placement." In J. Maxwell Atkinson and John Heritage (eds.) *Structures of Social Action: Studies in Conversation Analysis*. Cambridge: Cambridge University Press, pp. 299–345.

Heritage, John (1988). "Explanations as accounts: a conversation analytic perspective." In C. Antaki (ed.) *Understanding Everyday Explanation: A Casebook of Methods*. Beverly Hills: Sage, pp. 127–44.

Heritage, John (1997). "Conversation analysis and institutional talk: analyzing data." In D. Silverman (ed.) *Qualitative Analysis: Issues of Theory and Method*. London: Sage, pp. 161–82.

Heritage, John (1998). "Oh-prefaced responses to inquiry." *Language in Society* 27(3):291–334.

Heritage, John (2002a). "Ad hoc inquiries: two preferences in the design of 'routine' questions in an open context." In D. Maynard, H. Houtkoop-Steenstra, N. K. Schaeffer, and H. van der Zouwen (eds.) *Standardization and Tacit Knowledge: Interaction and Practice in the Survey Interview*. New York, Wiley Interscience, pp. 313–33.

Heritage, John (2002b). "Designing questions and setting agendas in the news interview." In P. Glenn, C. LeBaron, and J. Mandelbaum (eds.) *Studies in Language and Social Interaction*. Mahwah, NJ: Lawrence Erlbaum, pp. 57–90.

Heritage, John (2002c). "Oh-prefaced responses to assessments: a method of modifying agreement/disagreement." In C. Ford, B. Fox, and S. Thompson (eds.) *The Language of Turn and Sequence*. Oxford: Oxford University Press, pp. 196–224.

Heritage, John (2005). "Revisiting authority in physician-patient interaction." In M. Maxwell, D. Kovarsky, and J. Duchan (eds.) *Diagnosis as Cultural Practice*. New York: Mouton De Gruyter, pp. 83–102.

Heritage, John (forthcoming). "Justifying the medical visit: doctorability across the medical encounter." In Dale Brashers and Deana Goldsmith (eds.) *Managing Health and Illness, Relationships and Identity*. Mahwah, NJ: Erlbaum.

Heritage, John, Boyd, Elizabeth, and Kleinman, Lawrence (2001). "Subverting criteria: the role of precedent in decisions to finance surgery." *Sociology of Health and Illness* 23(5): 701–28.

Heritage, John and Greatbatch, David (1986). "Generating applause: a study of rhetoric and response at party political conferences." *American Journal of Sociology* 92(1):110–57.

Heritage, John and Greatbatch, David (1991). "On the institutional character of institutional talk: the case of news interviews." In Deirdre Boden and Don H. Zimmerman (eds.) *Talk and Social Structure*. Berkeley: University of California Press, pp. 93–137.

Heritage, John and Lindström, Anna (1992). "Advice-giving: terminable and interminable." Paper presented at the International Conference on Discourse and the Professions, Uppsala, Sweden, August 26–9.

Heritage, John and Lindström, Anna (1998). "Motherhood, medicine and morality: scenes from a medical encounter." *Research on Language and Social Interaction* 31(3/4):397–438.

Heritage, John and Raymond, Geoffrey (2005). "The terms of agreement: indexing epistemic authority and subordination in assessment sequences." *Social Psychology Quarterly* 68(1):15–38.

Heritage, John and Robinson, Jeffrey (forthcoming). "The structure of patients' presenting concerns opening questions." *Health Communication* 19(2):89–102.

Heritage, John and Roth, Andrew (1995). "Grammar and institution: questions and questioning in the broadcast news interview." *Research on Language and Social Interaction* 28(1):1–60.

Heritage, John and Sefi, Sue (1992). "Dilemmas of advice: aspects of the delivery and reception of advice in interactions between health visitors and first-time mothers." In P. Drew and J. Heritage (eds.) *Talk at Work: Interaction in Institutional Settings*. Cambridge: Cambridge University Press, pp. 359–417.

Heritage, John and Sorjonen, Marja-Leena (1994). "Constituting and maintaining activities across sequences: *and*-prefacing as a feature of question design." *Language in Society* 23:1–29.

Heritage, John and Stivers, Tanya (1999). "Online commentary in acute medical visits: a method of shaping patient expectations." *Social Science and Medicine* 49(11):1501–17.

Heritage, John and Watson, Rodney (1979). "Formulations as conversational objects." In G. Psathas (ed.) *Everyday Language: Studies in Ethnomethodology*. New York: Irvington, pp. 123–62.

Hewson, Mariana, J. Kindy, Phillips, Van Kirk, Judity, and Gennis, Virginia A. (1996). "Strategies for managing uncertainty and complexity." *Journal of General Internal Medicine* 11:481–5.

Hilbert, Richard (1984). "The acultural dimensions of chronic pain: flawed reality construction and the problem of meaning." *Social Problems* 31(4):365–78.

Hilbert, Richard (1992). *The Classical Roots of Ethnomethodology*. Chapel Hill: University of North Carolina Press.

Hopton, J., Hogg, R., and McKee, I. (1996). "Patients' accounts of calling the doctor out of hours: qualitative study in one general practice." *British Medical Journal* 313:991–4.

Horn, L. (1989). *A Natural History of Negation*. Chicago: University of Chicago Press.

Houtkoup-Steenstra, Hanneke (1987). *Establishing Agreement: An Analysis of Proposal-Acceptance Sequences*. Dordrecht, Holland: Foris Publications.

Houtkoop-Steenstra, Hanneke and Antaki, Charles (1997). "Creating happy people by asking yes–no questions." *Research on Language and Social Interaction* 30(4):285–313.

Hughes, David (1982). "Control in the consultation: organizing talk in a situation where co-participants have differential competence." *Sociology* 16:359–76.

Hughes, Everett C. (1951). "Mistakes at work." *Canadian Journal of Economics and Political Science* 17:320–7.

Hughes, Everett C. (1958). *Men and Their Work*. Glencoe: The Free Press.

Hughes, Everett C. (1963). "Desires and needs of a society." *Journal of the American Medical Association* 185:120–2.

Hunt, Linda, Jordan, Brigitte, and Irwin, Susan (1989). "Views of what's wrong: diagnosis and patients' concepts of illness." *Social Science and Medicine* 28(9):945–56.

Inui, Thomas and Carter, William B. (1985). "Problems and prospects for health service research on provider–patient communication." *Medical Care* 23(5):521–38.

Inui, Thomas S., Carter, William B., Kukull, Walter A., and Haigh, Virginia H. (1982). "Outcome based doctor-patient interaction analysis: 1. Comparison of techniques." *Medical Care* 20:535–49.

Jefferson, Gail (1973). "A case of precision timing in ordinary conversation: overlapped tag-positioned address terms in closing sequences." *Semiotica* 9:47–96.

Jefferson, Gail (1974). "Error correction as an interactional resource." *Language in Society* 2:181–99.

Jefferson, Gail (1979). "A technique for inviting laughter and its subsequent acceptance/declination." In G. Psathas (ed.) *Everyday Language: Studies in Ethnomethodology*. New York: Lawrence Erlbaum, pp. 79–96.

Jefferson, Gail (1980a). *End of Grant Report on Conversations in which "Troubles" or "Anxieties" are Expressed*, HR 4805/2. London: Social Science Research Council.

Jefferson, Gail (1980b). "On 'trouble-premonitory' response to inquiry." *Sociological Inquiry* 50:153–85.

Jefferson, Gail (1981a). "The abominable 'Ne?': a working paper exploring the phenomenon of post-response pursuit of response." Unpublished manuscript, Department of Sociology, University of Manchester.

Jefferson, Gail (1981b). "The rejection of advice: managing the problematic convergence of a 'troubles-telling' and a 'service encounter'." *Journal of Pragmatics* 5:399–422.

Jefferson, Gail (1984a). "Notes on the systematic deployment of the acknowledgement tokens 'yeah' and 'mm hm'." *Papers in Linguistics* 17:197–206.

Jefferson, Gail (1984b). "On the organization of laughter in talk about troubles." In J. Maxwell Atkinson and John Heritage (eds.) *Structures of Social Action: Studies in Conversation Analysis*. Cambridge: Cambridge University Press, pp. 346–69.

Jefferson, Gail (1984c). "On stepwise transition from talk about a trouble to inappropriately next-positioned matters." In J. Maxwell Atkinson and John Heritage (eds.) *Structures of Social Action: Studies in Conversation Analysis*. Cambridge: Cambridge University Press, pp. 191–221.

Jefferson, Gail (1985). "An exercise in the transcription and analysis of laughter." In Teun A. Dijk (ed.) *Handbook of Discourse Analysis*, vol. III. New York: Academic Press, pp. 25–34.

Jefferson, Gail (1986). "On the interactional unpackaging of a 'gloss'." *Language in Society* 14:435–66.

Jefferson, Gail (1987). "On exposed and embedded correction in conversation." In G. Button and J. Lee (eds.) *Talk and Social Organisation*. Clevedon: Multilingual Matters, pp. 86–100.

Jefferson, Gail (1988). "On the sequential organization of troubles-talk in ordinary conversation." *Social Problems* 35(4):418–41.

Jefferson, Gail (1989). "Preliminary notes on a possible metric which provides for a 'standard maximum' silence of approximately one second in conversation." In D. Roger and P. Bull (eds.) *Conversation: An Interdisciplinary Perspective*. Clevedon: Multilingual Matters, pp. 166–96.

Jefferson, G. (1990). "List construction as a task and interactional resource." In G. Psathas (ed.) *Interaction Competence*. Washington: International Institute for Ethnomethodology and Conversation Analysis/University Press of America, pp. 63–92.

Jefferson, Gail (1993). "Caveat speaker: preliminary notes on recipient topic-shift implicature." *Research on Language and Social Interaction* 26:1–30.

Jefferson, Gail (2004a). "'At first I thought': a normalizing device for extraordinary events." In G. Lerner (ed.) *Conversation Analysis: Studies from the First Generation*. Philadelphia: John Benjamins, pp. 131–67.

Jefferson, Gail (2004b). "Some orderly aspects of overlap in natural conversation." In G. Lerner (ed.) *Conversation Analysis: Studies from the First Generation*. Philadelphia: John Benjamins, pp. 43–59.

Jefferson, Gail and Lee, John (1992). "The rejection of advice: managing the problematic convergence of a 'troubles-telling' and a 'service encounter'." In P. Drew and J. Heritage (eds.) *Talk at Work: Interaction in Institutional Settings*. Cambridge: Cambridge University Press, pp. 521–48.

Jefferson, Gail, Sacks, Harvey, and Schegloff, Emanuel A. (1987). "Notes on laughter in the pursuit of intimacy." In Graham Button and John R. E. Lee (eds.) *Talk and Social Organisation*. Clevedon: Multilingual Matters, pp. 152–205.

Jick, H., Jick, S. S., and Derby, L. E. (1991). "Validation of information recorded on general practitioner based computerised data resource in the United Kindom." *British Medical Journal* (302): 766–8.

Johansson, M., Larsson, U. S., Säljö, R., and Svärdsudd, K. (1994). "Life style in the provision of health care: an empirical study of patient–physician interaction." In M. Johansson (ed.) *Perspectives on life style and post-operative complications*. Linköping Studies in Arts and Science 116, pp. 131–54.

Johansson, M., Larsson, U. S., Säljö, R., and Svärdsudd, K. (1995). "Life style in primary health care discourse." *Social Science and Medicine* 40:339–48.

John, E. and Curtis, P. (1988). "Physicians' attitudes to after-hours callers: a five year study in a university based family practice centre." *Family Practice* 5:168–73.

Johnson, Thomas M., Hardt, Eric J., and Kleinman, Arthur (1995). "Cultural factors in the medical interview." In Mack Lipkin, Samuel M. Putnam, and Aaron Lazare (eds.) *The Medical Interview: Clinical Care, Education, and Research*. New York: Springer-Verlag, pp. 153–62.

Kaplan, S., Greenfield, S. H., and Ware, J. E. (1989). "Assessing the effects of physician-patient interactions on the outcomes of chronic disease." *Medical Care* 27:S110–S126.

Kassirer, J. P. (1994). "Incorporating patients' preferences into medical decisions." *New England Journal of Medicine* 330:1895–6.

Katz, Jack (1983). "A theory of qualitative methodology: the social system of analytic fieldwork." In Robert M. Emerson (ed.) *Contemporary Field Research*. Boston: Little Brown.

Katz, Jay (1984). *The Silent World of Doctor and Patient*. New York: Free Press.

Kendon, A. (1967). "Some functions of gaze-direction in two-person conversation." *Acta Psychologica* 26:22–63.

Kleinman, Arthur (1980). *Patients and Healers in the Context of Culture*. Berkeley: University of California Press.

Kleinman, Arthur (1988). *The Illness Narratives: Suffering, Healing and the Human Condition*. New York: Basic Books.

Kleinman, Lawrence, Boyd, Elizabeth, and Heritage, John (1997). "Adherence to prescribed explicit criteria during utilization review: an analysis of communications between attending and reviewing physicians." *Journal of the American Medical Association* 278(6):497–501.

Kleinman, Arthur, Eisenberg, Leon, and Good, Byron (1978). "Culture, illness and care: clinical lessons from anthropologic and cross-cultural research." *Annals of Internal Medicine* 88:251–8.

Kollock, Peter, Blumstein, Philip, and Schwartz, Pepper (1985). "Sex and power in interaction: conversational privileges and duties." *American Sociological Review* 50:24–46.

Korsch, B., Gozzi, E. K., and Francis, V. (1968). "Gaps in doctor-patient communication." *Pediatrics* 42:855–71.

Korsch, Barbara M. and Negrete, V. F. (1972). "Doctor-patient communication." *Scientific American* 227:66–74.

Labov, William and Fanshel, David (1977). *Therapeutic Discourse: Psychotherapy as Conversation*. New York: Academic Press.

Lang, F., Floyd, M. R., and Beine, K. L. (2002). "Clues to patients' explanations and concerns about their illnesses: a call for active listening." *Archives of Family Medicine* 9:222–7.

Langewitz, Wolf, Denz, Martin, Keller, Anne, Kiss, Alexander, Ruttimann, Sigmund, and Wossmer, Brigitta (2002). "Spontaneous talking time at start of consultation in outpatient clinic: cohort study." *British Medical Journal* 325:682–3.

Larsson, U. S., Säljö, R., and Aronson, K. (1987). "Patient–doctor communication on smoking and drinking: lifestyle in medical consultations." *Social Science and Medicine* 25(10):1129–37.

Lazare, Aaron, Samuel M. Putnam, and Mack Lipkin (1995). "Three functions of the medical interview." In Mack Lipkin, Samuel M. Putnam, and Aaron Lazare (eds.) *The Medical Interview: Clinical Care, Education, and Research*. New York: Springer-Verlag, pp. 3–19.

Leppänen, Vesa (1998). *Structures of District Nurse-Patient Interaction*. Lund, Sweden: Department of Sociology, Lund University.

Lerner, Gene H. (1991). "On the Syntax of Sentences in Progress." *Language in Society* 20:441–58.

Lerner, G. H. (1996). "On the 'semi-permeable' character of grammatical units in conversation: conditional entry into the turn space of another speaker." In E. Ochs, E. A. Schegloff, and S. A. Thompson (eds.) *Interaction and Grammar*. Cambridge: Cambridge University Press, pp. 238–76.

Levine, M. N., Gafni, A., Markham, B., and MacFarlane, D. (1992). "A bedside decision instrument to elicit a patient's preference concerning adjuvant chemotherapy for breast cancer." *Annals of Internal Medicine* 117:53–8.

Levinson, Stephen C. (1983). *Pragmatics*. Cambridge: Cambridge University Press.

Levinson, Stephen C. (1992). "Activity types and language." In P. Drew and J. Heritage (eds.) *Talk at Work: Interaction in Institutional Settings*. Cambridge: Cambridge University Press, pp. 66–100.

Levinson, W., Roter, D., Mullooly, J. P., Dull, V. T., and Frankel, R. M. (1997). "Physician-patient communication: the relationship with malpractice claims among primary care physicians and surgeons." *Journal of the American Medical Association* 277(7):553–9.

Light, Donald W. (1988). "Toward a new sociology of medical education." *Journal of Health and Social Behavior* 29:307–22.

Light, Donald W. (1993). "Countervailing power: the changing character of the medical profession in the United States." In F. W. Hafferty and J. B. McKinlay (eds.) *The Changing Medical Profession: An International Perspective*. New York, Oxford University Press, pp. 69–80.

Light, Donald W. (2000). "The medical profession and organizational change: from professional dominance to countervailing power." In C. E. Bird, P. Conrad, and A. M. Fremont (eds.) *Handbook of Medical Sociology*. Upper Saddle River, NJ: Prentice Hall, pp. 201–16.

Lindström, Anna (1997). "Designing social actions: grammar, prosody and interaction in Swedish conversation." Unpublished PhD dissertation, Department of Sociology, University of California, Los Angeles.

Lipkin, Mack, Frankel, Richard, Beckman, Howard, Charon, Rita, and Fein, Oliver (1995). "Performing the interview." In Mack Lipkin, Samuel Putnam, and Aaron Lazare (eds.) *The Medical Interview: Clinical Care, Education, and Research*. New York: Springer Verlag, pp. 65–82.

Lipkin, Mack, Samuel Putnam, and Aaron Lazare (1995). *The Medical Interview: Clinical Care, Education and Research*. New York: Springer Verlag.

Luff, P., Heath, C. C., and Greatbatch, D. (1994). "Work, interaction and technology: the naturalistic analysis of human conduct and requirements analysis." In M. Jirotka and J. Goguen (eds.) *Requirements Engineering: Social and Technical Issues*. London: Academic Press, pp. 259–88.

Lutfey, Karen and Maynard, Douglas W. (1998). "Bad news in an oncology setting: how a physician talks about death and dying without using those words." *Social Psychology Quarterly* 61(4):321–341.

McCaig, L. F. and Hughes, J. M. (1995). "Trends in antimicrobial drug prescribing among office-based physicians in the United States." *Journal of the American Medical Association* 273:214–19.

McDonald, I. G., Daly, J., Jelinek, V. M., Panetta, F., and Gutman, J. M. (1996). "Opening Pandora's box: the unpredictability of reassurance by a normal test result." *British Medical Journal* 313:329–32.

McHoul, Alec (1978). "The organization of turns at formal talk in the classroom." *Language in Society* 7:183–213.

McKinlay, John B. (1999). "The end of the golden age of medicine." *New England Research Institutes Network* (Summer): 1, 3.

McKinley, R. K., et al. (1997a). "Comparison of out of hours care provided by patients' own general practitioners and commercial deputising services: a randomised control trial. II: the outcome of care." *British Medical Journal* 314:190–3.

McKinley, R. K., et al. (1997b). "Reliability and validity of a new measure of patient satisfaction with out of hours primary medical care in the United Kingdom: development of a patient questionnaire." *British Medical Journal* 314:193–8.

McWhinney, I. (1981). *An Introduction to Family Medicine*. New York: Oxford University Press.

McWhinney, I. (1989). "The need for a transformed clinical method." In M. Stewart and D. Roter (eds.) *Communicating with Medical Patients*. Newbury Park, CA: Sage.

Maguire, Peter, Fairbairn, Susan, and Fletcher, Charles (1986). "Most young doctors are bad at giving information." *British Medical Journal* 292: 1576–8.

Majeed, F. A., Cook, D. G., Hilton, S., Poloniecki, J., and Hagen, A. (1995). "Annual night visiting rates in 129 general practices in one family health services authority: association with patient and general practice characteristics." *British Journal of General Practice* 45:531–5.

Mangione-Smith, R., Elliott, M., McDonald, L., Stivers, T., and Heritage, J. (2004). "Doctor–parent communication: techniques for gaining parent acceptance of non-antibiotic treatment for upper respiratory infections." Pediatric Academic Societies' Meeting, APA Presidential Plenary Session, San Francisco, May 2004.

Mangione-Smith, Rita, McGlynn, Elizabeth, Elliott, Marc, Krogstadt, Paul, and Brook, Robert (1999). "The relationship between perceived parental expectations and pediatrician antimicrobial prescribing behavior." *Pediatrics* 103(4):711–18.

Mangione-Smith, Rita, McGlynn, Elizabeth, Elliott, Marc, McDonald, Laurie, Franz, C. E., and Kravitz, Richard (2001). "Parent expectations for antibiotics, physician-parent communication, and satisfaction." *Archives of Pediatrics and Adolescent Medicine* 155:800–6.

Mangione-Smith, Rita, Stivers, Tanya, Elliott, Marc, McDonald, Laurie, and Heritage, John (2003). "Online commentary during the physical examination: a communication tool for avoiding inappropriate prescribing." *Social Science and Medicine* 56:313–20.

Martin, Steven C., Arnold, Robert M., and Parker, Ruth M. (1989). "Gender and medical socialization." *Journal of Health and Social Behavior* 30:333–43.

Marvel, M. Kim, Epstein, Ronald M., Flowers, Kristine, and Backman, Howard B. (1999). "Soliciting the patient's agenda: have we improved?" *Journal of the American Medical Association* 281(3): 283–7.

Maynard, Douglas W. (1980). "Placement of topic changes in conversation." *Semiotica* 30:163–90.

Maynard, Douglas W. (1991a). "Citing the evidence vs. asserting the condition in the delivery of diagnostic news." Presented at the conference on Current Work in Ethnomethodology and Conversation Analysis, University of Amsterdam, July 1991.

Maynard, Douglas W. (1991b). "Deliveries of diagnosis and problems of meaning." Presented at the conference on Current Work in Ethnomethodology and Conversation Analysis, University of Amsterdam, July 1991.

Maynard, Douglas W. (1991c). "Interaction and asymmetry in clinical discourse." *American Journal of Sociology* 97(2):448–95.

Maynard, Douglas W. (1991d). "The perspective-display series and the delivery and receipt of diagnostic news." In D. Boden and D. Zimmerman (eds.) *Talk and Social Structure: Studies in Ethnomethodology and Conversation Analysis*. Cambridge, UK: Polity, pp. 164–92.

Maynard, Douglas W. (1992). "On clinicians co-implicating recipients' perspective in the delivery of diagnostic news." In P. Drew and J. Heritage (eds.) *Talk at Work: Social Interaction in Institutional Settings*. Cambridge: Cambridge University Press, pp. 331–58.

Maynard, Douglas W. (1996). "On 'realization' in everyday life: the forecasting of bad news as a social relation." *American Sociological Review* 61:109–31.

Maynard, Douglas W. (1997). "The news delivery sequence: bad news and good news in conversational interaction." *Research on Language and Social Interaction* 30:93–130.

Maynard, Douglas W. (2003). *Bad News, Good News: Conversational Order and Everyday Talk and Clinical Settings*. Chicago: University of Chicago Press.

Maynard, Douglas W. (2004). "On predicating a diagnosis as an attribute of a person." *Discourse Studies* 6:53–76.

Maynard, Douglas W. and Frankel, Richard M. (2003). "Indeterminacy and uncertainty in the delivery of diagnostic news in internal medicine: a single case analysis." In Phil Glenn, Curt LeBaron, and Jenny Mandelbaum (eds.) *Studies in Language and Social Interaction: Essays in Honor of Robert Hopper*. Mahwah, NJ: Lawrence Erlbaum, pp. 393–410.

Maynard, Douglas W. and Schaeffer, Nora C. (2002). "Opening and closing the gate: the work of optimism in recruiting survey respondents." In D. W. Maynard, H. Houtkoop-Steenstra, N. C. Schaeffer, and H. van der Zouwen (eds.) *Standardization and Tacit Knowledge: Interaction and Practice in the Survey Interview*.

Maynard, Douglas W. and Don H. Zimmerman (1984). "Topical talk, ritual and the social organization of relationships." *Social Psychology Quarterly* 47:301–16.

Mead, Nicola and Bower, Peter (2000). "Patient centredness: a conceptual framework and review of the empirical literature." *Social Science and Medicine* 51:1087–110.

Mechanic, David (1972). "Social psychologic factors affecting the presentation of bodily complaints." *New England Journal of Medicine* 286: 1132–9.

Meehan, Albert J. (1989). "Assessing the 'police-worthiness' of citizen complaints to the police: accountability and the negotiation of 'facts'." In D. Helm, W. T. Anderson, A. J. Meehan, and A. Rawls (eds.) *The Interactional Order: New Directions in the Study of Social Order*. New York: Irvington Press.

Mehan, Hugh (1985). "The structure of classroom discourse." In Teun A. Dijk (ed.) *Handbook of Discourse Analysis*, vol. III. New York: Academic Press, pp. 120–31.

Mehan, Hugh (1990). "Oracular reasoning in a psychiatric exam: the resolution of conflict in language." In Allen D. Grimshaw (ed.) *Conflict Talk: Sociolinguistic Investigations of Arguments in Conversations*. Cambridge: Cambridge University Press, pp. 160–77.

Mendonca, P. J. and Brehm, S. S. (1983). "Effects of choice on behavioral treatment of overweight children." *Journal of Social Clinical Psychology* 1:343–58.

Merton, Robert K., Reader, George G., and Kendell, Patricia (1957). *The Student Physician: Introductory Studies in the Sociology of Medical Education*. Cambridge, MA: Harvard University Press.

Miller, Gale and Holstein, James A. (1993). "Reconsidering social constructionism." Hawthorne, NY: Aldine De Gruyter.

Millman, Marcia (1977). *The Unkindest Cut: Life in the Backrooms of Medicine*. New York: William Morrow.

Mishler, Elliot G. (1984). *The Discourse of Medicine: Dialectics of Medical Interviews*. Norwood, NJ: Ablex.

Mishler, Elliot G. (1986). *Research Interviewing: Context and Narrative*. Cambridge, MA: Harvard University Press.

Mittleman, R. E. and Wetli, C. V. (1982). "The fatal cafe coronary: foreign-body airway obstruction." *Journal of the American Medical Association* 247(9):1285–8.

Mizrahi, Terry (1986). *Getting Rid of Patients: Contradictions in the Socialization of Physicians*. New Brunswick, NJ: Rutgers University Press.

National Center for Health Statistics (1994). "National Ambulatory Medical Care Survey 1989, 1992." Washington, DC: National Technical Information Service.

Nava, J. M., Bella, F., Garau, J., Lite, J., Morera, M. A., Marti, C., Fontanals, D., Font, B., Pineda, V., Uriz, S., et al. (1994). "Predictive factors for invasive disease due to penicillin-resistant Streptococcus pneumoniae: a population-based study." *Clinical Infectious Diseases* 19:884–90.

Nazareth, I., King, M., Baines, A., Rangel, L., and Myers, S. (1993). "Accuracy of diagnosis of psychosis on general practice computer systems." *British Medical Journal* 307:32–4.

Neu, H. C. (1992). "The crisis in antibiotic resistance." *Science* 257:1064–73.

Novack, Dennis (1995). "Therapeutic aspects of the clinical encounter." In Mack Lipkin, Jr., Samuel M. Putnam, and Aaron Lazare (eds.) *The Medical Interview: Clinical Care, Education, and Research*. New York: Springer-Verlag, pp. 32–49.

Novack, Dennis, Suchman, Anthony, Clark, William, Epstein, Ronald, Najberg, Eva, and Kaplan, Craig (1997). "Calibrating the physician: personal awareness and effective patient care." *Journal of the American Medical Association* 267:502–9.

O'Dowd, T. and Sinclair, H. (1994). "Open all hours: night visits in general practice." *British Medical Journal* 308:386.

Ochs, E., Schegloff, E. A., and Thompson, S. A. (eds.) (1996). *Interaction and Grammar*. Cambridge: Cambridge University Press.

Orth, J. E., Stiles, W., Scherwitz, L., Hennrikus, D., and Valbonna, C. (1987). "Patient exposition and provider explanation in routine interviews and hypertensive patients' blood pressure." *Health Psychology* 6:29–42.

Paget, Marianne A. (1988). *The Unity of Mistakes: A Phenomenological Interpretation of Medical Work*, vol. VI. Philadelphia: Temple University Press.

Palmer, D. A. and Bauchner, H. (1997). "Parents' and physicians' views on antibiotics." *Pediatrics* 99(6):862–3.

Parsons, Talcott (1951). *The Social System*. New York: Free Press.

Parsons, Talcott (1964). *Social Structure and Personality*. New York: Free Press.

Parsons, Talcott (1975). "The sick role and the role of the physician reconsidered." *Milbank Memorial Fund Quarterly* 53:257–78.

Parsons, Talcott and Bales, Robert F. (1955). *Family, Socialization and Interaction Process*. New York: Free Press.

Pendleton, David (1983). "Doctor-patient communication: a review." In D. Pendleton and J. Hasler (eds.) *Doctor-Patient Communication*. New York: Academic, pp. 5–53.

Peräkylä, Anssi (1998). "Authority and accountability: the delivery of diagnosis in primary health care." *Social Psychology Quarterly* 61(4): 301–20.

Peräkylä, Anssi (2002). "Agency and authority: extended responses to diagnostic statements in primary care encounters." *Research on Language and Social Interaction* 35(2):219–47.

Peräkylä, Anssi and David Silverman (1991). "Owning experience: describing the experience of other persons." *Text* 11:441–80.

Pescosolido, B. and Kronenfeld, J. J. (1995). "Sociological understandings of health, illness and healing: the challenge from and for medical sociology." *Journal of Health and Social Behavior* 35 (extra issue): 5–33.

Pescosolido, B., McLeod, J., and M. Alegria (2000). "Confronting the second social contract: the place of medical sociology in research and policy for the twenty-first century." In C. E. Bird, P. Conrad, and A. M. Fremont (eds.) *Handbook of Medical Sociology*. Upper Saddle River, NJ: Prentice Hall, pp. 411–26.

Peyrot, M., Alperstein, N. M., van Doren, D., and Poli, L. G. (1998). "Direct-to-consumer ads can influence behavior: advertising increases consumer knowledge and prescription drug requests." *Marketing Health Services* (Summer):27–32.

Physicians' Working Group for Single-Payer National Health Insurance (2003). *Journal of the American Medical Association* 290:798–805.

Pinto, M. B., Pinto, J. K., and Barber, J. C. (1998). "The impact of pharmaceutical direct advertising: opportunities and obstructions." *Health Marketing Quarterly* 15(4):89–101.

Platt, Frederic W. (1995). *Conversation Repair: Case Studies in Doctor–Patient Communication*. Boston: Little, Brown.

Polanyi, Michael (1958). *Personal Knowledge: Towards a Post-Critical Philosophy*. Chicago: University of Chicago Press.

Pollner, Melvin (1987). *Mundane Reason*. Cambridge: Cambridge University Press.

Pomerantz, Anita M. (1980). "Telling my side: 'limited access' as a 'fishing' device." *Sociological Inquiry* 50:186–98.

Pomerantz, Anita (1984a). "Agreeing and disagreeing with assessments: some features of preferred/dispreferred turn shapes." In J. Maxwell Atkinson and John Heritage (eds.) *Structures of Social Action: Studies in Conversation Analysis*. Cambridge: Cambridge University Press, pp. 57–101.

Pomerantz, Anita (1984b). "Giving a source or basis: the practice in conversation of telling 'how I know.'" *Journal of Pragmatics* 8:607–25.

Pomerantz, Anita (1984c). "Pursuing a response." In J. M. Atkinson and J. Heritage (eds.) *Structures of Social Action*. Cambridge: Cambridge University Press, pp. 152–64.

Pomerantz, Anita (1986). "Extreme case formulations: a way of legitimizing claims." *Human Studies* 9:219–29.

Pomerantz, Anita (1988). "Offering a candidate answer: an information seeking strategy." *Communication Monographs* 55:360–73.

Pomerantz, Anita, Ende, Jack, and Erickson, Frederick (1995). "Precepting in a general medicine clinic: how preceptors correct." In G. H. Morris and R. J. Chenail (eds.) *The Talk of the Clinic*. New York: Lawrence Erlbaum.

Pomerantz, Anita, Fehr, B. J., and Ende, Jack (1997). "When supervising physicians see patients: strategies used in difficult situations." *Human Communication Research* 23(4):589–615.

Ptacek, J. T. and Eberhardt, Tara L. (1996). "Breaking bad news: a review of the literature." *Journal of the American Medical Association* 276: 296–502.

Quill, Timothy E. (1995). "Barriers to effective communication." In M. Lipkin, S. M. Putnam, and A. Lazare (eds.) *The Medical Interview: Clinical Care, Education, and Research*. New York: Springer-Verlag, pp. 110–21.

Quill, Timothy E. and Townsend, Penelope (1991). "Bad news: delivery, dialogue, and dilemmas." *Archives of Internal Medicine* 151:463–8.

Raevaara, Liisa (1996b). "Puheenaiheiden esittely ja jatkaminen lääkärin vastaanotolla." ("The introduction and the continuation of topics of talk in medical consultations.") *Virittäjä* 3:357–74.

Raevaara, Liisa (1996a). "Patients' diagnostic utterances in Finnish doctor-patient encounters." Presented at the Eleventh World Congress of Applied Linguistics, Jyväskylä, Finland, 4–9 August.

Raevaara, Liisa (1998). "Patients' etiological explanations in Finnish doctor-patient consultations." Presented at the Netherlands Institute for Primary Health Care conference on Communication in Health Care, The Free University, The Netherlands, June 1998.

Raevaara, Liisa (2000). "Potilaan diagnoosiehdotukset lääkärin vastaanotolla." ("Patients, candidate diagnoses in the medical consultation.") Helsinki: SKS.

Raymond, Geoffrey (2003). "Grammar and social organization: yes/no interrogatives and the structure of responding." *American Sociological Review* 68:939–67.

Reichardt, C. S. and Cook, T. D. (1969). "Beyond qualitative versus quantitative methods." In C. S. Reichardt and T. D. Cook (eds.) *Qualitative and Quantitative Methods in Evaluation Research*. Beverly Hills, CA: Sage.

Reichler, M. R., Allphin, A. A., Breiman, R. F., Schreiber, J. R., Arnold, J. E., McDougal, L. K., Facklam, R. R., Boxerbaum, B., May, D., and Walton, R. O., et al. (1992). "The spread of multiply resistant *Streptococcus pneumoniae* at a day care center in Ohio." *Journal of Infectious Diseases* 166:1346–53.

Reiser, David and Schroder, Andrea Klein (1980). *Patient Interviewing: The Human Dimension*. Baltimore, MD: Williams and Wilkins.

Robinson, Jeffrey D. (1998). "Getting down to business: talk, gaze, and body orientation during openings of doctor-patient consultations." *Human Communication Research* 25(1):97–123.

Robinson, Jeffrey D. (1999). "The organization of action and activity in general-practice, doctor–patient consultations." Unpublished Ph.D. dissertation, University of California, Los Angeles.

Robinson, Jeff (2001a). "Asymmetry in action: sequential resources in the negotiation of a prescription request." *Text* 21:19–54.

Robinson, Jeffrey D. (2001b). "Closing medical encounters: two physician practices and their implications for the expression of patients' unstated concerns." *Social Science and Medicine* 53(5):639–56.

Robinson, Jeffrey D. (2003). "An interactional structure of medical activities during acute visits and its implications for patients' participation." *Health Communication* 15(1):27–59.

Robinson, Jeffrey and Heritage, John (2003). "The structure of patients' presenting concerns: the completion relevance of current symptoms." *Social Science and Medicine* 61:481–93.

Robinson, Jeffrey and Stivers, Tanya (2001). "Achieving activity transitions in primary-care consultations: from history taking to physical examination." *Human Communication Research* 27(2):253–98.

Rodwin, Marc A. (1993). *Medicine, Money and Morals: Physicians' Conflicts of Interest*. New York: Oxford University Press.

Roter, Debra (1977). "Patient participation in the patient–provider interaction: the effects of patient question asking on the quality of interaction, satisfaction and compliance." *Health Education Monographs* 5:281.

Roter, Debra (2000). "The enduring and evolving nature of the patient–physician relationship." *Patient Education and Counseling* 39:5–15.

Roter, Debra (2004). *The Roter Interactional Analysis (RIAS) Coding Manual.* Baltimore, MD: Johns Hopkins University. http://www.rias.org/manual.html

Roter, Debra and Frankel, Richard M. (1992). "Quantitative and qualitative approaches to the evaluation of the medical dialogue." *Social Science and Medicine* 34(10):1097–103.

Roter, Debra and Hall, Judith (1992). *Doctors Talking with Patients/Patients Talking with Doctors: Improving Communication in Medical Visits*. Westport, CT: Auburn House.

Roter, Debra L., Hall, Judith A., and Katz, N. R. (1988). "Physician–patient communication: a descriptive summary of the literature." *Patient Education and Counseling* 12:99–109.

Roter, Debra and Larson, Susan (2001). "The relationship between residents' and attending physicians' communication during primary care visits: an illustrative use of the Roter Interaction Analysis System." *Health Communication* 13(1):33–48.

Roter, Debra and Larson, Susan (2002). "The Roter Interaction Analysis System (RIAS): utility and flexibility for analysis of medical interactions." *Patient Education and Counseling* 42:243–51.

Roter, Debra and McNeilis, Kelly S. (2003). The nature of the therapeutic relationship and the assessment of its discourse in routine medical visits." In T. Thompson, A. Dorsey, K. Miller, and R. Parrott (eds.) *Handbook of Health Communication*. Mahwah, NJ: Lawrence Erlbaum, pp. 121–40.

Roter, D., Stewart, M., Putnam, S., Lipkin, M., Stiles, W., and Inui, T. S. (1997). "Communication patterns of primary care physicians." *Journal of the American Medical Association* 227(4):350–6.

Roth, Andrew (1998). "Who makes news: descriptions of television news interviewees' public personae." *Media ,Culture and Society* 28(1):79–107.

Russel N. K. and Roter, D. L. (1993). "Health promotion counselling of chronic-disease patients during primary care visits." *American Journal of Public Health* 83(7):979–82.

Ruusuvuori, Johanna (2000). "Control in the medical consultation: practices of giving and receiving the reason for the visit in primary health care." Unpublished Ph.D. dissertation, University of Tampere, Finland.

Sacks, Harvey (1972). "An initial investigation of the usability of conversational data for doing sociology." In D. Sudnow (ed.) *Studies in Social Interaction*. New York: Free Press.

Sacks, Harvey (1974). "An analysis of the course of a joke's telling in conversation." In Richard Bauman and Joel Sherzer (eds.) *Explorations in the Ethnography of Speaking*. Cambridge: Cambridge University Press, pp. 337–53.

Sacks, Harvey (1975). "Everyone has to lie." In B. Blount and M. Sanches (eds.) *Sociocultural Dimensions of Language Use*. New York: Academic Press, pp. 57–80.

Sacks, Harvey (1984). "On doing 'being ordinary'." In J. Maxwell Atkinson and John Heritage (eds.) *Structures of Social Action*. Cambridge: Cambridge University Press, pp. 413–29.

Sacks, H. (1987). "On the preferences for agreement and contiguity in sequences in conversation." In G. Button and J. R. Lee (eds.) *Talk and Social Organisation*. Clevedon: Multilingual Matters, pp. 54–69.

Sacks, Harvey (1989). "On members' measurement systems." *Research on Language and Social Interaction* 22:45–60.

Sacks, Harvey (1992a). *Lectures on Conversation*, vol. I, ed. G. Jefferson, introduction E. A. Schegloff. Oxford: Blackwell.

Sacks, Harvey (1992b). *Lectures on Conversation*, vol. II, ed. G. Jefferson, introduction E. A. Schegloff. Oxford: Blackwell.

Sacks, Harvey and Schegloff, Emanuel A. (1979). "Two preferences in the organization of reference to persons and their interaction." In G. Psathas (ed.) *Everyday Language: Studies in Ethnomethodology*. New York: Irvington Publishers, pp. 15–21.

Sacks, Harvey, Schegloff, Emanuel A., and Jefferson, Gail (1974). "A simplest systematics for the organization of turn-taking for conversation." *Language* 50:696–735.

Salisbury, C. (1993). "Visiting through the night." *British Medical Journal* 306:762–4.

Salisbury, C. (1997). "Observational study of a general practice out of hours cooperative: measures of activity." *British Medical Journal* 314:182–6.

Sankar, A. (1986). "Out of the clinic into the home: control and patient–doctor communication." *Social Science and Medicine* 22(9):973–82.

Scarry, E. (1985). *The Body in Pain.* Oxford: Oxford University Press.

Schegloff, Emanuel A. (1968). "Sequencing in conversational openings." *American Anthropologist* 70:1075–95.

Schegloff, Emanuel A. (1972). "Notes on a conversational practice: formulating place." In David Sudnow (ed.) *Studies in Social Interaction.* New York: Free Press, pp. 75–119.

Schegloff, Emanuel A. (1979). "The relevance of repair for syntax-for-conversation." In T. Givon (ed.) *Syntax and Semantics*, vol. XII, *Discourse and Syntax.* New York: Academic Press, pp. 261–88.

Schegloff, Emanuel A. (1980). "Preliminaries to preliminaries: 'Can I ask you a question?'" *Sociological Inquiry* 50(3/4):104–52.

Schegloff, Emanuel A. (1982). "Discourse as an interactional achievement: some uses of 'uh-huh' and other things that come between sentences." In D. Tannen (ed.) *Analyzing Discourse: Text and Talk.* Washington, DC: Georgetown University Press, pp. 71–93.

Schegloff, Emanuel A. (1986). "The routine as achievement." *Human Studies* 9: 111–51.

Schegloff, Emanuel A. (1987). "Recycled turn beginnings: a precise repair mechanism in conversation's turn taking organization." In Graham Button and John Lee (eds.) *Talk and Social Organisation.* Clevedon: Multilingual Matters, pp. 70–85.

Schegloff, Emanuel A. (1988). "On an actual virtual servo-mechanism for guessing bad news: a single case conjecture." *Social Problems* 35(4): 442–57.

Schegloff, Emanuel A. (1990). "On the organization of sequences as a source of 'coherence' in talk-in-interaction." In B. Dorval (ed.) *Conversational Organization and its Development.* Norwood, NJ: Ablex, pp. 51–77.

Schegloff, Emanuel A. (1992). "Repair after next turn: the last structurally provided defense of intersubjectivity in conversation." *American Journal of Sociology* 97(5):1295–1345.

Schegloff, Emanuel A. (1993). "Reflections on quantification in the study of conversation." *Research on Language and Social Interaction* 26:99–128.

Schegloff, Emanuel A. (1995). "Sequence organization." Unpublished ms, Department of Sociology, University of California, Los Angeles.

Schegloff, Emanuel A. (1996a). "Confirming allusions: toward an empirical account of action." *American Journal of Sociology* 102(1):161–216.

Schegloff, Emanuel A. (1996b). "Issues of relevance for discourse analysis: contingency in action, interaction, and co-participant context." In

E. Hovy and D. Scott (eds.) *Computational and Conversational Discourse: Burning Issues – An Interdisciplinary Account*. Berlin: Springer-Verlag, pp. 3–35.

Schegloff, Emanuel A. (1996c). "Some practices for referring to persons in talk-in-interaction: a partial sketch of a systematics." In B. Fox (ed.) *Studies in Anaphora*. Amsterdam/Philadelphia: John Benjamins, pp. 437–85.

Schegloff, Emanuel A. (1996d). "Turn organization: one intersection of grammar and interaction." In E. Ochs, E. Schegloff, and S. Thompson (eds.) *Interaction and Grammar*. Cambridge: Cambridge University Press, pp. 52–133.

Schegloff, Emanuel A. (2000a). "On granularity." *Annual Review of Sociology* 26:715–20.

Schegloff, Emanuel A. (2000b). "On turns' possible completion, more or less: increments and trail-offs." Paper presented at the National Communication Association Convention, Seattle, WA.

Schegloff, Emanuel A. (2000c). "Overlapping talk and the organization of turn-taking for conversation." *Language in Society* 29(1):1–63.

Schegloff, Emanuel A. (2001). "Increments: where they are and what they do." Paper presented at the Linguistic Institute, Santa Barbara, California.

Schegloff, Emanuel A. (in press). *Sequence Organization in Interaction: A Primer in Conversation Analysis*. Cambridge: Cambridge University Press.

Schegloff, Emanuel A., Jefferson, Gail, and Sacks, Harvey (1977). "The preference for self-correction in the organization of repair in conversation." *Language* 53(2):361–82.

Schegloff, Emanuel A. and Sacks, Harvey (1973). "Opening up closings." *Semiotica* 7:289–327.

Schulman, B. A. (1979). "Active patient orientation and outcomes in hypertensive treatment." *Medical Care* 17:267–80.

Schutz, Alfred (1962). *Collected Papers*, vol. I, *The Problem of Social Reality*. The Hague: Martinus Nijhoff.

Schwartz, B. (1999). "Preventing the spread of antimicrobial resistance among bacterial respiratory pathogens in industrialized countries: the case for judicious antimicrobial use." *Clinical Infectious Diseases* 28: 211–13.

Schwartz, R. H., Freij, B. J., Ziai, M., and Sheridan, M. J. (1997). "Antimicrobial prescribing for acute purulent rhinitis in children: a survey of pediatricians and family practitioners." *Pediatric Infectious Disease Journal* 16:185–90.

Schwartz, R. K., Soumerai, S. B., and Avorn, J. (1989). "Physician motivations for non-scientific drug prescribing." *Social Science and Medicine* 28:577–82.

Seidel, Henry M., Ball, Jane W., Dains, Joyce E., and Benedict, G. W. (1995). *Mosby's Guide to Physical Examination*, 3rd edition. St. Louis, MO: Mosby Year Book.

West, Candace and Frankel, R. (1991). "Miscommunication in medicine." In N. Coupland, H. Giles and J. M. Wiemann (eds.) *Miscommunication and Problematic Talk*. Newbury Park, CA: Sage, pp. 166–94.

West, Candace and Garcia, Angela (1988). "Conversational shift work: a study of topical transitions between women and men." *Social Problems* 35(5):551–75.

West, Candace and Zimmerman, Don H. (1983). "Small insults: a study of interruptions in cross-sex conversations with unacquainted persons." In B. Thorne, C. Kramarae, and N. Henley (eds.) *Language, Gender and Society.* Rowley, MA: Newbury House, pp. 102–17.

Whalen, Marilyn and Zimmerman, Don H. (1987). "Sequential and institutional contexts in calls for help." *Social Psychology Quarterly* 50:172–85.

Whalen, Marilyn and Zimmerman, Don H. (1990). "Describing trouble: practical epistemology in citizen calls to the police." *Language in Society* 19:465–92.

Whalen, Jack and Zimmerman, Don H. (1998). "Observations on the display and management of emotion in naturally occurring activities: the case of 'hysteria' in calls to 9-1-1." *Social Psychology Quarterly* 61:141–59.

Whalen, Jack, Zimmerman, Don H., and Whalen, Marilyn R. (1988). "When words fail: a single case analysis." *Social Problems* 35(4): 335–62.

White, J., Levinson, W., and Roter, D. (1994). "'Oh, by the way . . .': the closing moments of the medical visit." *Journal of General Internal Medicine* 9 (January):24–8.

White, J. C., Rosson, C., Christensen, J., Hart, R., and Levinson, W. (1997). "Wrapping things up: a qualitative analysis of the closing moments of the medical visit." *Patient Education and Counselling* 30:155–65.

Whitney, C. G., Farley, M. M., Hadler, J., Harrison, L. H., Lexau, C., Reingold, A., Lefkowitz, L., Cieslak, P. R., Cetron, M., Zell, E. R., Jorgensen, J. H., and Schuchat, A. (2000). "Increasing prevalence of multidrug-resistant Streptococcus pneumoniae in the United States." *New England Journal of Medicine* 343:1917–24.

Williams, B. (1993). "Night visits in general practice: an acceleration, with the new contract, of an underlying trend." *British Medical Journal* 306:734–5.

Williams, Geoffrey C., Frankel, Richard M., Campbell, Thomas L., and Deci, Edward L. (2003). "The science of the art of medicine: research on the biopsychosocial approach to health care." In R. M. Frankel, T. E. Quill, and S. H. McDaniel (eds.) *The Biopsychosocial Approach: Past, Present, Future.* Rochester, NY: University of Rochester Press, pp. 108–22.

Wise, R., Hart, T., Cars, O., Streulens, Helmuth R., Huovinen, P., and Sprenger, M. (1998). "Antimicrobial resistance is a major threat to public health." *British Medical Journal* 317:609–10.

Wittgenstein, Ludwig (1953). *Philosophical Investigations*. New York: Macmillian Publishing Co.

Wittgenstein, Ludwig (1964). *The Blue and Brown Books*. Oxford: Basil Blackwell.

Zimmerman, Don H. (1988). "On conversation: the conversation analytic perspective." In J. Anderson (ed.) *Communication Yearbook*, vol. II. Newbury Park, CA: Sage, pp. 406–32.

Zimmerman, Don H. (1992). "The interactional organization of calls for emergency assistance." In P. Drew and J. Heritage (eds.) *Talk at Work: Social Interaction in Institutional Settings*. Cambridge: Cambridge University Press, pp. 418–69.

Zimmerman, Don H. and Pollner, Melvin (1971). "The everyday world as phenomenon." In J. Douglas (ed.) *Understanding Everyday Life*. London: Routledge and Kegan Paul, pp. 80–104.

Zimmerman, Don H. and Wakin, Michelle (1995). "'Thank you's' and the management of closings in emergency calls." Paper presented at the 90th Annual Meeting of the American Sociological Association, Washington, DC, August 19–23.

Zimmerman, Don H. and West, Candace (1975). "Sex roles, interruptions and silences in conversation." In B. Thorne and N. Henley (eds.) *Language and Sex: Difference and Dominance*. Rowley, MA: Newbury House, pp. 105–29.

Zola, Irving K. (1964). "Illness behavior of the working class: implications and recommendations." In A. Shostak and W. Gomberg (eds.) *Blue-Collar World*. Englewood Cliffs, NJ: Prentice Hall, pp. 350–61.

Zola, Irving K. (1973). "Pathways to the doctor: from person to patient." *Social Science and Medicine* 7:677–89.

Zola, Irving K. (1981). "Structural constraints on the doctor-patient relationship: the case for non-compliance." In Leon Eisenberg and Arthur Kleinman (eds.) *The Relevance of Social Science for Medicine*. Dordrecht, The Netherlands: Reidel, pp. 242–52.

Zoppi, Kathleen A. (1997). "Interviewing as clinical conversation." In M. B. Mengel and S. A. Fields (eds.) *Introduction to Clinical Skills: A Patient-Centered Textbook*. New York: Plenum Medical Book Company, pp. 41–55.

Subject index

Name index